Normal and Abnormal Prepuce

Mohamed A. Baky Fahmy

Normal and Abnormal Prepuce

Springer

Mohamed A. Baky Fahmy
Pediatric Surgery
Al Azher University
Cairo
Egypt

ISBN 978-3-030-37620-8   ISBN 978-3-030-37621-5 (eBook)
https://doi.org/10.1007/978-3-030-37621-5

This Springer imprint is published by the registered company Springer Nature Switzerland AG
The registered company address is: Gewerbestrasse 11, 6330 Cham, Switzerland

It is my honour to dedicate this unique book to my beloved wife Rula for her unremitting physical and spiritual advocacy and support.

Foreword

The prepuce has never been studied before as a separate structure, as in many societies it is simply excised during circumcision. However, it is an organ as other body parts do have its structure, pathologies and value.
This books aims to illuminate in details this rarely studied body part where it is described as “a complex of specialized erogenous structures that work in sympathy with adjacent penile structures”.

The historic review of the prepuce with the comparative anatomy to animal prepuce may be the first literature ever comparison published. Many surgeons who are interested in genital surgery and its reconstruction do pay attention to the prepuce anatomy, histology and its use to reconstruction of nearby genital organs.

The different pathologies of the prepuce have never been collected before in the literature in one place, whether those associated with meatal or penile anomalies. Other pathologies might not have been seen by many specialized surgeons due to the prevalence of circumcision in their societies and an adult or child prepuce pathology is really rare.

Female prepuce is another rarely discussed skin structure that is expanded in this book. The anatomy or variations are rarely addressed or discussed in the literature, adding to that its pathologies set up the important information that is needed and searched for by anyone who needs to perform surgery on this body part.

The photographic illustrations of each pathology, whether male or female, give a clearer description of these rare problems and add great value to this book.

In conclusion, what is really new about this book is that it addresses an important body part that many surgeons may excise at least once during their career and discuss its value and related diseases with an extensive illustrative photos.

Ahmed Medhat Zaki
Pediatric Surgery
Ain Shams University
Cairo, Egypt

Contents

Part VI Female Prepuce

Contributors

Amilal Bhat Department of Urology, Jaipur National University Institute for Medical Sciences and Research Centre, Jaipur, Rajasthan, India

Dr. S.N. Medical College Jodhpur, Jodhpur, Rajasthan, India

S.P. Medical College, Bikaner, Rajasthan, India

Medical Council of India, New Delhi, India

Academic and Research Council of RUHS, Jaipur, Rajasthan, India

Mahakshit Bhat NIIIMS, Jaipur, Rajasthan, India

Massimo Garriboli Department of Paediatric Nephro-Urology, Evelina London Children's Hospital, London, UK

Mohamed A. Baky Fahmy Pediatric Surgery, Al Azher University, Cairo, Egypt

Nikhil Khandelwal VIMS, Ballari, Karnataka, India

Irene Paraboschi Department of Paediatric Surgery, IRCCS Giannina Gaslini Children's Hospital, Genoa, Italy

V. Raveenthiran Department of Pediatric Surgery, SRM Medical College, Chennai, India

Alexander Springer Department of Pediatric Surgery, Center for Pediatric Urology, General Hospital/Medical University of Vienna, Vienna, Austria

1 Introduction

The argument is continuous along the history, whether this piece of skin is a vestigial redundant part of human body and deserves removal, or it is rather a complex of specialised erogenous structures that work in sympathy with adjacent penile structures and merits reverence? Is the prepuce is a superfluous tag of skin, or it is a large platform for the reception and expression of sensual and sexual sensation?

Nowadays the universe divided into territories discarding the prepuce along the process of circumcision, and another concerned to preserve it in an optimal healthy condition.

We have to admit that the prepuce as an exquisitely designed, it is highly innervated and vascularised complex of specialised erogenous structures and it could be affected by different acquired diseases and congenital anomalies; but as it is removed in about 40% of men along the mankind history, so there is no previously convenient opportunity to study thoroughly the preputial diseases and anomalies. There is no accurate classification exists for preputial anomalies in children and adults, and some of these anomalies are difficult to define or diagnose, while it may significantly alter penile appearance.

Most relevant medical texts contain no or little information regarding the anatomy and physiology of the prepuce, even some do not even include the prepuce in diagrams of the penis, so our goal through this illustrative textbook is to elaborate the normal embryology, anatomy, functions, normal variations and diseases affecting this dialectical organ, without any discussion about its removal in circumcision, preserving or reconstructing it. Discussion will not only concern with male prepuce, but also it will be extended to deal with female prepuce (hood) to elucidate some lights in its normal and abnormal situations. Many new items which were not previously discussed are elaborated like microposthia (Congenital incomplete preputial development), macroposthia (akroposthia, or redundant prepuce) and the normal variations of preputial meatus will be illustrated, also the dilemma of phimosis and its confusion with other anomalies and diseases will be addressed.

During the last two decades the prevalence of circumcision declined dramatically, specially in Europe, Canada, Australia and many Asian countries. Previous trend to take off the prepuce for management of many penile and preputial diseases is moved recently for more preservation of the prepuce, and on the background of its importance, as an essential organ, we are now seeing many centers offering several procedures to restore the previously removed prepuce; so these enforce the importance of this textbook; which will collect most data available about the prepuce in health and diseases along my experience in dealing with genital anomalies during the last 35 years.

According to Oster [1], there are three fundamental dates in the history of the foreskin: at

M. A. B. Fahmy, *Normal and Abnormal Prepuce*, https://doi.org/10.1007/978-3-030-37621-5_1

1713 BC, when Abraham was circumcised as a sign of his covenant with God; 43 AD, when the apostle Paul stated that circumcision of the heart and not that of the flesh was the only way to salvation; and AD 1949, when Gairdner published, first hand, the typical preputial development. The first two events are historically notable and have influenced millions of people, while the third seems not to have been so remarkable so far.

Bokai [2] was the first to direct attention to the physiological adherence of the foreskin. Schweigger-Seifd [3] gave the first description of the development of the prepuce in the human, but Retterere [4]was the first to describe development of the prepuce.

Problems with the prepuce are usually presented with pain, micturition difficulties, nonretractibility, infection or cosmesis, which are the common reasons for referral to out-patients clinics. Surgeons from many different subspecialties frequently consulted for boys and adults with preputial problems including specialist paediatric surgeons, general surgeons, urologists, dermatologists and plastic surgeons. In addition to the operative workload, a considerable amount of outpatient work is involved, often seeing children who do not need surgical intervention.

Generally, late and misdiagnoses of rare disease patients are common and often result in medical, physical and mental burden for the patient, and financial and emotional encumbrance for the patient's family and community. Low level of awareness about rare diseases among physicians is believed to be one of the reasons for late and misdiagnoses of either congenital or acquired diseases which affect prepuce [5].

Definition and Terminology

Gary L. Harryman [6], identify and analyse the accuracy of the anatomical source materials regarding the human penis that are immediately available to medical school students and medical professionals. Ninety sources were vetted for entries and images of the penile definitions, photos, illustrations, and drawings. He found 67% of the depictions of the human penis are anatomically incorrect. Of the primary images of the human penis, 71% are incorrect, while 54% of the secondary are incorrect. It is evident that the penis is misrepresented in the medical literature used in medical schools.

The word Prepuce originally came from the old French word "prepuce", and from Latin "praeputium", which means "præ-" before and "putos" means "penis", but in Greeks language the word prepuce composed of two distinct structures: the *posthe* (ποσθη) and the *akroposthion* (ακροπσθτου). *Posthe* referred to that part of the prepuce that covers the glans penis, and "Akroposthion" designates the tapered, tubular, visually defining portion of the prepuce that extends beyond the glans and terminates at the preputial orifice.

Current dictionaries use the terms foreskin and prepuce interchangeably. It is now possible to make a clear distinction between them. According to Roberts [7], the prepuce, or sheath, is a double invagination of skin which contains and covers the free portion of the penis when not erect (italics mine) and covers the body of the penis behind the glans when the penis is erect. A foreskin is a double invagination of skin that covers the glans when the penis is erect and is retracted over the body of the penis with intromission.

I think the term "prepuce" is the scientific analogue for the demotic word "foreskin", also foreskin represents the outer sheath covering the glans, but prepuce represent the whole structure of the skin and mucous membrane (inner layer).

Foreskin is colloquial term while prepuce is anglicized technical term. Prepuce/ˈpriːpjuːs/, or as an adjective, preputial/prɪˈpjuːʃəl/, refers to two homologous structures of male and female genitals.

References

1. Oster J. Further fate of the foreskin. Incidence of preputial adhesions, phimosis, and smegma among Danish schoolboys. Arch Dis Child. 1968;43(228):200–3. https://doi.org/10.1136/adc.43.228.200.
2. Bokai J. A fityma (preputium) sejtes adatapadgsa a makkoz gyermakel-n61. Orv Hetil. 1860;4:583.

3. Schweigger-Seifd F. Zur eiitwickelung des praeputium. Arch. de Vir-chow. 1866;37:219.
4. Retterere. Note sur le development du prepuce, de la coronue du gland et du col du penis chez l'embryo humain. Compt. rend. Soc de Biol. 1890;2:528.
5. Vandeborne L, van Overbeeke E, Dooms M, De Beleyr D, Huys I. Information needs of physicians regarding the diagnosis of rare diseases: a questionnaire-based study in Belgium. Orphanet J Rare Dis. 2019;14:99. https://doi.org/10.1186/s13023-019-1075-8.
6. Harryman GL. An analysis of the accuracy of the presentation of the human penis in anatomical source materials. In: Denniston GC, Hodges FM, Milos MF, editors. Flesh and blood. Boston: Springer; 2004. https://doi.org/10.1007/978-1-4757-4011-0_2.
7. Roberts SJ. Veterinary obstetrics and genital diseases (Theriogenology). Ithaca, Ann Arbor: Edwards Brothers; 1971. p. 610.

Part I

Normal Prepuce

History of the Prepuce

2

Evolutionary Prepuce

Although the penises of all mammalian males are protected by the prepuce, they considerably differ from that of the man. In quadrupeds, it is represented by a long tunnel called *preputial sheath* that forms part of the abdominal wall. A penis hanging outside the body of quadrupeds is clearly at risk of injury while hunting or escaping from predators. For this reason, in flaccid state the entire penis, not merely the glans, is safely retracted into the preputial sheath. However, when man assumed bipedality preputial sheath was no longer required because the flaccid penis has been safeguarded by thighs on either side. Hence the long preputial sheath of primitive mammals is replaced by simple prepuce in man. Evolutionary retaining of the prepuce indicates that it is intended to protect the glans. In a simulation experiment Taves demonstrated that rolling back of prepuce during intercourse facilitates easy penetration of the glans [1]. Foreskin rich in erogenous nerve endings is also a source of foreplays that are unique to human race (Chap. 5).

It will be interesting to explore as to who demonized the innocent prepuce and recommended its excision [2].

Prehistoric Prepuce

Baculiform artifacts of Paleolithic period have been excavated from various caves of France, Spain, Germany and Ukraine [3]. They belong to Gravettian (more than 20,000 years ago) and Magdalenian (20,000–16,000 years ago) periods. The oldest of them was a 30,000 years-old ivory phallic replica excavated from Vogelherd. Characteristically many of these artifacts resemble 'circumcised penis with exposed glans' (Fig. 2.1). This prompted some researchers to claim that circumcision must have been practiced by prehistoric man. In the absence of conclusive proof, such a view is simply untenable. There are strong reasons to believe that early man would not have preferred deliberate circumcision because ensuing wound infection would have proved to be a survival disadvantage [4, 5]. In an era when antibiotics and microbial origin of diseases were not known primitive man must have avoided self infliction of wounds in fear of infection and its consequences. Further, the primitive man, who venerated genital organs, would not have dared mutilating them [6]. If so, what do those artifacts actually represent? Hypothetical suggestions such as dildos, drumsticks and tent holders appear to be incorrect because they need not have to be so painstakingly carved. The celebrated archeologist Gabriel de Mortillet called them "*bâton de commandement*". In ancient days erect penis was considered a sign

M. A. B. Fahmy, *Normal and Abnormal Prepuce*, https://doi.org/10.1007/978-3-030-37621-5_2

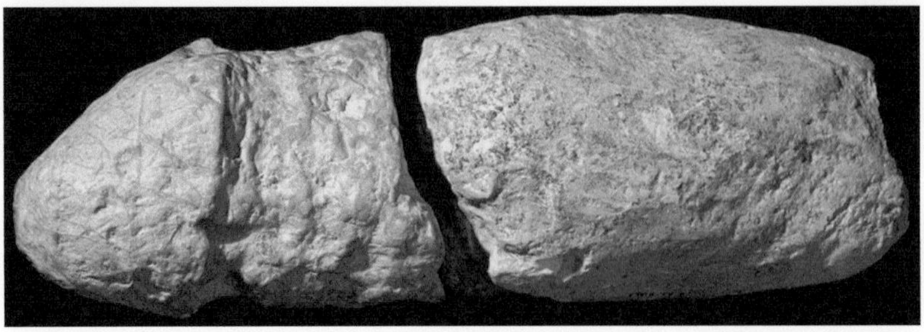

Fig. 2.1 Baculiform stone artifacts of 30,000 years old excavated from Maumbury rings. It is now exhibited at the Dorset County Museum. (Unknown photographer)

of authority and prosperity [6]. Therefore, these baculiform replicas were perhaps batons held by clan leaders which they passed on to their successors as a symbol of power and authority. Exposed glans-like appearance probably represents erect penis rather than circumcised member. In those primitive days exquisite carvings were expectedly difficult, which is why the retracted frills of foreskin could not be seen in them. Alternatively, if such delicate carvings had been done, they might have got corroded over thousands of years. It is safe to assume that prehistoric man did not practice circumcision, yet unaware of the role of prepuce in coitus.

Egyptian Prepuce

Egyptians are known to have practiced circumcision for over 5000 years [6, 7]. Herodotus, the Greek historian who visited Egypt in circa 450 BCE has noted it being practiced among the upper-class citizens. He remarked, "They place cleanliness ahead of comeliness" [8]. It gives an impression as if Egyptians preferred this procedure mainly to maintain hygiene. But the saga of prepuce and circumcision was more complex which, for the sake of descriptive convenience, can be divided into 4 overlapping eras of imprecise time scale [4].

Era of Punitive Circumcision

At the dawn of human civilization, circumcision must have been considered a punishment and a substitute for emasculation. In primitive days it was common for victors to mutilate the genitals of their enemies as a mark of humiliation. For example, Saturn castrated his father Uranus as a punishment of killing his siblings (Fig. 2.2). According to the inscriptions near the sixth pylon of Karnak temple, Generals of the 70-year-old Pharaoh Merneptah (1212–1203 BCE), when they invaded Libya, brought back 13,240 penises of enemies as war trophy [8]. At some undefined period of time, Egyptian Pharaohs instead of killing defeated soldiers preferred to emasculate them as they proved to be useful slaves in fields and harems. Since penile amputation carried high mortality from wound infection and bleeding, it must have been substitute by circumcision as a symbolic humiliation. This assumption is supported by the descriptions of Diodorus Siculus (circa 100 BC) in his magnum opus '*Bibliotheca Historica*'. He claimed to have seen a bas-relief in the Tomb of Ozymandias that depicted chain-bound war prisoners being lined up in preparation for penile amputation or circumcision and the excised organs being piled up in the foreground [9]. Thus, only slaves appeared to have been circumcised during this era, which was probably the pre-dynasty period (before 3000 BCE).

Era of Emulative Circumcision

Circumcision that was originally considered a humiliating punishment of slaves, soon transformed into divine sacrifice and a religious rite of nobles. This radical change was perhaps prompted by the myth of Osiris cult which originated circa 2600–2100 BCE [10]. Osiris was considered the God of fertility and agriculture in Egyptian mythology. Possibly Osiris could have

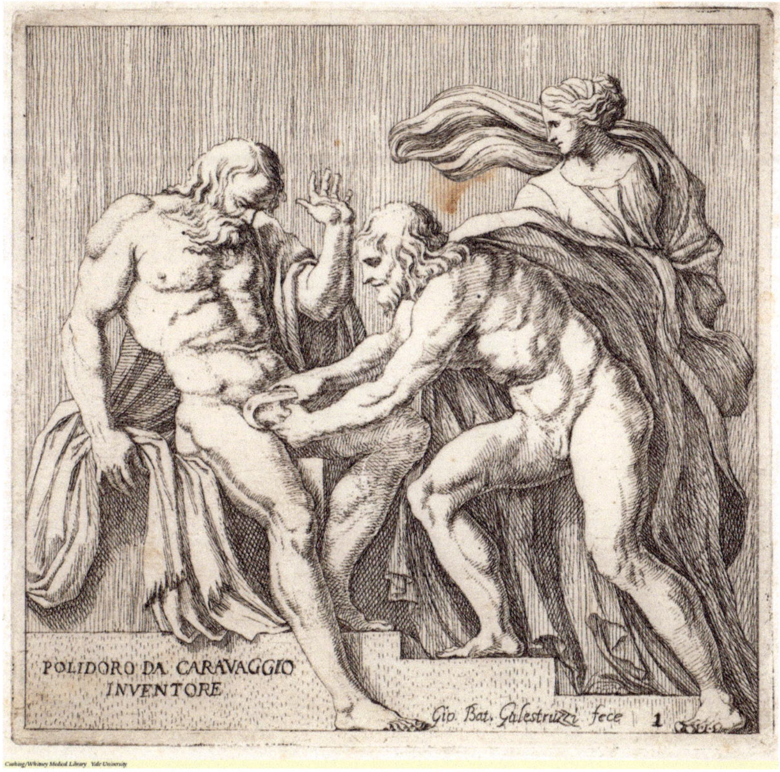

Fig. 2.2 Saturn castrating his father Uranus as a punishment of killing his siblings. Etching by Polidoro de Caldara (circa 1540 CE) now exhibited at the Cushing—Whitney Medical Library of Yale University

been a primeval king of prehistoric Egypt rather than a pure mythical character because in ancient world the rulers were considered as God incarnations and were deified after death. According to the mythology, Osiris was the brother of Isis, Seth and Nephthys. Brothers Osiris and Seth married their sisters Isis and Nephthys respectively. Such incestuous marriages are not uncommon in those days. According to Plutarch, Seth envied the throne of Osiris. Further, Seth was infuriated when Osiris had illicit intercourse with his wife Nephthys (Fig. 2.3). Enraged Seth cut the body of Osiris into 42 pieces and scattered them all over the country. According to the tradition of punitive emasculation, Seth mutilated the penis of his enemy-brother and drowned it in the Nile. Aggrieved Isis, the goddess of rivers and night, searched for the body parts of her husband with the help of Thoth, the god of healing and her sister Nephthys. She could retrieve all of them except his penis which had been eaten by Medjed, the mythical fish of Nile. Isis sewed and embalmed the collected parts of Osiris' body and supplemented the missing penis with a golden replica. Priests of Osiris cult probably adopted circumcision as a symbolic emulation of Osiris' emasculation. Thus, circumcision which was previously restricted to slaves became a sign of aristocracy [11]. Priests, kings and nobles must have had felt compelled to get circumcised. In fact, Pharaohs were not allowed to ascend throne unless they get circumcised [12].

There are two surviving evidences of priestly circumcision being practiced during this era: (1) Bas-relief at the necropolis of Saqqara dedicated to Akhmahor, the Ka-Priest of the sixth dynasty king Teti (circa 2300 BCE); (2) The carvings at the Karnak Temple of Mut commissioned during the reign of the 12th dynasty Pharaoh Senusret-I (circa 1971–1926 BCE). They are often interpreted to depict priesthood initiation ceremony [11]. In both of them men are seen to undergo some ritual concerning their genitals (Fig. 2.4). Art historian Ann Macy Roth contends that it could simply be ritual shaving of pubic hair. However, the need of an assistant to hold the

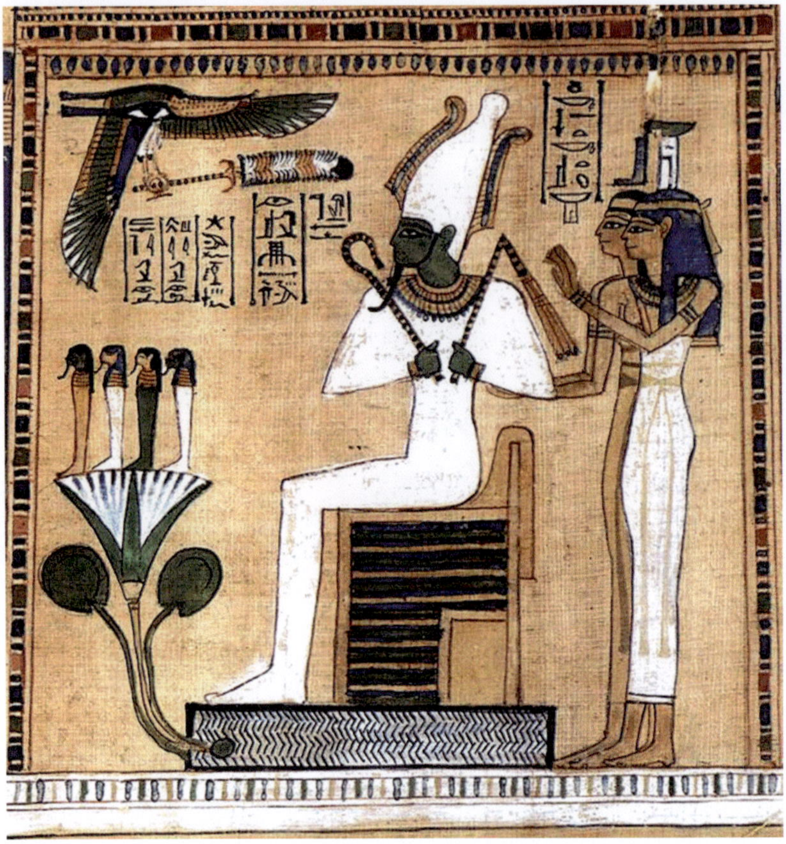

Fig. 2.3 Papyrus painting depicting Osiris in his judgment throne flanked by his sister-wives Isis and Nephthys. (British Museum Pap., No. 10470; Public domain figure)

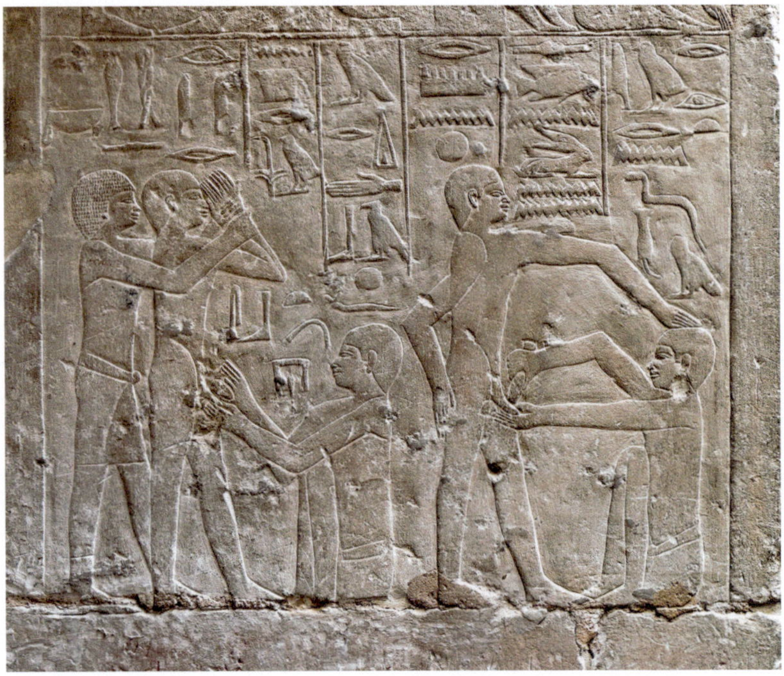

Fig. 2.4 Bas-relief from Mastaba of Ankhmahor depicting a genital procedure being performed on priesthood initiates. It is popularly interpreted to represent circumcision. (Public domain figure from Wikimedia)

subjects as well as the reassurance of the operator recorded in hieroglyphics indicate that it was a painful procedure, most likely to be circumcision. Thus, during the era of emulation, which probably lasted during the early dynasty period (circa 3100–2200 BCE), circumcision was adopted as a religious ritual and had become a sign of aristocracy [11].

Era of Religious Revolt

During the era of religious revolt, circumcision was, perhaps, once again degraded to be a sign of slavery. In old kingdom high priests, especially those of *Amun* cult, enjoyed privileges equivalent to that of Pharaohs. They increasingly became autocratic and started interfering with the regal powers of Pharaohs. Priestly supremacy was apparently prominent during the times of New Kingdom (circa 1600–1100 BCE). Many Pharaohs disliked the high-handed behavior of priests and the bitterness reached its zenith during the 18th dynasty. An internal revolt against the priestly dominance started during this period. As a symbolic gesture of disobedience some of the Pharaohs refused to undergo circumcision that was insisted by priests. This is supported by the fact that the mummy of Ahmose-I (circa 1549–1524 BCE) is found uncircumcised [13]. The revolt reached its peak during the reign of Amenhotep-IV (circa 1353–1334 BCE), popularly known as the Amarna period [14]. The Pharaoh changed his name as Akhenaten, thereby deleting the reference to the God Amun from his original name (Fig. 2.5). He banned the polytheistic Amun cult and clipped the wings of priests. In his final years, he aggressively destroyed all Amun temples which were the source of income for the priests. He imposed the monotheistic worship of Aten, the sun disc. Royal decree prohibited citizens from following Amun cult rituals including circumcision. Presumably, circumcision rituals were a source of income to priests which the Pharaoh curbed. Akhenaten's reforms infuriated Amun priests as they were deprived of their former prestige and livelihood. It is rumored that Akhenaten could have been murdered by them. Thus, during the Amarna period circumcision was once again reduced to debauchery; fearing royal scorn nobles and laity refrained from it. Only slaves and Amun priests appeared to have undergone the procedure during this era.

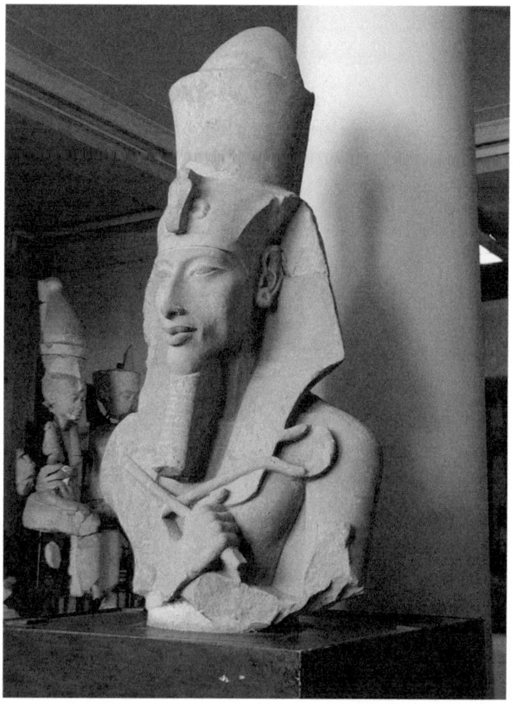

Fig. 2.5 Statue of Akhenaten from his Aten Temple at Karnak; now displayed at the Egyptian Museum of Cairo. (Photo credit Gérard Ducher, reproduced under creative common license of Wikipedia)

Era of Chaos and Common Adaptation

Akhenaten's son Tutankhaten (circa 1332–1323 BCE) was only 9 years when his father died. So, he was anointed, with his general Ay as regent. Exploiting the situation, Ay made compromising pacts with the repressed priests and built back the Amun temples destroyed by Akhenaten. He even managed to change the boy-kings name as Tutankhamun with reference to the God Amun. As a part of these restorative measures, circumcision must have also been brought back. Assumably, mass circumcision carnivals were organized. According to Sigmund Freud this is the time when

Biblical Exodus must have happened [15]. Unlike the previous eras, there was no clear distinction as to who can undergo circumcision. Both elites as well as slaves must have got circumcised during this era. Exploiting this chaotic situation, Moses, in the name of God, prompted en masse circumcision of Israeli slaves; and at an opportune moment escaped with them under the disguise of being nobles. At the end of the 18th dynasty circumcision appears to have been practiced by everyone irrespective of their social status.

Although the foregoing description is largely conjectural based on circumstantial evidences, there are no better explanations as regard to the conflicting reports on the social status of circumcision in ancient Egypt [7]. Interestingly, this alternating status of circumcision between pride of nobles and shame of slaves is reflected though out history. For example, Mogul rulers of India considered circumcision as a proud religious rite. They insisted Ehlu Yale, the founder of Yale University, to get circumcised when he wanted to meet Mogul Emperor for bussiness pacts. But when young Warren Hastings, who destined to become the first Governor General of British India, was arrested after his defeat in Kasimbazar war of 1756 CE, he was stripped, sodomized and publically humiliated by circumcising [16]. Understanding the Egyptian eras of circumcision perhaps explains as to why one would use what they consider as pious ritual for humiliating their enemy.

Greek Prepuce

At the same time when circumcision was fervently practiced in ancient Egypt, Greeks and Romans expressed great aversion towards it. Ancient Greeks recognized two distinct component of the prepuce: the portion that covers the glans was known as posthe and the tapering portion that hangs beyond the limits of glans was called akroposthion [17]. They considered akroposthion aesthetically pleasing and depicted their heroes with small penis and megaprepuce (Chap. 10).

Keeping up with the tradition, even renaissance artists like Michelangelo (1475–1564 CE) sculpted David and Jesus with intact prepuce contrary to the unambiguous Biblical description of their circumcision [18] (Fig. 2.6).

In ancient Greece, public exposure of the glans, but not the penis per se, was condemned as indecent. Olympic athletes took part in competitive games in full nudity; but they cautiously protected their modesty by wearing 'kynodesme', a string that strapped the tip of prepuce with waist band thereby preventing accidental exposure of glans [17]. An intact prepuce was considered a proof of male virginity much analogous to an intact hymen of females. As a long prepuce was commended a sign of aristocracy, men wanted to elongate their 'akroposthion' by infibulation, a method of stretching prepuce [19]. Greek physicians such as Aulus Cornelius Celsus (25 BCE to 50 AD) and Oribasius (325–403 AD) described meticulous techniques of infibulations wherein the prepuce is stretched, pierced and transfixed with a strut (fibula). Lengthening of the prepuce was facilitated by suspending specially designed graded weights (Pondus Judaeus) from the fibula or by periodic proximal relocation of the fibula (Fig. 2.7).

Close to the end of Common Era, Greco-Roman intolerance towards circumcision reached a new dimension. Antiochus IV Epiphanes (circa 215–164 BCE), the Hellenistic king of the Seleucid Empire made circumcision a punishable offence. Jewish parents who circumcised their wards were flogged, crucified or hanged along with the circumcised child. This repression is said to be the cause of Maccabean Revolt (167 to 160 BCE) and the ensuing 7 battles which eventually led to the victory of Jews [13]. Hanukkah is the Jewish festival that celebrates this victory. Titus Flavius Vespasian (9–79 CE) the Roman emperor outlawed ritual circumcision as he considered it barbaric. This resulted in the Great Jewish Revolt (66–73 CE). However, Vespasian suppressed it with brutal force and revenged by imposing Fiscus Judaicus, a new tax to be paid by all circumcised Jewish men [16]. For the purpose of tax collection, every year Jewish men had to strip before an appointed officer who ascertained their circumcision status. For this reason, it is popularly known as *circumcision tax*. Vespasian's

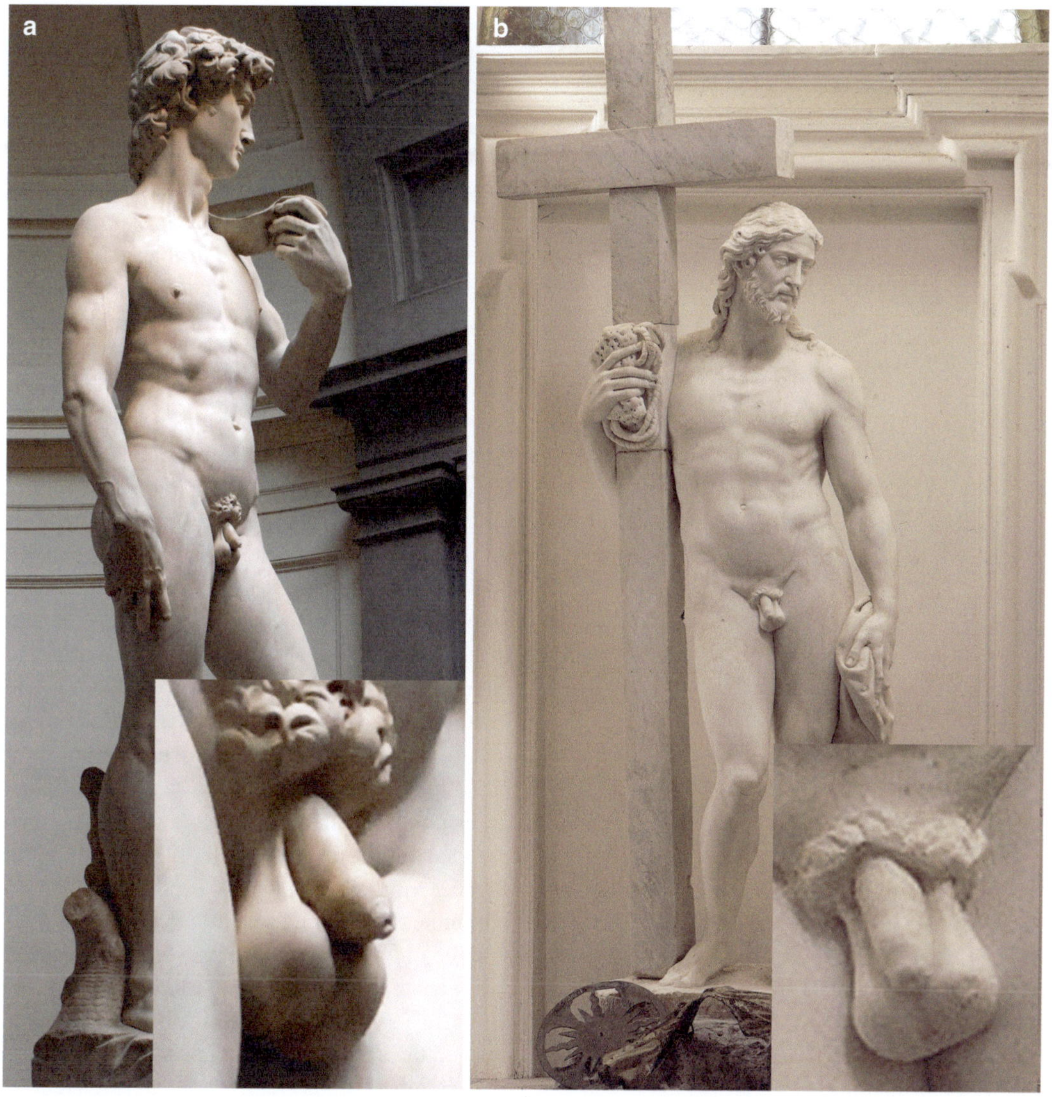

Fig. 2.6 Michelangelo's sculptures depicting intact prepuce of Biblical characters. (**a**) David and (**b**) Jesus Christ (photo credit to Mr. Jörg Bittner Unna and Mr. Don Giacinto respectively). Insets show close-up views of genitals of corresponding sculptures. (Both photographs are edited and reproduced from Wikipedia under Creative Common license)

hatred towards circumcision was such that he even executed his own nephew Titus Flavius Clemens for undergoing the Jewish ritual. Bar Kokhba revolt (circa 132–136 CE) was precipitated when Publius Aelius Hadrianus (76–138 CE), the Roman emperor enacted laws to abolish circumcision. In all these confrontations, prepuce and circumcision symbolically represented Jewish pride.

The Jewish Prepuce

Jews performed circumcision in two different ways: *Brit Milah* is just nicking or amputating the protruding tip of the prepuce while *Periah* is complete excision of the prepuce up to the coronal sulcus. Historicity of *brit milah* dates back to Biblical times, while the practice of *periah* appears to have become popular much

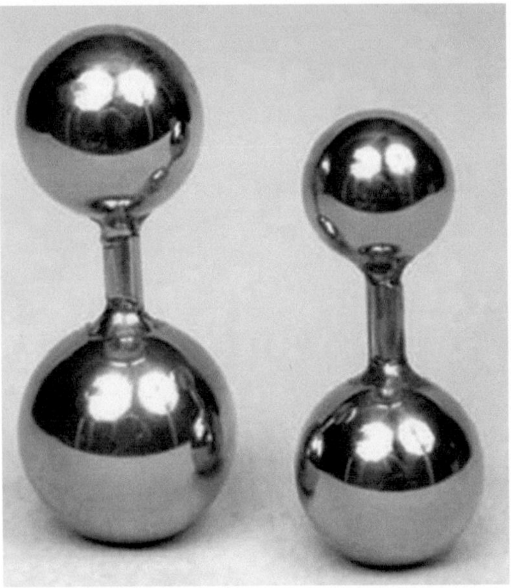

Fig. 2.7 A modern replica of Pondus Judaeus manufactured by Wayne Griffiths. Each set of them contain ball-studs of varying weights raging from 200 g to 350 g. (From Canadian Medical Association Journal 2011)

later, perhaps after the war of Bar Kokba in 140 CE.

According to Bible, Abraham got himself and his entourage circumcised at an advanced age of 99 (Fig. 2.8). It is said that the God insisted it as a sign of covenant. It is intriguing as to why would the Lord ask to cut an organ hidden from public gaze. Circumcision was perhaps a secret tool of clan identification that was necessary in an era when ethnic conflict between Israelites and Egyptians was enormous [15]. Even as late as the twentieth century, when large scale violence erupted following the Indian partition, men were stripped to ascertain their religious identity thereby either got killed or let go accordingly. The same was also true of Nazi concentration camps and Bosnian conflicts. The period of Abraham probably corresponds to the era of emulative circumcision when only the elite practiced it in Egypt. Abraham being a slave was not originally circumcised and he was thrown out of Egypt when he deceived Pharaoh by misrepresenting his wife Sarai as his sister [20]. Abraham's circumcision could well be a desperate ploy of re-entering Egypt under the disguise of being a noble. This assumption is supported by the fact that the God's covenant was not followed after Abraham until it was revived by Moses.

Moses was also not circumcised; but was said to have born with aposthia (congenital absence of the prepuce). He probably lived during the Egyptian era of chaos and common adoptation. Death of first born royal child mentioned in the book of Exodus probably refers to the murder of the boy-king Tutankhamun. Jewish slaves have long discontinued the Abrahamic custom of circumcision. Exploiting the chaotic situation that then prevailed, Moses must have hatched a plan to escape Egypt by getting his men circumcised. In effect, Moses appears to have reversed the plan of Abraham who perhaps used circumcision to enter Egypt. In fact, Moses was also thought to be a priest of Aten cult who escaped Egypt following the death of its benefactor Akhenaten and propagated the legacy of monotheism among Jews [15]. It is also rumored that Moses was none other than the Pharaoh Akhenaten himself who escaped Egypt in disguise. Following the great escape, Moses did not show keen enthusiasm to continue the custom of circumcision which is why he did not circumcise his son until the God intervened and threatened to kill him.

Forty years after the death of Moses, Joshua revived the custom by organizing mass circumcision camps at a place called Gilgal. The Hebrew word Gilgal actually means 'removed' and the mountain is popularly known as *'circumcision hill'* [20]. Notwithstanding the holy nature of the procedure, intermittently circumcision was also used to shame enemies. For example, Soul who wanted to avenge both David and Philistines, asked David to bring 100 foreskins of Philistines as dowry to marry his daughter Michael. He expected both of them to be killed in the battle; but David came back with 200 of foreskins and took Michael's hand in wedlock. In another story, Jacob's sons Simeon and Levi wanted to revenge Shechem for the disgraceful rape of their sister Dinah. Pretending to get him married with Dinah,

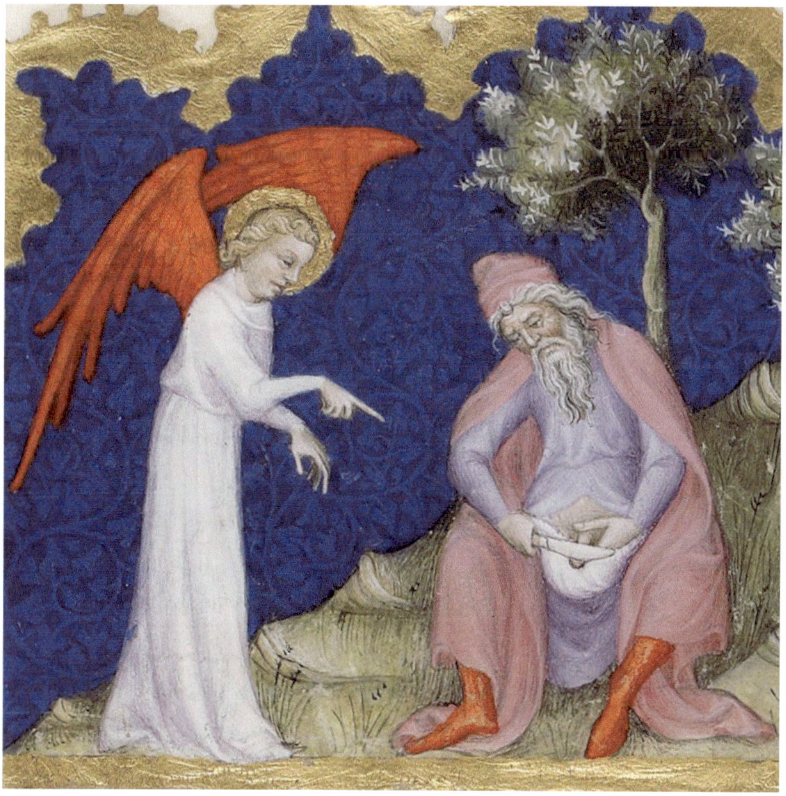

Fig. 2.8 Self-circumcision of Abraham. (From the Bible de Jean de Sy - circa 1355–1357 CE; Public domain figure from Wikimedia)

her brothers preconditioned that Shechem and his men should first get circumcised. While their enemies were still incapacitated by the circumcision sore, Simeon and Levi ravaged their camps and killed all of them. Thus, the ancient Egyptian legacy of viewing circumcision as both a sacred ritual and a humiliating punishment continued during Biblical times.

During the times of the Old Testament *brit milah* was the method of circumcision. As only the tip of prepuce was removed in this method, Jewish young men easily grew back the foreskin by infibulation. They primarily did it to appear uncircumcised to the Greeks so as to secure opportunities of job, trade and participation in Olympic Games. Rabbies, who did not like this, introduced *periah* (complete excision of the prepuce) thereby making reversal of circumcision difficult. In their frenzy to prevent reversal of circumcision, rabbies advocated a procedure called synechotomy in which considerable amount of shaft skin was also excised.

The Holy Prepuce of Jesus

Being born a Jew, as per the prevailing custom, Jesus Christ was circumcised on the 8th day of life (Octave). In fact, Catholic Churches celebrated the first day of January (the 8th day of Christmas as per Julian calendar) not as 'New Year day' but as 'Circumcision Day' [21]. Only in 1960 the second Vatican council re-designated it as Solemnity of Mary. Mother Mary, who was aware of the supernatural qualities of her son, preserved the excised prepuce in a marble alabaster and gifted it to Mary Magdalene who is variously described as friend, patient, disciple or wife of Jesus. Mary Magdalene gave it back to Peter (pun unintended). After changing many hands the Holy prepuce reached Byzantine Empress Irene, who gave it as her wedding gift to Emperor Charlemagne (742–814 CE), of Germany (Fig. 2.9). The Saint's prepuce was finally kept in Charroux Abbey of France for public worship. During middle ages, this relic

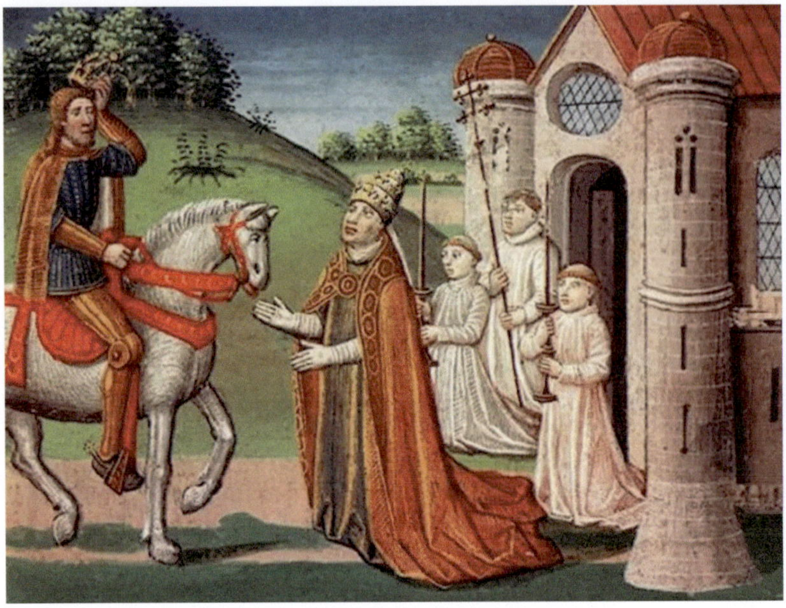

Fig. 2.9 Charlemagne and Pope Adrian I: painting by Antoine Vérard (circa 1493). The Frankish king was said to have inherited the Holy prepuce as a wedding gift from Byzantine empress Irene in circa 768 CE. (Public domain figure from Wikipedia)

drew large number of pilgrims who believed that touching it will cure infertility and will make childbirth painless. Popularity of the relic soon prompted as many as 21 cathedrals to announce that they were holding the original Holy foreskin. Pope Clement VII (1523–1534 CE) certified that the Charroux Abbey relic was the genuine one. Magical powers of the foreskin were so strongly believed that King Henry V, who wished a painless labor of his French wife, arranged to steal the Holy prepuce when the church authorities refused to part with it. Saint Brigida brought another copy of the relic to the Scala Santa of Rome which was also stolen in 1527 CE when Charles V besieged Rome.

Claims of Lord's preputial relics caused deep embarrassment to theologists of the Church. Unlike other prophets who left behind their human body, Jesus was said to have resurrected and ascended to heaven with his human body. Thus, acknowledging the earthly existence of his foreskin clearly contradicted the theological principles. Distressed Vatican increasingly denied '*Preputium Domini*' and explained that the Lord's prepuce had reunited with him on his resurrection. By 1900 CE, Pope even threatened to excommunicate those who talk of the Holy prepuce.

Irrespective of what happened to the excised Holy prepuce, Jesus did not approve circumcision. Was he troubled by any long-term complication of the procedure will be an interesting question to explore. He recommended replacing circumcision with baptism. When few churches of Gelatia refused to deviate from the custom of circumcision, Paul, the disciple of Jesus was said to have told, "When we are in union with Christ Jesus, neither circumcision nor the lack of it makes any difference at all; what matters is faith that works through love". The word 'circumcision' semantically means 'cutting all around'. Thus, it does not exclusively mean excision of the prepuce but in spiritual sense the isolation of oneself from all surrounding evils. When the Book of Ezekiel mention, "You have brought in strangers, uncircumcised in heart and uncircumcised in flesh, to be in my sanctuary, to pollute it", it clearly identifies two types of circumcision – one is physical pertaining to the foreskin and the other one is spiritual concerning the heart (conscience). Jesus must have interpreted the word 'circumcision' of the Old Testament in spiritual sense. Thus, the long tradition of the ritual was disrupted during the Anno Domini, only to be revived 500 years later by Prophet Mohammed.

The Islamic Prepuce

Like Jews, Muslims are known to be fanatical of circumcision. Surprisingly the ritual is nowhere mentioned in the Holy *Quran* and the reference to it comes from the books of prophetic traditions called *Hadiths* [22]. Circumcision, known as *Khitan* to Arabs, was practiced even during pre-Islamic times. An interesting hypothesis suggests that it must have been done to prevent accumulation of desert sand within the preputial sac [2]. Circumcision is merely a *Sunnah* (optional) rather than a *Wajib* (obligatory). Shiites and Sunnites differ considerably in their interpretation and implementation of Islamic rules. Consequently, among the six schools of Islamic theology (Hanafite, Jafarite, Malikite, Hanbalite, Shafiite and Zaidite) only the Shafiite consider it obligatory. In other sects, a child born to Muslim parents or a convert from other religions will not be considered a non-Muslim just because he is uncircumcised.

As circumcision is a prophetic tradition in Islam, it would be curious to know when and how Prophet Mohammed (570–632 CE) was circumcised. Ibin Kathir (1300–1373 CE), the authentic biographer of Mohammed, mentioned that the prophet was born without prepuce [23]. He quoted Mohammed's grandfather *Abd-al-Muttalib* saying, "The messenger of God was born circumcised and his umbilical cord severed. This son of mine is sure to be important." Even prophet Mohammed himself was once said to have told, "One way God honored me was in my being born already circumcised so that, no one saw my private parts." Such congenital absence of foreskin is now called in modern medical science as aposthia. Owing to its extreme rarity, Arabs must have considered aposthia as a divine miracle [24]. Contrary to these statements, *Abu Bakr*, the father-in-law of Mohammed, maintained that his son-in-law was circumcised by the archangel Gabriel. Irrespective of the foregoing controversy, followers of Islam appears to emulate the circumcised state of their leader much similar to the priests of Osiris cult imitating their God.

The Prepuce of French Revolution

Causative connection between phimotic prepuce and the French revolution is underemphasized in the pages of world history [25]. Louis XVI, the crown prince of France married the Austrian Archduchess Marie Antoinette on the 16th May 1770 (Fig. 2.10). However the royal marriage was not consummated for 8 long years. The dauphin obviously avoided the archduchess and pretended to be engaged in full-time hunting. Even on the day of nuptial night, he has remarked a single word "nothing" in his journal. Even when Marie approached him amorously, Louis simply excused himself by asking more time to overcome his fear. Everyone convulsed as to what could be the cause. Rumors abound among general public as to the potency of the young prince. On 16 July 1770, the dauphin fell ill with severe cough and cold. Taking advantage of the situation, Louis XV asked his court physicians to examine his grandson for any genital defects that might preclude intercourse. La Martiniere, the

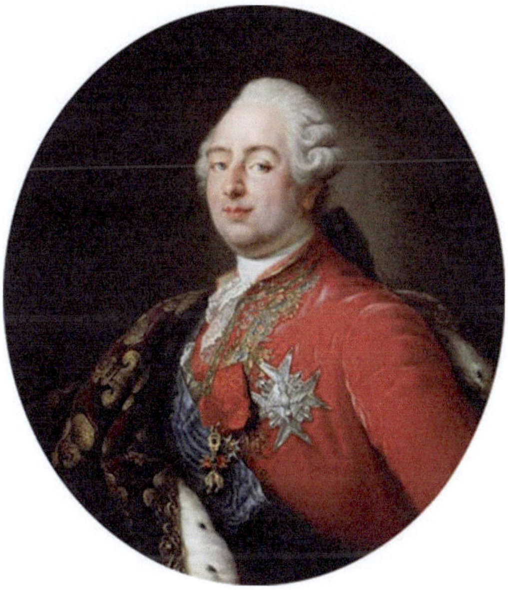

Fig. 2.10 Portrait of Louis XVI by Antoine-François Callet, 1786. Phimosis and the consequential sexual inadequacy of the dauphin are said to have indirectly influenced the origin of French revolution. (Public domain figure from Wikipedia)

chief physician diagnosed impotence that does not require any surgical correction. A second opinion was sought. Although the famous urologists Jacques Louis Moreau of Hotel Dieu diagnosed phimosis, he - like the celebrated author of surgical textbook Pierre Dionis - opined that it will resolve spontaneously over time. Two years elapsed, when the young prince confided to his father that he was suffering severe pain whenever he attempted penetration. In 1777, Joseph-II, brother of Antoinette visited the couple and made enquiry about their barrenness. It is supposed that he arranged for a secret circumcision of his brother-in-law and even offered to hold him during the procedure. Following the operation, Louis XVI confessed to his aunt, "I delight in pleasure and I regret that I was not aware of it for so long". The intervening 7 years proved devastating to the frustrated young couple. They engaged themselves in notorious frivolity and spendthrift which, according to the Austrian psychiatrist Zweig, may be the psychic reaction to their sexual frustration. Public were infuriated by the extravaganzas of Antoinette which ultimately culminated in French Revolution in 1789. Had the prepuce of Louis XVI been guillotined earlier, his head would have escaped. Centuries later Sigmund Freud emphasized the psychosexual implication of circumcision.

The Freudian Prepuce

Sigmund Freud, the founder of psychoanalysis, appears to have been excessively influenced by the circumcision that he underwent as a Jewish boy. Like Jesus, Freud must have been troubled by an untold complication of circumcision. He hypothesized that every young boy develops libidinal attachment to his mother and hatred towards father who is a jealous competitor of his love [26]. During the Oedipal phase of psychosexual development the boy fears that his father may punish him by castration because of his incestuous relationship with mother. Freud, in his theory of castration complex, proposed circumcision as a symbolic substitute of emasculation. "When our children come to hear of ritual circumcision, they equate it with castration", wrote the distraught Freud in *Totem and Taboo*. Freud's theory is nothing new, but a remix of the ancient Egyptian custom wherein slaves were circumcised in lieu of castration. Freud incriminated circumcision-related anxiety as the cause of neurosis.

In the background of Freudian theory, it is essential to examine if childhood circumcision, especially during the phallic phase of psychosexual development, will cause any permanent psychological scar. Some evidence suggests that those who underwent the procedure in childhood are likely to recommend it to others [27]. Psychologists refer to this phenomenon as 're-enactment or re-victimization of childhood trauma' which is perhaps a sado-masochist trait [28].

The Prepuce of Aboriginal Tribes

Freud hypothesized that every female is envious of male for possessing a penis. This '*penis envy*' theory of Freud drew sharp criticism from feminists. Bruno Bettelheim retaliated by proposing a theory of '*vagina envy*', according to which every male is said to be envious of female vagina and menstruation [29]. He suggested that circumcision practiced as initiation rites among Australian aboriginals could be an expression of male desire to imitate menarcheal bloodshed of females (Fig. 2.11). Men of Wogeo, Murngin and Dwoma tribes of New Guinea incise their prepuce not only once but periodically and allow monthly flow of blood akin to menstruation. Although psychologists may eccentrically attribute it to 'vagina envy' reaction, the real anthropological reason behind such "male menstruation" is to get rid of evil forces that are believed to accumulate and cause diseases [30, 31]. In this context, it is worth remembering that as late as in the nineteenth century bloodletting was a popular treatment of many maladies.

Anthropologists have noted that another interesting reason for tribal circumcision. According to the beliefs of certain African tribes such as the Dogon, Bambara and Lobi, every newborn child

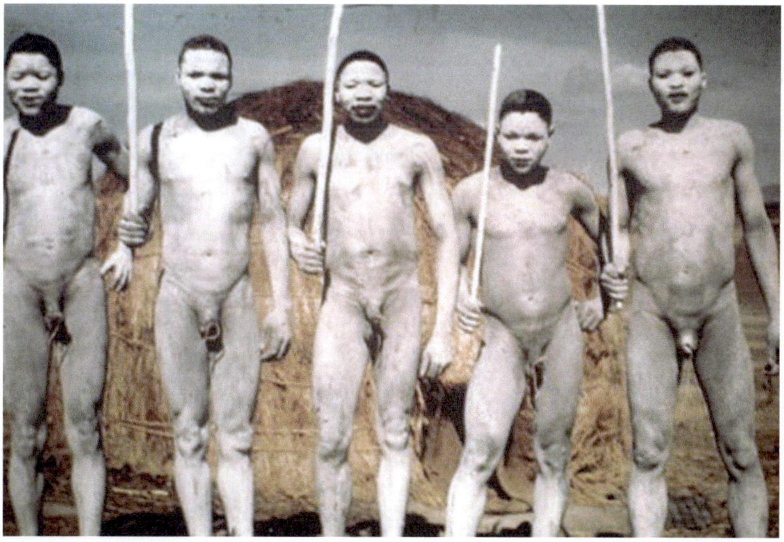

Fig. 2.11 A group of circumcision initiates of Xhosa tribe. Symbolic wounds testing the ability to endure pain are the underlying principle of passing rites. (Reproduced from WHO document on African circumcision)

is considered to be androgynous having both male and female spirit in them; freeing one of them is essential for the developmental completion of the individual. Thus they contemplate circumcision will release female spirit from males while clitoridectomy (popularly known as female circumcision) will release male spirit from females [13].

In addition to circumcision, initiation rites followed in different tribes include tooth pulling, tattooing, body piercing, whipping and stab incisions [32]. The central theme of all these is testing the ability to endure pain. In worrier tribes, tolerating pain is an essential attribute needed to protect its members from foreign attacks. Thus, aboriginal circumcision is rooted in both superstitious beliefs as well as symbolic test of integrity.

The Victorian Prepuce

Freudian anxiety of foreskin got escalated during the Victorian era (1837–1901 CE), the period when personal morality was excessively emphasized. There was a great panic among the public about male masturbation as it was considered a form of self abuse [33]. Ingenuously engineered devices and surgical procedures were employed to deter young men from masturbating. Among them, the method that most consistently worked was circumcision. Sooner the focus was turned on to smegma, the irritation of which was hypothesized to cause excessive venery and masturbation.

Smegma, the new found felon, was enthusiastically incriminated in every other disease of unknown etiology. For example, Lewis Sayre (1820–1900 CE) the famous orthopedic surgeon of New York and the founder of American Medical Association, attributed hip ankylosis to neuronal reflex of preputial irritation by smegma [34]. For 30 years Sayre travelled extensively on either side of the Atlantic and propagated circumcision as the cure of many weird conditions such as scoliosis, hip contractures, backache and hernia. Nathaniel Heckford extended the reflex neurosis theory and recommended circumcision to cure epilepsy and cholera. The famous gynecologist James Sims, influenced by his friend Sayre, recommended female circumcision as the treatment of female nervousness, an imprecise term which may mean anything from insomnia to premenstrual symptoms to depression. Circumcision soon became a panacea. Hurd used it to cure whooping cough, chronic crying, unexplained weight loss and even fever in children. Norman Chapman, a student of Sayre and noted professor of neurology, extended the indications of circumcision to wide range of neurological disorders including paralysis, mental retardation, schizophrenia and neurasthenia. In a 1894 review article, Merrill Ricketts listed 29 indications of circumcision [13].

In 1858 Rudolph Virchow proposed his carcinogenic theory of chronic irritation. Peter Charles Remondino, vice-president of the California Medical Society and an ardent advocate of circumcision, saw a link between Sayre's theory of reflex neurosis and Virchow's theory of chronic irritation. He suggested that chronic irritation of smegma could be the cause of penile cancers and substantiated it by citing its low incidence among Jews who routinely circumcise [35]. Remondino took circumcision to another level, promoting it for the first time as a prophylactic procedure. Impact of his views is so strong that traces of them are still seen in modern textbooks despite lack of rigorous scientific proofs [36]. By the turn of the twentieth century, prepuce was successfully demonized and circumcision got the scientific endorsement of being a legitimate treatment and prophylaxis.

The Modern Prepuce

In 1949, Douglas Gairdner, the brilliant pediatrician of United Cambridge Hospital published a seminal paper in the British Medical Journal [37]. Until then physicians diagnosed all non-retractable foreskins of infants as phimosis; circumcision was obviously the logical treatment of it. Thus, millions of circumcisions were done which added to the economic burden of world wars. Gairdner in his paper entitled, "On the fate of the foreskin" announced that the preputial adhesion of infancy is quite physiological and nothing need to be done for it. His paper was instrumental in removing circumcision from the list of operations that were eligible for NHS funding and insurance reimbursement. This paper also mooted the concept that infantile circumcision could be a form of human rights violation. 'Intactivists', the social activists against circumcision, soon sprung into action and succeeded in getting anti-circumcision laws enacted in some states. They work under the motto, "Pain should not be the first experience of the penis". Alternating between proscription and prescription is not new to circumcision ever since the days of Eyptian Pharaohs and this millennium-old operation will continue to intrigue laity as well as scientists.

References

1. Taves D. The intromission function of the foreskin. Med Hypotheses. 2002;59:180–2.
2. Darby R. A surgical temptation: the demonization of the foreskin and the rise of circumcision in Great Britain. Chicago: University of Chicago Press; 2005.
3. Angulo JC, García-Díez M. Male genital representation in paleolithic art: erection and circumcision before history. Urology. 2009;74:10–4.
4. Raveenthiran V. On the origin of circumcision. J Pediatr Surg. 2018;53:1877–8.
5. Raveenthiran V. Tracing the origins of circumcision. J Pediatr Surg. 2019;54:360–1.
6. Raveenthiran V. The penis in history. In: Fahmy M, editor. Congenital anomalies of the penis. Cham: Springer International; 2017. p. 15–31.
7. Raveenthiran V. The evolutionary saga of circumcision from a religious perspective. J Pediatr Surg. 2018;53:1440–3.
8. Friedman DM. A mind of its own: a cultural history of the penis. London: Robert Hale; 2001.
9. Dunsmuir WD, Gordon EM. The history of circumcision. BJU Int. 1999;83(Suppl):s1–12.
10. Griffiths JG. The origins of Osiris and his cult. Leiden: EJ Brill; 1980.
11. Hodges FM. Phimosis in antiquity. World J Urol. 1999;17:133–6.
12. Kaicher DC, Swan KG. A cut above: circumcision as an ancient status symbol. Urology. 2010;76:18–20.
13. Gollaher DL. Circumcision: a history of the world's most controversial surgery. New York: Basic Books; 2000.
14. Shaw I, editor. The Oxford history of ancient Egypt. Oxford: Oxford University Press; 2000.
15. Freud S. Moses and Monotheism (English translation by Jones K). Hertfordshire: Hogarth Press; 1939.
16. Aggleton P. A social history of male circumcision. Reprod Health Matters. 2007;15:15–21.
17. Hodges FM. The ideal prepuce in ancient Greece and Rome: male genital aesthetics and their relation to lipodermos, circumcision, foreskin restoration, and the kynodesme. Bull Hist Med. 2001;75:375–405.
18. Ciaglia P. The "David" of Michelangelo or (why the foreskin?). JAMA. 1971;218:1304.
19. Schultheiss D, Mattelaer JJ, Hodges FM, et al. Preputial infibulation: from ancient medicine to modern genital piercing. BJU Int. 2003;92:758–63.
20. The Holy Bible (King James Version). www.davinci.com/bible. Accessed 4 Aug 2019.

21. Mattelaer JJ, Schipper RA, Das S. The circumcision of Jesus Christ. J Urol. 2007;178:31–4.
22. Rizvi SA, Naqvi SA, Hussain M, Hasan AS. Religious circumcision: a Muslim view. BJU Int. 1999;83(Suppl 1):13–6.
23. Kathir I. The life of the prophet Muhammad (English translation of Al Sira al Nabawiyya by Gassick TL), vol. 1. Reading: Garner Publishing; 1998.
24. Amin Ud Din M. Aposthia - a motive of circumcision origin. Iran J Public Health. 2012;41:84.
25. Androustsos G. Le phimosis de Louis XVI (1754-1793) aurait-il été à l'origine de ses difficultés sexuelles et de sa fécondité retardée? Prog Urol. 2002;12:132–7.
26. Freud S. Totem and taboo (English translation by Brill AA). New York: Moffat-Yard; 1918.
27. Muller AJ. To cut or not to cut? Personal factors influence primary care physicians' position on elective circumcision. J Men's Health. 2010;7:227–32.
28. van der Kolk BA. The compulsion to repeat the trauma. Re-enactment, re-victimization, and masochism. Psychiatr Clin North Am. 1989;12:389–411.
29. Bettelheim B. Symbolic wounds: pubertal rites and envious male. New York: Collier Books; 1962.
30. Brekell J. A dissertation upon the subject of circumcision containing an inquiry into the original of this religious rite. London: Waugh; 1763.
31. Charles W. Motives for male circumcision among preliterate and literate peoples. J Sex Res. 1966;2:69–88.
32. Vardanyan AV. Socially constructed phallus: an anthropological inquiry of male circumcision. M.A. Thesis in Anthropology. Northridge: California State University; 2007.
33. Hunt A. The great masturbation panic and the discourses of moral regulation in nineteenth- and early twentieth-century Britain. J Hist Sex. 1998;8:575–615.
34. Sayre LA. Circumcision versus epilepsy, etc. Med Rec. 1870;71(5):233–4.
35. Remondino PC. History of circumcision from the earliest times to the present. London: F. A. Davis; 1891.
36. Van Howe RS, Hodges FM. The carcinogenicity of smegma: debunking a myth. J Eur Acad Dermatol Venereol. 2006;20:1046–54.
37. Gairdner D. The fate of the foreskin, a study of circumcision. Br Med J. 1949;2(4642):1433–7.

3 Animal Prepuce

Animal prepuce is usually called the penile sheath, which is a skin surrounding and protecting the head of the penis, but the term foreskin is not in common use for animal.

Some animals had a brightly coloured prepuce like Cercopithecus, Mandrillus, Papio, and Pongo.

Vervet monkeys that have black faces and grey bodies, but a turquoise or cyan coloured scrotal skin, which is extended to the penile sheath, but actually the preputial ring is more or less fleshy red (Fig. 3.1).

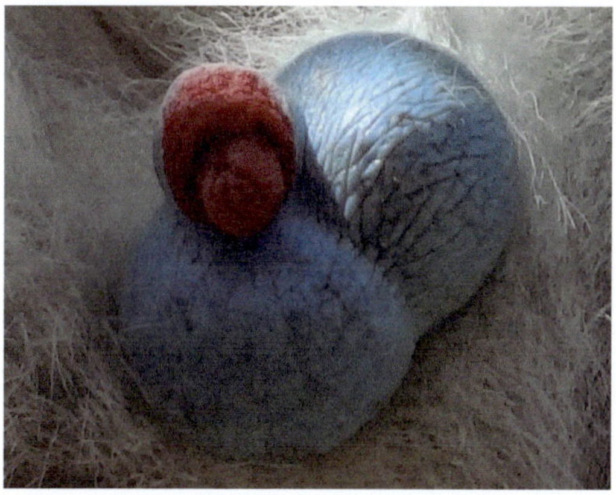

Fig. 3.1 External male genitalia of Papio hamadryas and Chlorocebus pygerythrus, with the characteristic blue scrotum and red penis of the vervet monkey. "https://upload.wikimedia.org/wikipedia/commons/a/a8/Chlorocebus-pygerythrus-private-parts.JPG"

Other animals had a horny papillae of the prepuce as chimpanzees and baboons. A distinctive penile curvature is seen in some species [1].

Some animals had a smaller penile sheath which may not reach half the length of the phallus, which looks prolapsed during erection, like the bellied slider turtles.

In most mammals, the male prepuce is important for normal copulatory function, because its surgical removal disturbs normal copulatory behaviour in male mammal [2].

Preputial glands are exocrine glands that are located in the folds of skin in front of the genitals of some mammals including mice, ferrets, rhinoceroses, and even-toed ungulates and it produce pheromones. The glands play a role in the urine-marking behaviour of canids such as gray wolves and African wild dogs. The preputial glands of female animals are sometimes called clitoral glands. The preputial glands of male musk deer produce strong-smelling deer musk which is of economic importance, as it is used in perfumes production [3].

Long time ago there is a debate about whether humans have a functional homologues to preputial glands, but it is now settled that human don't have such glands (Chap. 17).

Several congenital external genital anomalies related to the prepuce have been documented in animals.

M. A. B. Fahmy, *Normal and Abnormal Prepuce*, https://doi.org/10.1007/978-3-030-37621-5_3

Animal Smegma

In healthy animals, smegma helps clean and lubricate the genitals. In veterinary medicine, analysis of this smegma is sometimes used for detection of urogenital tract pathogens, such as Tritrichomonas foetus. Accumulation of smegma in the equine preputial folds and the urethral fossa and urethral diverticulum can form large "beans" and promote the carriage of Taylorella equigenitalis, the causative agent of contagious equine metritis. Some equine veterinarians have recommended periodic cleaning of male genitals to improve the health of the animal.

The Prepuce of the Stallion (Fig. 3.2)

It is formed by a double fold of skin and resembles scrotal skin in that it is essentially hairless and well supplied with sebaceous and sweat glands. It functions to contain and protect the non-erected penis. The external part of the prepuce, or sheath, begins at the scrotum and displays a marked raphe that is continuous with the scrotal raphe. This external layer extends some distance cranially before reflecting dorsocaudad to the abdominal wall to form the preputial orifice. The internal layer of the prepuce extends caudally from the orifice to line the internal side of the sheath, then reflects cranially toward the orifice again before reflecting to form the internal preputial fold and preputial ring. It is this additional internal fold that allows the marked lengthening (approximately by 50%) of the stallion's penis during erection, where the preputial orifice is visible at the base of the penis just in front of the scrotum, and the preputial ring is visible approximately midshaft of the penis. Located distal to the preputial ring during erection is the internal layer of the internal preputial fold.

Horse sheath cleaning occasionally needed by male horses both geldings and stallions, it is recommended that the sheath be cleaned once or twice a year. Cleaning the sheath is a specialized task requiring a mild cleaner with grease-cutting properties, generally designed specifically for the process, along with warm water and many clean (usually disposable) towels. Rubber gloves for the handler are recommended, as the job is rather smelly and messy [4].

Monkey Prepuce

Only Macaque species of monkeys do not have foreskins. There is a prosimian species described as having an ample prepuce which narrows over the apex glandis in singularly human fashion' but the size of the flaccid penis looks small and seems unlikely to remain covered during an erection [5].

The corpora cavernosa and the prepuce are the only two universally common characteristics of the primate penis. Although it is stated that the chimpanzee shares 98.4 percent of its genetic material (similar DNA) with humans, it is unclear why chimpanzees and Bonobos do not retain bulbous glans penis while rhesus monkeys and baboons do 'have a distinctive glans penis' [6] (Fig. 3.3).

Canine Prepuce

Canine prepuce is a hairy structure accommodating the flaccid penis (Fig. 3.4). During erection the preputial sheath is retracted completely

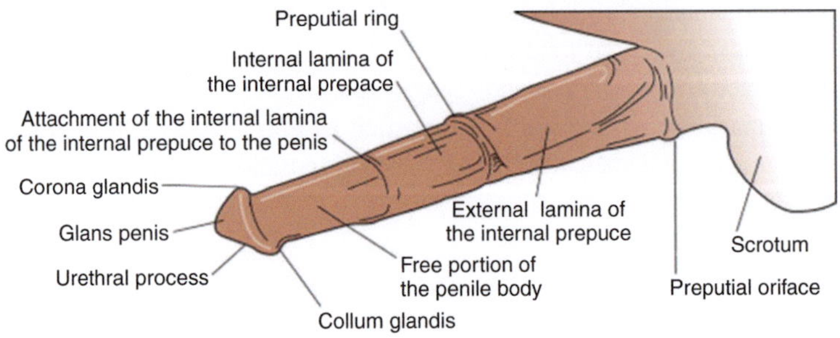

Fig. 3.2 Structures of the stallion's penis and prepuce

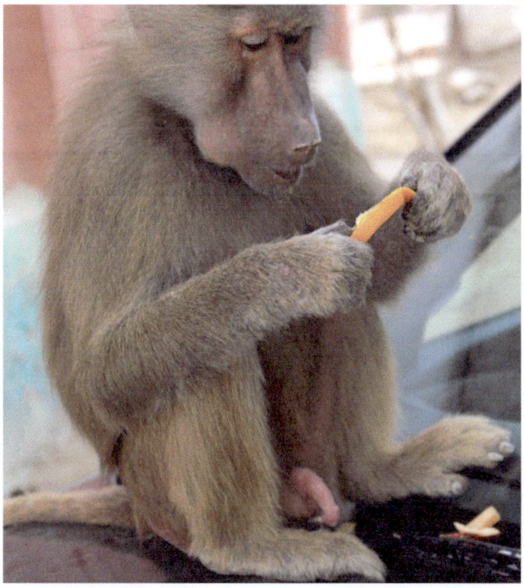

Fig. 3.3 Papio hamadryas adult penis erected outside the sheath

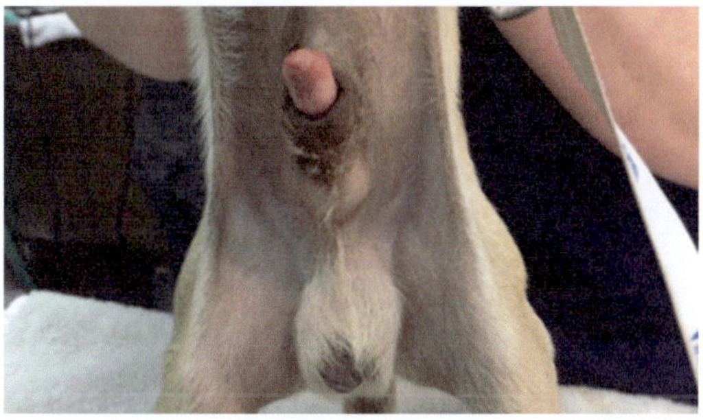

Fig. 3.4 Canine prepuce during erection

and the whole penis; the elongated cranial part (pars longa) and a round basal part (bulbus glandis) is exposed without any visible covering (Fig. 3.5).

The prepuce may be underdeveloped, absent or may not fuse normally because of failure of the genital folds to close normally during fetal life. Clinical signs are attributed to chronic exposure of the penis leading to inflammation, balanitis and balanoposthitis, which is not rare in dogs and may be presented with a purulent discharge (Fig. 3.6).

Paraphimosis is quite common among dogs, which if not treated early may results in

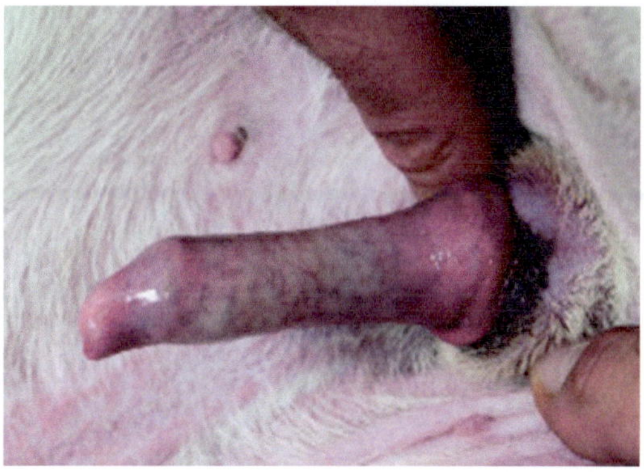

Fig. 3.5 The distal portion of the penis (glans penis) of the dog consists of an elongated cranial part (pars longa) and a round basal part (bulbus glandis)

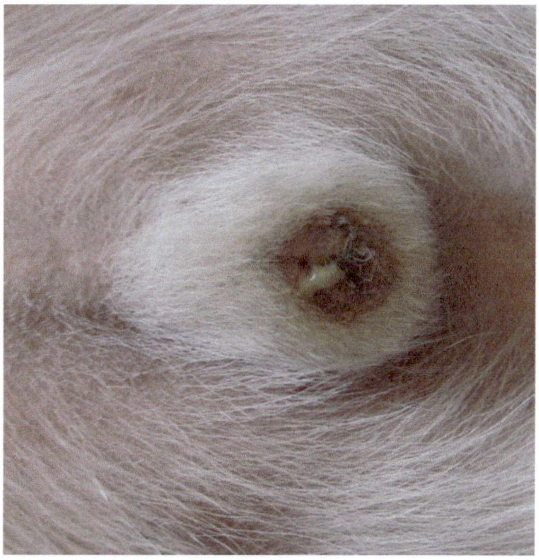

Fig. 3.6 Balanoposthitis of canine prepuce with purulant discharge. https://upload.wikimedia.org/wikipedia/commons/9/90/Balanoposthitis_canine_prepuce_discharge. Thesis4Eva at English Wikipedia [CC BY 3.0]

penile tissue necrosis and urinary retention (Fig. 3.7).

Abnormal preputial fusion can be seen in dogs in association with hypospadias. Preputial advancement may be performed to correct small penile exposures. Severe hypoplasia may be managed with penile amputation. Abnormal preputial fusion may be treated by removal of the exposed preputial mucosa, penile amputation and scrotal or perineal urethrostomy [7].

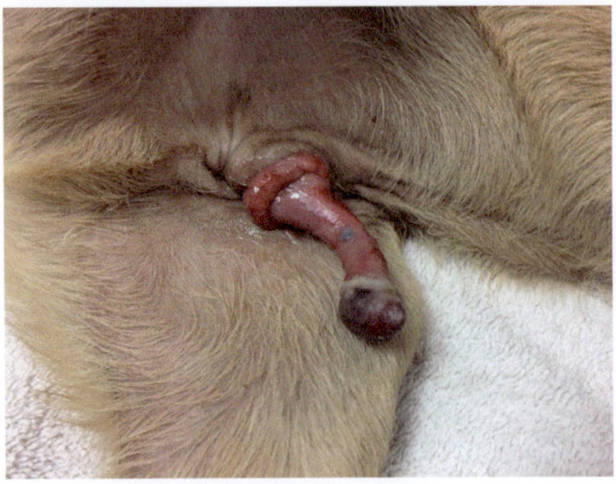

Fig. 3.7 Paraphimosis of dog prepuce with an obvious ischaemia at the tip of the penis

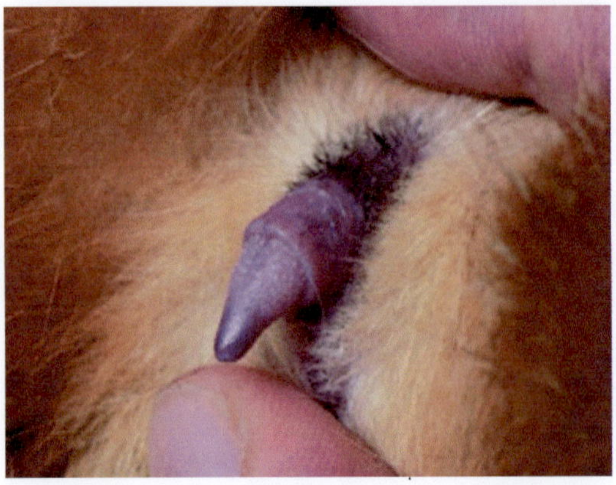

Fig. 3.8 The cone-shaped penis of the male cat has keratinized papillae, which are androgen dependant and disappear after castration

Cats Prepuce

The prepuce is comparatively short, and with a narrow preputial orifice that makes extrusion of the penis very difficult, specially in the conscious cat. The urethral orifice is small and present on the tapered tip of the glans.

When not erect, the penis is completely enclosed within the prepuce. The glans of the penis of a mature tom cat is covered with 120–150 penile spines that are directed caudally. The spines are testosterone-dependent and start to appear at about 12 weeks of age, are fully developed at puberty, and are absent in neutered males, disappeared by about 6 weeks after castration (Fig. 3.8).

House Mice

Deermice and house mice have a relatively long prepuces. Additionally, the tip of the house mouse prepuce possesses many long hairs which may act as brushes during urination.

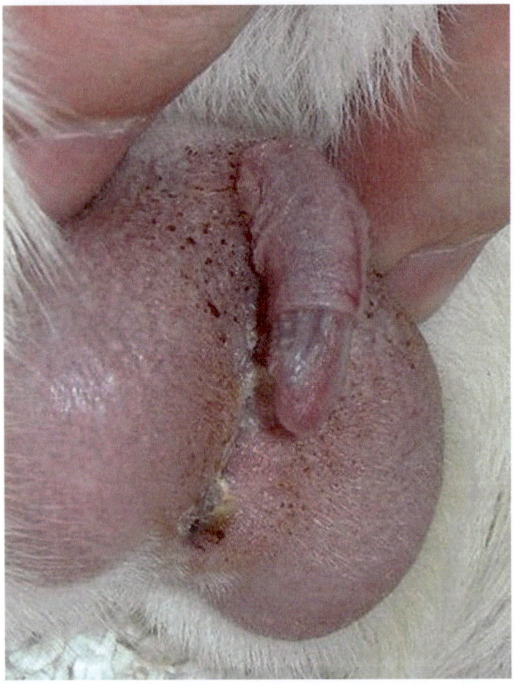

Fig. 3.9 Guinea pig penis with a long prepuce

The distal regions of the lumen of the house mouse prepuce are convoluted to a much greater extent than in the other species and the tip of the penis lies well within the interior of the sheath, providing a reservoir for urine accumulation. By contrast, the lumen of the hamster's prepuce has few convolutions, and the tip of the penis lies in close proximity to the luminal terminus. The prepuce of the gerbil and of the deermouse seems intermediate, but -like the house mouse- the tip of the deermouse penis appears to reside well inside the sheath (Fig. 3.9).

Maruniak et al. [8] postulate that a potential morphological adaptation of the penis sheath in rodents is one enabling it to act as a wick for the deposition of urine and, hence, urinary pheromones. It is possible that a long preputial sheath, relative to height above the ground, would be an energy-conserving adaptation allowing frequent deposition of urine while engaging in normal home-range or territorial activities, and the requirement for specific muscular involvement during such marking would be less.

Preputial anatomy also differs markedly in mice versus humans. The external portion of the mouse penis (called the glans) resides within an extensive preputial space defined by the attachment of the prepuce to the glans, which occurs proximally near the internal/external or glans/body junction in the mouse. Distally the mouse prepuce is represented as the prominent hair-bearing elevation in the perineum [9]. This terminology makes sense as the space created by this "external prepuce" houses the penis. In contrast, the human prepuce is attached to and covers only the distal aspect of the penis, namely the glans. Thus, the hair-bearing "traditional mouse prepuce" is clearly not homologous to the human prepuce.

References

1. Harrison RM, Lewis RW. The male reproductive tract and its fluids. In: Dukelow WR, Erwin J, editors. Comparative primate biology: reproduction and development, vol. 3. New York: Liss; 1986.
2. Desrochers A, St. Jean G, Anderson DE. Surgical management of preputial injuries in bulls: 51 cases (1986–1994). Can Vet J. 1995;36:553–6.
3. Van Heerden J, The role of integumental glands in the social and mating behaviour of the hunting dog Lycaon pictus (Temminck), 1820; 1981.
4. Crabbe B. Cleaning a horse's sheath. Archived 2012-02-05 at the Wayback Machine. Equisearch.com;2000. Reprinted from Horse & Rider, June, 2000. Accessed 17 July 2007.
5. Hill WCO. Primates: comparative anatomy and taxonomy: II Haplorhini: Tarsioidea. Edinburgh: The University Press; 1955. p. 136–7.
6. Izor W, Walchuk SL, Wilkms L. Anatomy and systematic significance of the penis of the pygmy chimpanzee. Folia Primatologica. 1981;35:218–24.
7. Boothe HW. Penis, prepuce and scrotum. In: Slatter D, editor. Textbook of small animal surgery. Philadelphia: Saunders; 2003. p. 1531–42.
8. Maruniak JA, Desjardins C, Bronson FH. Adaptation for urinary marking in rodents: prepuce length and morphology. J reprod Fert. 1975;44:567–70.
9. Rodriguez E Jr, Weiss DA, Ferretti M, Wang H, Menshenia J, Risbridger G, Handelsman D, Cunha G, Baskin L. Specific morphogenetic events in mouse external genitalia sex differentiation are responsive/dependent upon androgens and/or estrogens. Differentiation. 2012;84:269–79.

4 Embryology of Prepuce

Abbreviations

AR	Androgen receptor
DHT	Dihydrotestosterone
GT	Genital tubercle
wpc	Weeks post conceptional

Historical Background

Bokai at 1860 [1] was the first to direct attention to the physiological adherence of the foreskin. Schweigger and Seidel [2] gave the first description of the development of the prepuce in human, but Glenister [3] cited Retterer (1885–1915) as the first to show that the prepuce was formed by a combination of preputial folding and the ingrowth of a cellular lamella, Glenister is first one to examine thirty-eight human fetuses and he concluded that the prepuce results from a combination of preputial fold formation and ingrowth of a cellular lamella, these processes are closely linked with the formation and fusion of the urethral folds on the glans. This fact accounts for the formation of the frenulum in normal males and the disposition of the prepuce in females and in cases of hypospadias. During the last 10 years there are many valuable researches and illustrations published by Laurence Baskin and his colleagues [4, 5] from University of California, San Francisco about the human development of genitalia and urethra.

Sequential Development of Prepuce

Fetal sex development involves a series of sequential stages, and both differentiation and formation of internal and external genitalia are late-developmental steps in human ontogeny which are regulated by the action of testicular hormones [6]. The formation of the male and female sexual phenotype is initiated at the sixth week of gestation. At this time, a small rudimentary bud called the genital tubercle initially appears, and differentiation between the two sexes only begins at the ninth week. The genital tubercle, urethral (urogenital) folds, and labioscrotal swellings are formed by the cloacal membrane and under the influence of dihydrotestosterone (DHT) produced by the testis, genital tubercle growth is stimulated and the glans is formed at 9–11 weeks (Fig. 4.1).

The glanular urethra develops from a nearly solid urethral plate at the tip of the genital tubercle apparent on the thirteenth week, 25 mm embryo, when the mesenchyme is still diffuse and not differentiated into glans and corpora cavernosa. At this time, a well-marked urethral groove at the tubercle's undersurface, that does not reach the tip, represents the origin of the penile urethra. On the fourteenth week embryo, a

M. A. B. Fahmy, *Normal and Abnormal Prepuce*, https://doi.org/10.1007/978-3-030-37621-5_4

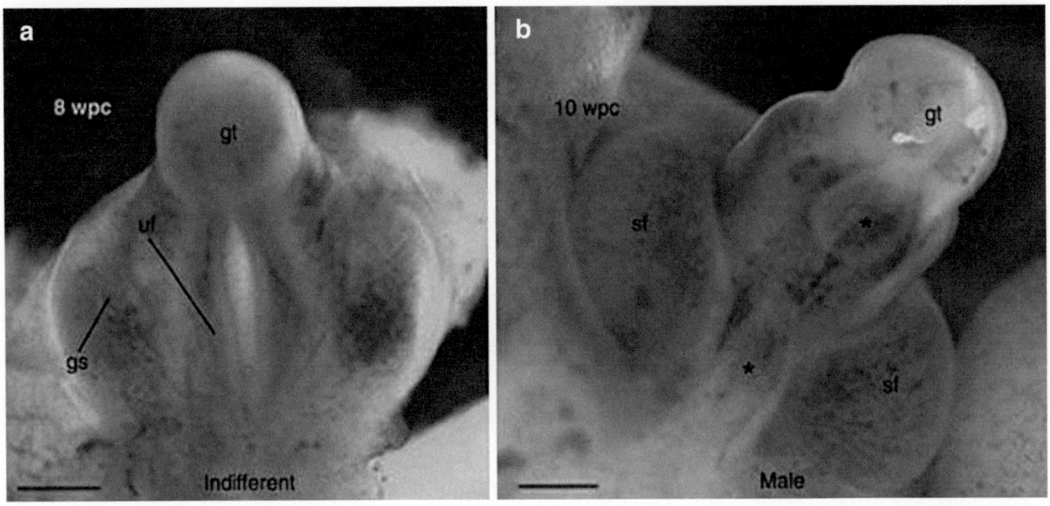

Fig. 4.1 (**a**) Undifferentiated human external genitalia at 8 wpc. (**b**) Male differentiation of scrotal folds and fusion of the urethral folds (asterisks mark patent regions, either side) at 10 wpc. *gs* genital swelling, *gt* genital tubercle, *sf* scrotal folds, *uf* urethral folds. Scale bars: 500 μm [12]

glans penis can be identified, with a fine solid indentation at the tip representing the epithelial plate which extends proximally into the glans penis. At the mid glans, the epithelial plate is vacuolated forming a glanular canal. At the level of the proximal glans, the vacuolization reaches the undersurface and thus, a deep glanular urethral groove is created. The distal migration of the glanulo-preputial lamella, which forms the prepuce, causes the fusion of the edges of the glanular groove as well, forming the floor of the glanular urethra under the frenulum [7] (Figs. 4.2 and 4.3).

The prepuce develops from two components at the junction between the glans and the shaft penis (the corona): (a) a major component from the shaft (dartos fascia and superficial stroma) and (b) a minor component from the glans stroma. Between the glans stroma of the glans itself and the preputial glans component grows the solid glanulopreputial lamella outwards in a concerted growth. That growth is outward because the position of the deepest part of the lamella remains the same in relation to the underlying nerves to the glans and corpora cavernosa [8].

The formation of the median ventral part of the prepuce is due to rapid forward (distal) proliferation of the median ventral raphe and synchronously the medial ventral part of the growing prepuce more than the dorsal part of the prepuce. The formation of the frenulum is due to an expansion of the corona of the glans and glanulopreputial lamella proximal to the urethral orifice. As a result, the median ventral raphe and septum form the floor of the glanular urethra and remain as the

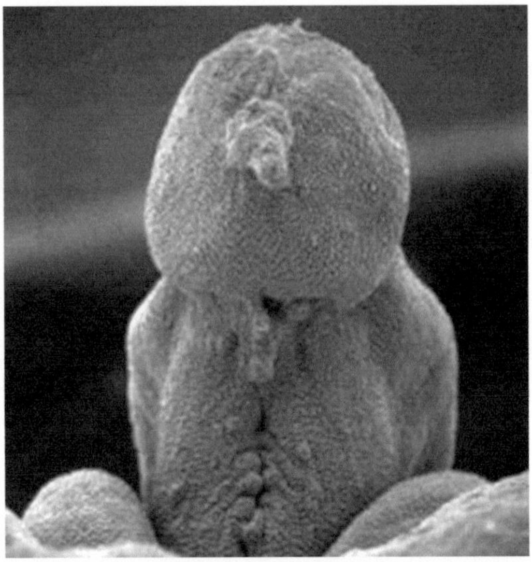

Fig. 4.2 Prominent genital tubercle forming penis with glans, coronal sulcus, but prepuce not yet developed, labioscrotal folds migrate slightly down, but still surrounding the root of the phallus in 12 weeks fetus

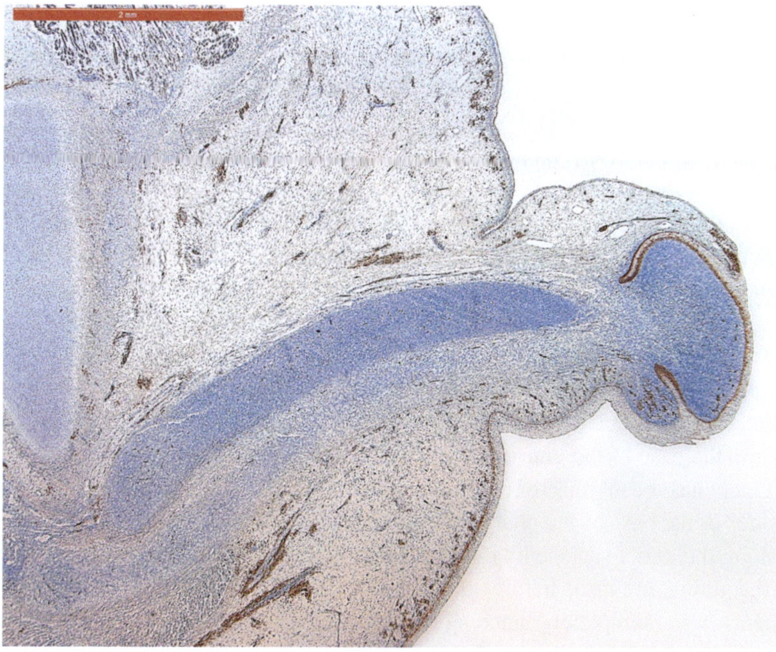

Fig. 4.3 Sagittal section of human fetal penis at the age of 12.5 weeks male genital tract, K14 1.6×. The glans penis can be recognized, but there is no evidence of preputial development

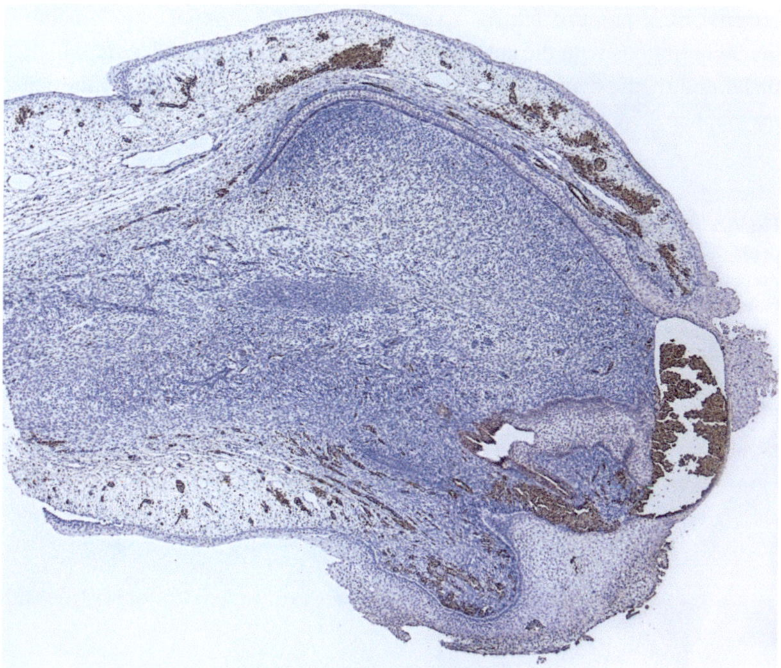

Fig. 4.4 13.5 weeks male penis S40 2.5× 0001. The preputial lamina is seen dorsally, but it is absent ventrally

frenulum inside the medial ventral part of the prepuce which covers the ventral surface of the glans [9].

The embryological development of the prepuce begins when the embryo measures about 65 mm, and when it reaches 100 mm, the prepuce completely covers the glans dorsally (Fig. 4.4).

Prior to 11 weeks of gestation there is no evidence of preputial development (Figs. 4.2 and 4.3). Shortly after, the preputial placode forms, it delaminates from the epidermis with appearance of a layer of mesenchymal cells between the preputial lamina and the epidermis. With time the preputial lamina expands ventrally to cover the glans gradually [10].

In a 55-mm. embryo, the glans is delimited from the shaft on its dorsal and lateral walls by a constricting coronal sulcus, with a prominent epithelia tag at the dome of the glans, which will canalise to give raise of the glanular urethral, perpetual lamella start to grow from the coronal sulcus to form the prepuce, which start to develop in the 57 mm human fetus (8 weeks of gestation from the base of the glans, as a preputial lamella which has been raised round the dorsum and sides of the base of the glans, but it is interrupted along the under surface by the urogenital ostium (the future urethra), before that time the glans penis was completely uncovered and splitted with the urethral plate at its depth (Fig. 4.3).

In a 75-day foetus, the end of the penis is not covered by a prepuce but by a thick epidermal layer continuous with the anterior body wall. The distal end of the penis, represents the glans, but no prepuce is in evidence.

In the 65 mm fetus (fourth month of intrauterine life) the urogenital ostium is confined to the under surface of the glans and the preputial fold has rolled over the base of the glans except in the region of the urogenital ostium where it is deficient at that stage, with the further distal development of the glandular urethra and closure of its edges, the perpetual fold close ventrally to form the frenulum (which is attached to the undersurface of the glans) at the inner mucosal aspect and preputial raphe at the outer surface, with the dorsal portion growing at a more rapid rate than the ventral component, this fold covers the glans progressively, and the epithelium covering the deep aspect of the fold fusing with the epithelium covering the glans (Fig. 4.5).

The closure of the ventral portion of the prepuce is completed by the fifth month of gestation after the closure of the glanular urethra, In relation to the distal part of the glans the lower margins of the lamella fuse to form a complete epithelial cuff which, by breaking down, gives rise to the cylindrical terminal part of the prepuce. Phimosis could be explained in terms of the

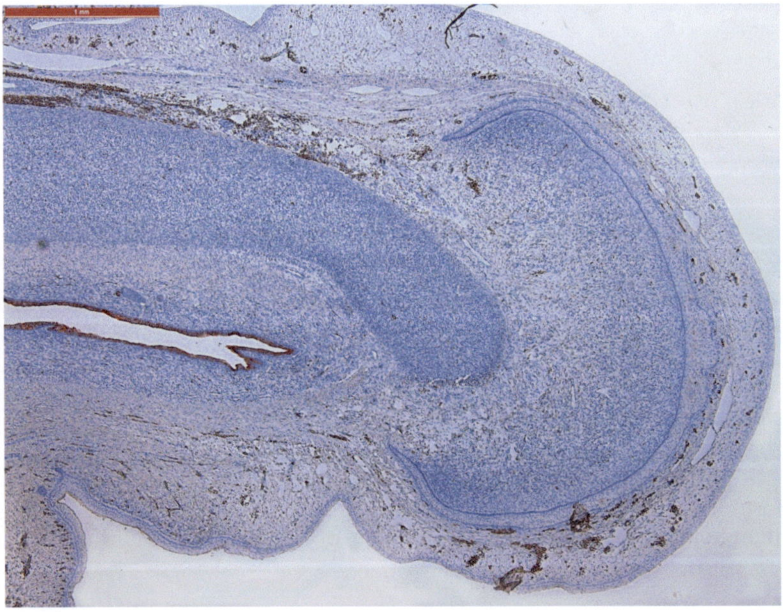

Fig. 4.5 16 week male penis, K7 2.5×. The preputial lamina is extensive dorsally and reduced in size ventrally, still there is no formation of the glandular urethra

preputial fold continuing to grow forward too far beyond the tip of the glans and failure of the glandar lamella to disintegrate (Chap. 18).

The Evolution of the Prepuce from Infancy to Maturity

Only 4% of newborn males have a fully retractable prepuce, the remaining 96% are non-retractable secondary to two normal physiological conditions; the adherence between the inner prepuce and the glans due to the presence of the glandopreputial membrane and secondly the tightness of the preputial meatus. During preputial development into adolescence and its maturity the tubular, tapered, and elongated prepuce of the young boy are not commonly seen at adulthood; as the corpora cavernosa develop in adolescence, the penis will enlarge to "take up the slack." A prepuce that in childhood appears long, may, at maturity, fail to completely cover the glans. A study published in the Journal of Urology finds that by ages 8–10, 50% of boys will have a fully retractable prepuce [11].

Development of Female Prepuce

Observations made on female embryo lead to the conclusion that the same processes are involved in the formation of the clitorial prepuce, but persistence of the urethral groove in female and hypospadiac penis in male prevent the fusion of the margins of the preputial folds and of the glandar lamella [12]. This again emphasises the close association of the preputial anlage with the urethral folds, this association explains the presence of a hood-like prepuce in cases of hypospadias. The only non explainable exception of this concept is the intact prepuce megameatus anomaly and the very rare cases of epispadias with intact prepuce; where the prepuce developed completely to the tip of the glans, but the underneath glandular urethra is still not completed, but the common membrane formed (balanopreputial membrane) attaches the prepuce tightly to the glans.

Figures 4.3, 4.4, and 4.5, are kindly offered by Prof. Laurence S. Baskin, MD, Director UCSF KURe, Chief Pediatric Urology UCSF Benioff Children's Hospitals, University of California, San Francisco

References

1. Bokai J. A fityma (preputium) seites adatapadasa a makkoe gyermakelnel. Orv Heill. 1860;4:583–7.
2. Schweigger-Seidel F. Zur Entwickelung des Praeputium. Virchows Archiv. 1866;37:219–28.
3. Glenister TW. A consideration of the process involved in the development of the prepuce in man. Br J Urol. 1956;28:243–9.
4. Baskin L, Shen J, Sinclair A, Cao M, Liu X, Liu G, Isaacson D, Overland M, Li Y, Cunha J. Development of the human penis and clitoris. Differentiation. 2018;103:74.
5. Isaacson D, Shen J, Overland M, Li Y, Sinclair A, Cao M, McCreedy D, Calvert M, McDevitt T, Cunha GR, Baskin L. Three-dimensional imaging of the developing human fetal urogenital-genital tract: indifferent stage to male and female differentiation. Differentiation. 2018;103:14. https://doi.org/10.1016/j.diff.2018.09.003.
6. Renfree MB, Wilson JD, Shaw G. The hormonal control of sexual development. Novartis Found Symp. 2002;244:136–52; discussion 152–136, 203–136, 253–137.
7. Hadidi AT, Roessler J, Coerdt W. Development of the human male urethra: a histochemical study on human embryos. J Pediatr Surg. 2014;49(7):1146–52.
8. Hadidi AT. Normal development of the penis and urethra. In: Carachi R, Doss S, editors. Clinical embryology. Cham: Springer; 2019. https://doi.org/10.1007/978-3-319-26158-4_44.
9. Gleniste TW. A consideration of the processes involved in the development of the prepuce in man. Br J Urol. 1956;28:243–9.
10. Liu X, Liu G, Shen J, Yue A, Isaacson D, Sinclair A, Cao M, Liaw A, Cunha GR, Baskin L. Human glans and preputial development. Differentiation. 2018;103:86. https://doi.org/10.1016/j.diff.2018.08.002.
11. Kayaba H, Tamura H, Kitajima S, Fujiwara Y, Kata T, Kata T. Analysis of shape and retractability of the prepuce in 603 Japanese boys. J Urol. 1996;156:1813–5.
12. Goto M, et al. In humans, early cortisol biosynthesis provides a mechanism to safeguard female sexual development. J Clin Invest. 2006;116(4):953.

Anatomy of the Prepuce

5

Preputial Distinction

Most of the textbooks or research papers describing prepuce are not inclusive, and usually deal with the prepuce only from the point of either its removal along circumcision or preservation to compete against this deeply rooted procedure. Steve Scott indicated that most physicians were ignorant of the anatomy and physiology of the genital structures they were routinely removing from infants and children [1]. The prepuce is remarkably thin, dark, and loosely connected to the rest of penile skin. It has features of true skin but is devoid of subcutaneous adipose tissue, without associated hair follicles and few sweat glands are present in the superficial dermis.

Prepuce is an impressive organ, as a segment of the penis, it has a unique structure from many aspects:

- Despite its delicate appearance, the inner surfaces of foreskin are built to withstand frictional trauma along the whole life; hence it is called "frictional mucosa" it also a waterproof structure to withstand damp conditions.
- Its outer surface is not well demarcated from the rest of the penile skin (the landmark between the prepuce and penile skin in flaccid penis is sometimes recognised by the coronal ridge projection) (Fig. 5.1).

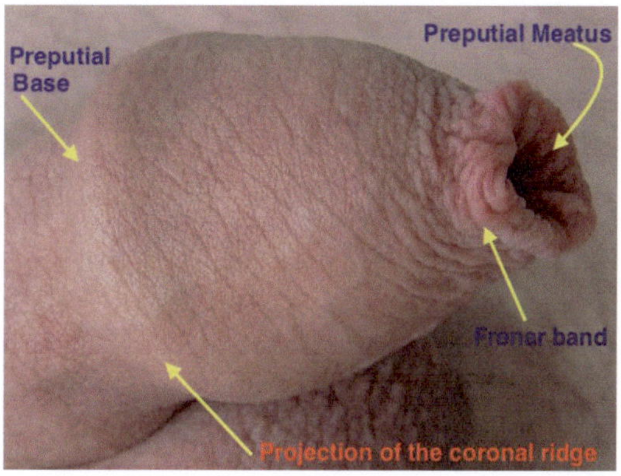

Fig. 5.1 Preputial structures with a prominent coronal ridge demarcating preputial skin from the penile skin

- Prepuce is a conical structure, with three folds over itself:
  - The outer skin folded distally at the preputial meatus, where we can recognize the mucocutaneous junction and frenar band (Fig. 5.2).
  - The inner mucous membrane is folded sagittally at the ventral surface to attach the wings of glans to form the frenulum (Fig. 5.3).
  - The inner mucous membrane attached and incorporated circumferentially to the coronal sulcus, with slight slopping, below the coronal ridge, except at the ventral surface

M. A. B. Fahmy, *Normal and Abnormal Prepuce*, https://doi.org/10.1007/978-3-030-37621-5_5

where it is incorporated in the sagittal folds of the frenulum (Fig. 5.4).

- Retractable prepuce sliding proximally to expose the glans, while it is still attached circularly at the coronal sulcus and sagittally at the frenulum. The elastic tissue of the preputial dermis, along with the dartos muscle and frenulum, tether the prepuce and help its return to the anatomically correct position after deployment during erection or after manual retraction.
- The frenulum should normally be sufficiently long and supple to allow for the full retraction of the prepuce, so that it lies smoothly back on the shaft of the erected penis. The penile frenulum is comparable to the tongue's frenulum between the tongue's lower surface and the lower jaw (Fig. 5.5).
- Baby delivered with a prepuce completely different from the adult's one in many aspects, which will be discussed latter (Fig. 5.6).
- Most of the skin that covers the human body is attached to underlying structures, but the skin covering the eyes and the penis are exceptions.
- Foreskin is a highly vascularised and densely innervated bilayer tissue, with a surface area of up to 60 cm^2, and potentially larger in adult.

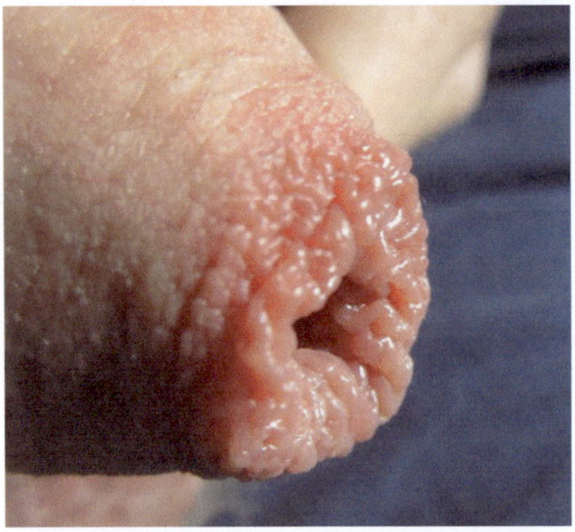

Fig. 5.2 Preputial meatus with the mucocutaneous junction

Preputial Surface Anatomy and Morphology

If prepuce is inspected while the penis uplifted or erected, it is commonly conical in shape and formed of five subsections (Fig. 5.7):

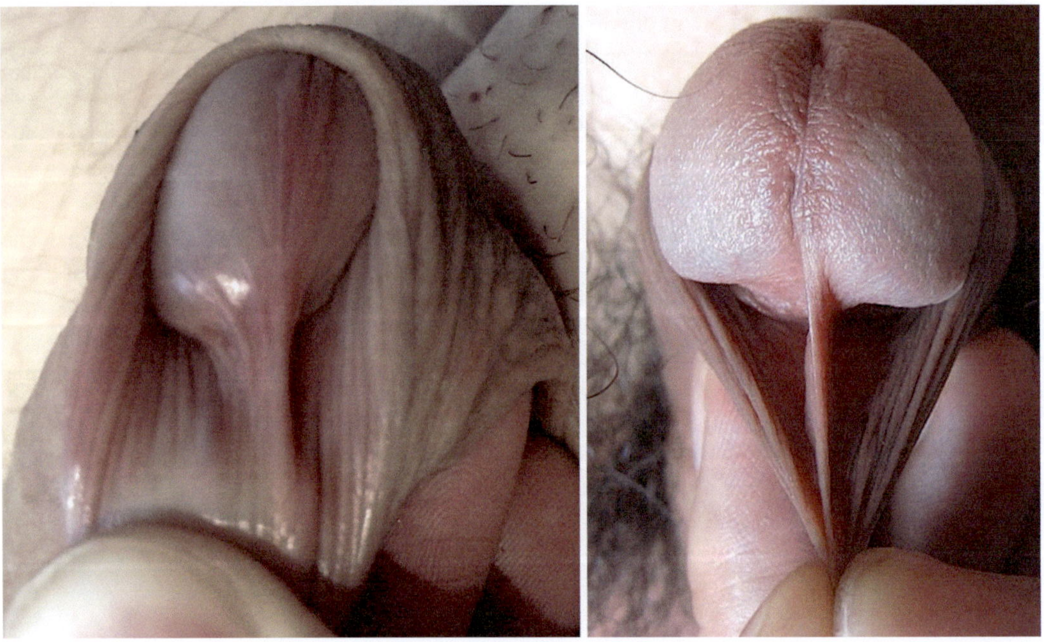

Fig. 5.3 Sagittal folding of the preputial mucosa to form the frenulum

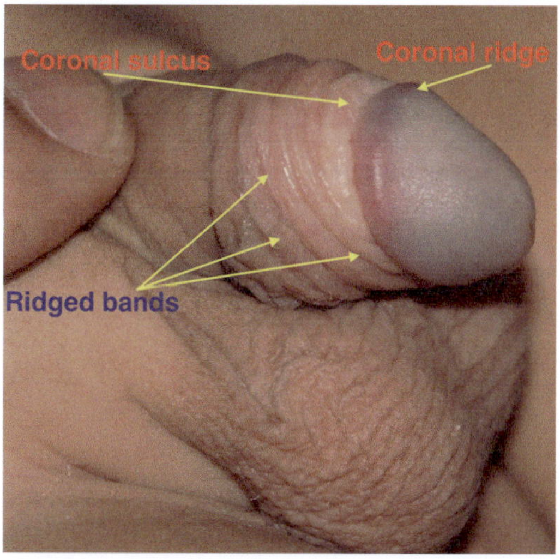

Fig. 5.4 Sloping circumferential attachment of the inner mucosal to the glans at the coronal sulcus, with obvious ridged mucosal bands

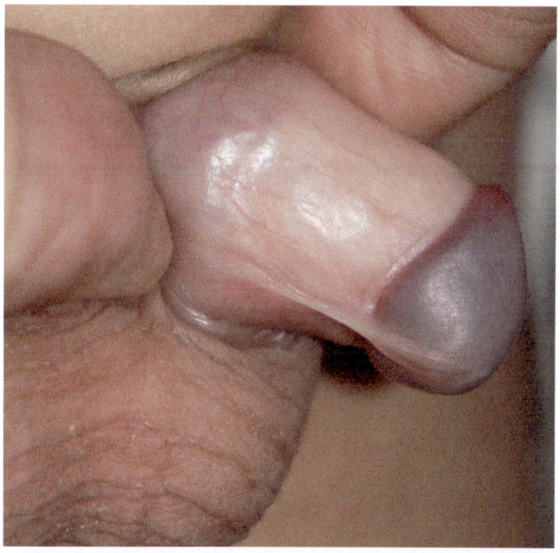

Fig. 5.5 Stretched frenulum allowing the prepuce to retract proximally, and to be included in the penile skin during erection

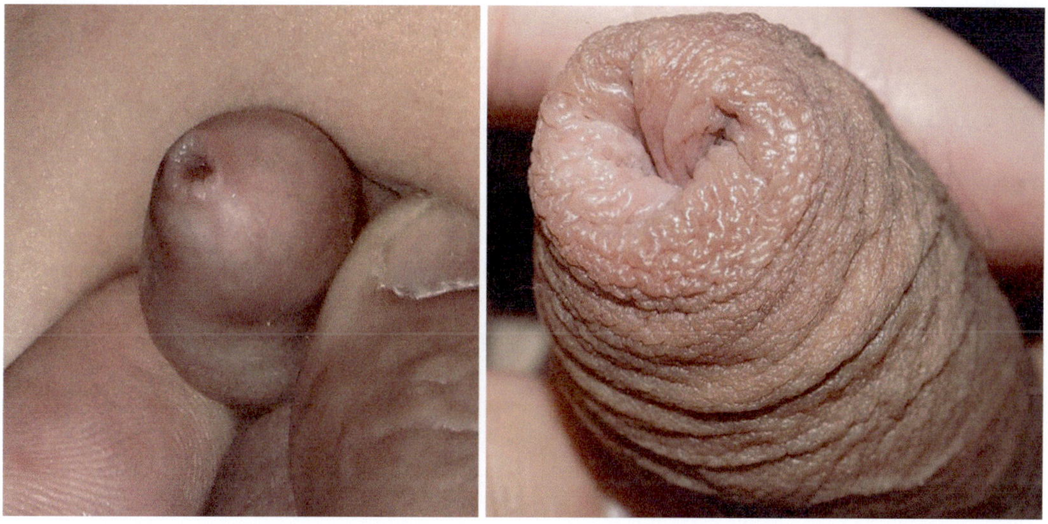

Fig. 5.6 Wide difference between infantile small preputial opening and the adult hiatus

1. Outer skin:
   - Base
   - Body
   - Free tip
2. Preputial Meatus
3. Inner mucosa:
   - Smooth mucosa
   - Ridged band
4. Frenulum
5. Preputial sac

Outer Preputial Skin

The preputial skin system is unique in its structure and function. No other part of the human anatomy possesses the ability to evert and invert like the movable penile skin sheath.

Preputial skin is hairless (glabrous skin), this could be an attempt to make it suitable for good taste or simply superfluous to requirements. It is remarkable for its thinness, its darker colour, and

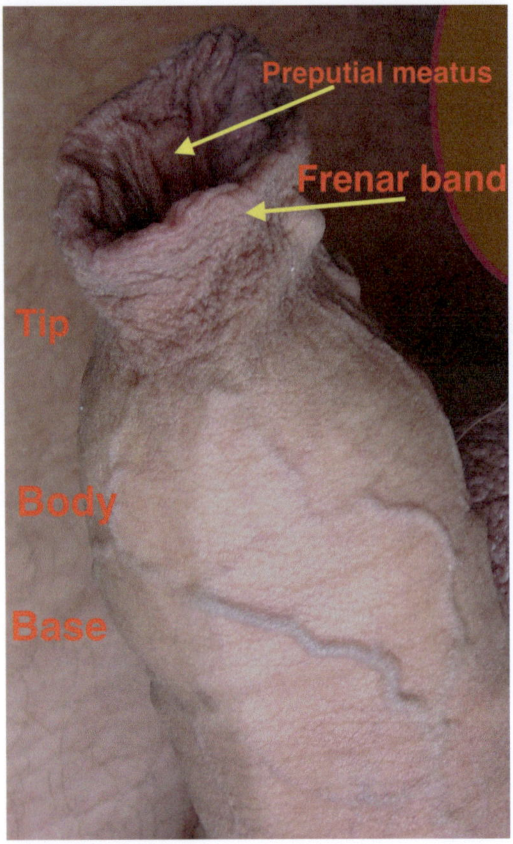

Fig. 5.7 Different structures and subsections of the adult prepuce

its looseness of connexion with the fascial sheath of the organ.

Preputial skin is lined by a squamous mucosal epithelium in its inner aspect and a glabrous skin in its outer surface, and the two layers of the preputial fold are separated by the dartos fascia. Because of its retractile properties, the prepuce provides adequate mucosa and skin to cover the entire penis during full erection.

Base of the Prepuce

At young age, and also in many adults, it is difficult to distinguish the end of the prepuce from the rest of the penile skin in a flaccid penis, commonly the preputial base is in continuity with the penile skin externally, but in some adults and rarely in children; the prominence of coronal ridge demarcating the end of the prepuce and the start of the boundaries of penile skin (Fig. 5.1), but during erection the whole prepuce becomes a single-layered cylinder; mucosa regress proximally between the mucocutaneous junction proximally and the coronal sulcus distally, so the mucosa will be seen behind the corona, skin regress distally enclosing about half of the shaft, sometimes the base of the prepuce may goes proximally to the root of the penis (depending upon the length of the prepuce) (Fig. 5.8).

Body of the Prepuce: (Posthe)

It is the outer skin layer of the prepuce, which represent the main magnitude of the prepuce and extend from the base to the tip, it may acquire the same corrugations of the scrotum; due to attachment of the underneath dartos muscle fibers directly to the dermis, this corrugations is variable from man to man, it is clearly seen in coloured children and sometimes it is invisible at adulthood; specially during erection, these rogues usually confined only to the tip of the prepuce and the rest is similar to the penile texture (Fig. 5.9).

Preputial rugae is androgen dependant [2]. So children with other genital anomalies (mainly microphallus) who had been managed with topical testosterone may show an increased area of preputial corrugations, which also became more darker (Fig. 5.10).

The mean length of prepuce in some studied samples of normal healthy adults was 6.4 cm (range from 4.8 to 9.2 cm), preputial skin and mucosa form about 51% of the length of the mean adult penile shaft (Fig. 5.11).

Werker [3] reported a mean surface area of 46.7 sq. cm of the combined inner and outer layers with a range of 18.1 sq. cm to 67.5 sq. cm.

At young age the length of the prepuce is near equal to the penile length (with a wide variations between individuals), with progress in age and at adolescent; the penile shaft progressively increase in size to exceed the preputial development, so the prepuce getting shorter, but in some individuals the prepuce may progressively incriminates to exceed the penile growth.

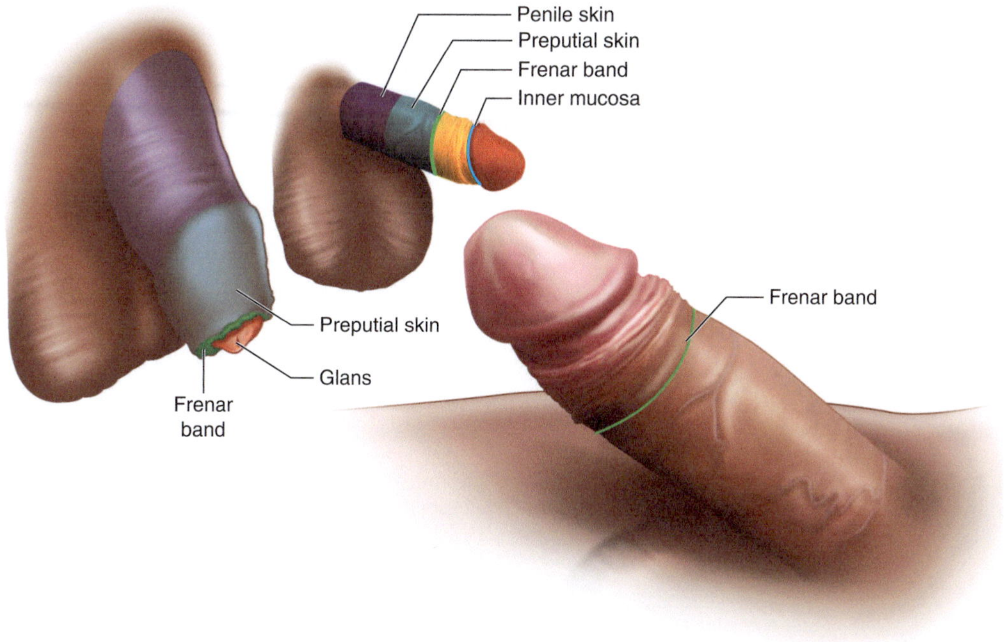

Fig. 5.8 Normal positioning of the preputial structures during erection, with incorporation of preputial skin and mucosa in the penile skin behind the coronal sulcus

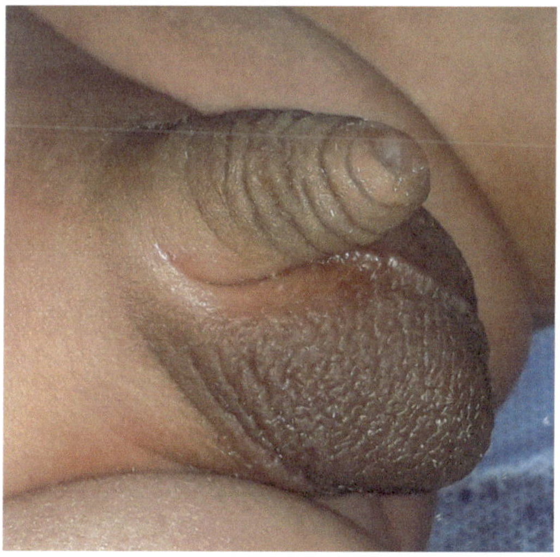

Fig. 5.9 Prominant preputial corrugations, with a great similarly to the scrotal skin

Excessive long prepuce (*Macroposthia)* will be discussed in Chap. 11, and abnormally short prepuce, which we called *Microposthia* will be discussed in Chap. 9.

Dorsal preputial skin is longer than the ventral skin, this is may be in correspondence to the same difference between dorsal and ventral length of the glans.

Ventral preputial skin is deficient in almost all cases of hypospadias except cases of MIP, the dorsal preputial skin is usually plenty in hypospadias cases, and it may acquaints the shape of copra head appearance (Chap. 12).

Rarely the ventral prepuce is completely deficient with a normal urethra and meatus, and in such cases the prepuce forming a hood to semblance the female prepuce, this cases called "Hooded prepuce without hypospadias" (Chap. 12).

In men with darker and coloured skin the median raphe could be recognised at the ventral surface of the body of the prepuce extending from the penile raphe till the preputial meatus, this raphe continue proximally with penile, scrotal and perineal raphe, sometimes the median raphe of the prepuce poses some anomalies like the rest of the penile raphe [4] (Fig. 5.12).

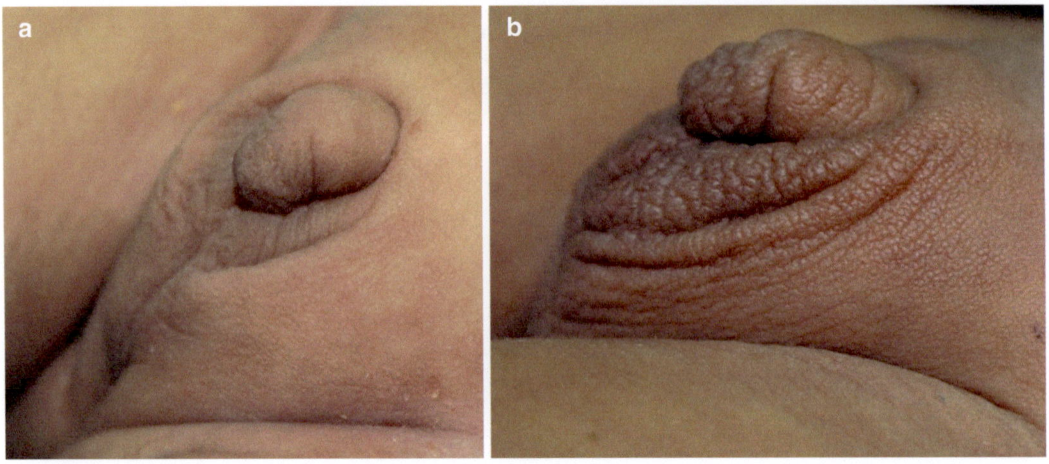

Fig. 5.10 Increased numbers of corrugations of the prepuce and brown darkening after local application of testosterone ("a" before testosterone management and "b" 3 weeks after daily application)

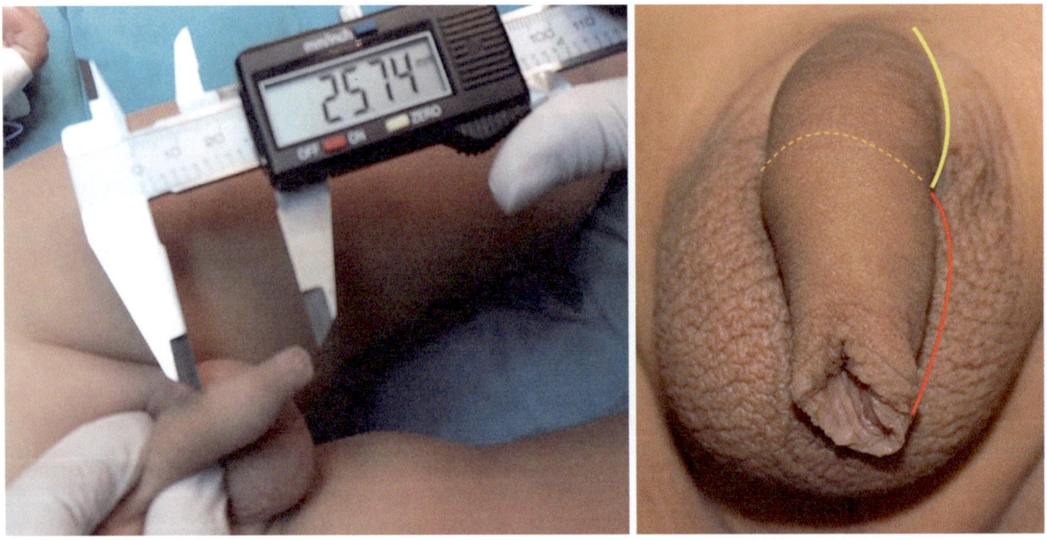

Fig. 5.11 Measuring the length of the prepuce in children; which sometimes exceeding the penile length, as we can see in this case

Preputial raphe anomalies may be an indicator for an underlying urethral anomalies like megameatus intact prepuce [5] (Fig. 5.13).

Preputial Tip (Fig. 5.14)

Preputial skin proximal to the meatus is tapered and wrinkled, resembling the scrotal skin in its corrugations and darker colour, the wrinkled skin gives a large surface area. This corrugations will disappear during stretching of the prepuce and during erection, this tip had a variable length and configurations, and in some individuals it is completely absent, where the preputial meatus continuous directly with the body of the prepuce, this commonly seen in cases with short prepuce, of course this tip is absent in cases of microposthia and also in hypospadias (Fig. 5.15).

Preputial tip is a common scene for all types of dermatitis at young age and the sexually transmitted diseases in adults [6]. It is sometimes

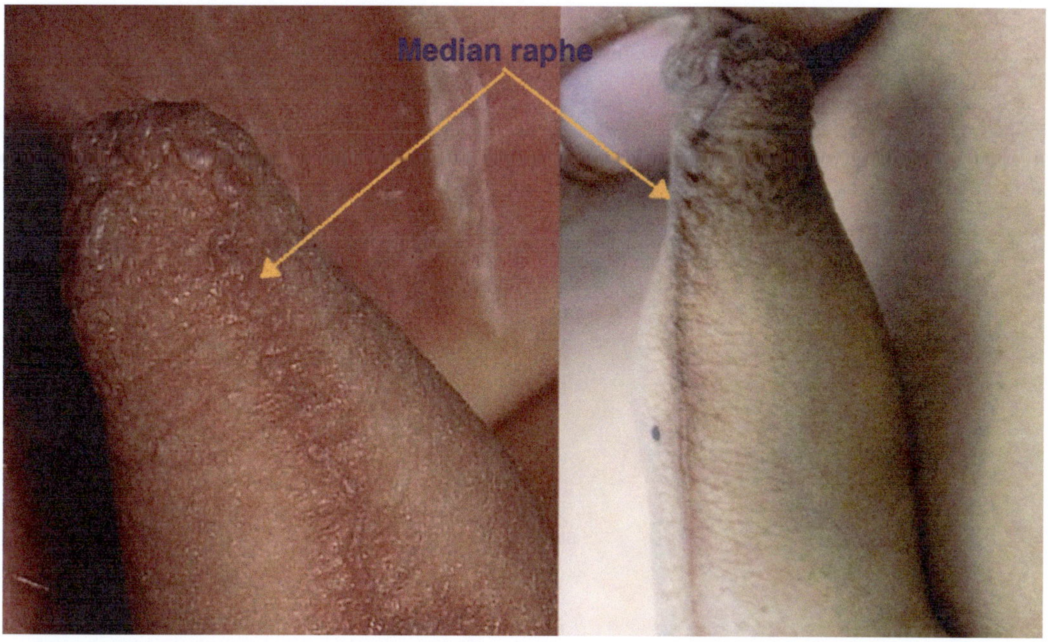

Fig. 5.12 Continuation of penile raphe in the ventral surface of the prepuce

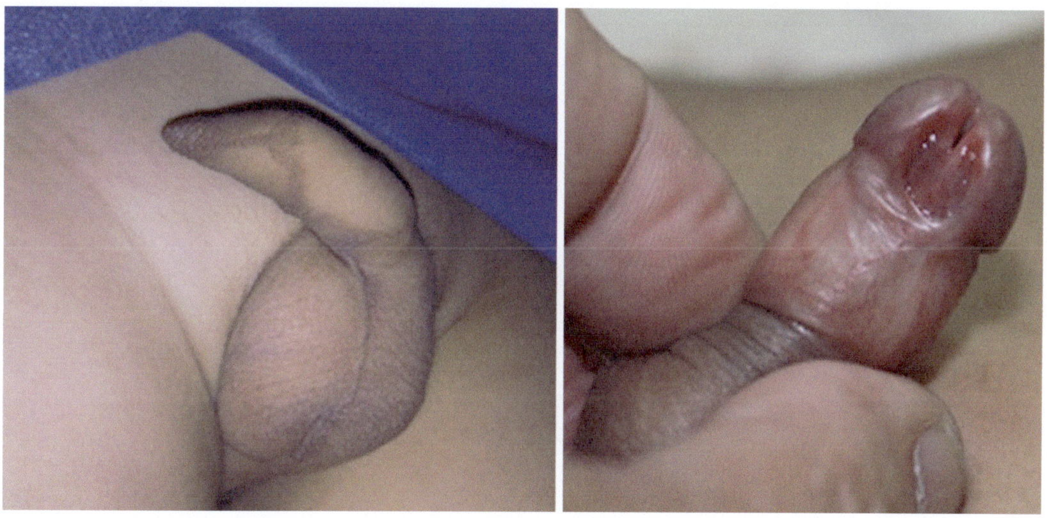

Fig. 5.13 Deeply dark deviated preputial raphe as an indicator for the presence of a megameatus anomaly, which covered by an intact prepuce (MIP)

termed wrongly as akroposthion or acroposthion, but akropothia represents an abnormal long preputial tip; which is a congenital anomaly or a sort of anatomical variation, and will be discussed later with macroposthia, so normally long tip of the prepuce is not a synonyms to akroposthion.

Preputial Meatus (Figs. 5.1, 5.2, 5.6, and 5.7)

Nomenclature

Frenar band, preputial aperture, preputial hiatus, and preputial ostium.

The muscle fibres of the dartos fascia under the preputial skin form a mosaic pattern along the penile shaft skin and arrange themselves in a circular sphincter-like configuration at the tip of the prepuce, this natural narrowing is called Frenar band, which lies just proximal to the preputial meatus (Fig. 5.16). This band forming a sphincteric closing mechanism, beyond the urinary meatus, allows for the passage of urine while guarding against the entrance of foreign pathogens into the preputial space (one-way valve), these muscle fibers work to keep the tip of the preputial meatus closed when the child is not urinating, also this sphincteric action of this muscle can inhibit preputial retraction early in infancy, the intertwined and mosaic like pattern of the arrangement of subcutaneous dartos muscle is responsible for the pucker look of the preputial tip and meatus, but its over spasm may contributes to the occurrence of phimosis (Fig. 5.17).

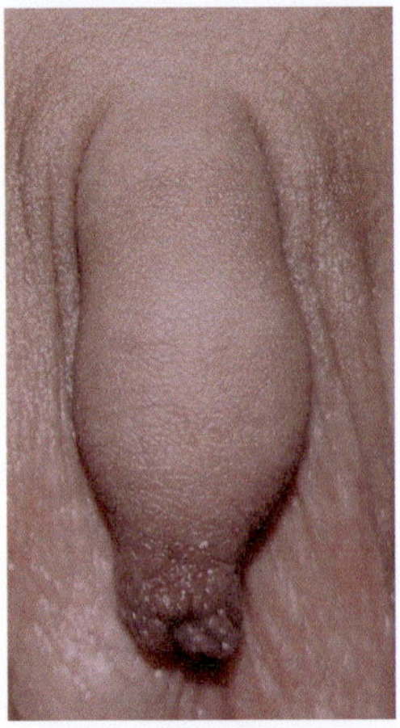

Fig. 5.14 Normally corrugated preputial tip

This meatus represents the mucocutaneous junctional zone, and sometimes the mucous membrane could be seen protruding in a different degrees from this apparatus, which is rich in specialized nerve endings (Figs. 5.18 and 5.19).

The transitional region from the external to the internal prepuce is the most sensitive region of the uncircumcised penis and more sensitive than the most sensitive region of the circumcised penis [7].

Gairdner [8] showed that the external urethral meatus was not exposed in approximately 40% of the newborns, and Kayaba et al. [9] found a tight ring, which inhibited exposure of the meatus in approximately half of the boys aged below half a year.

Hiraoka et al. [10] suggest that an external urethral meatus tightly covered with prepuce may

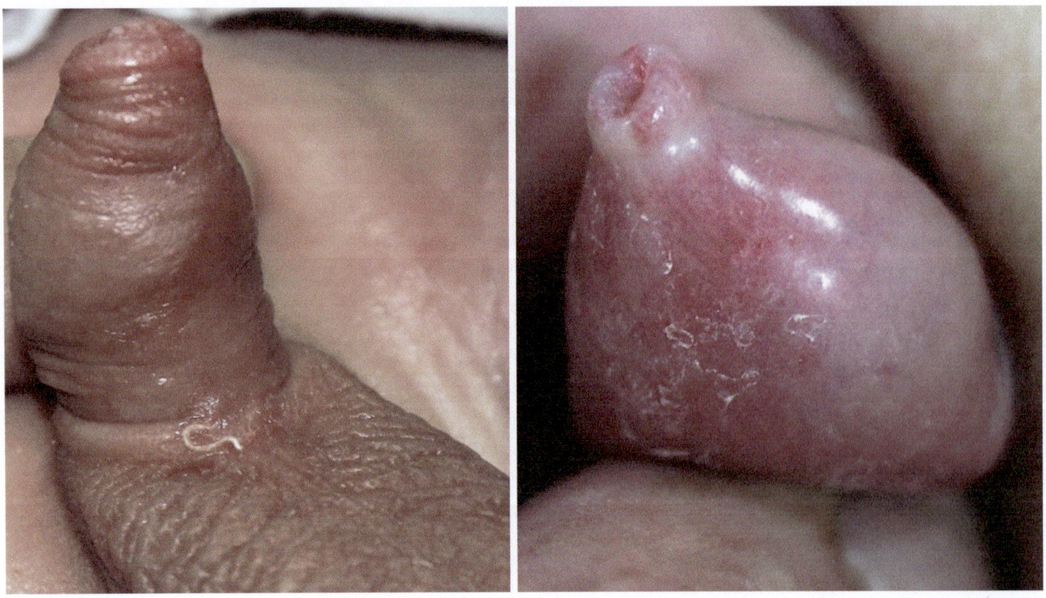

Fig. 5.15 Preputial tip in rest and on stretching, which usually abolish the puckered tip

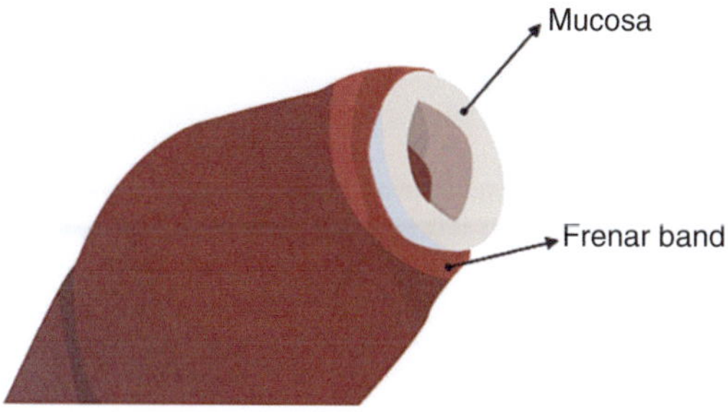

Fig. 5.16 Preputial meatus and frenar band

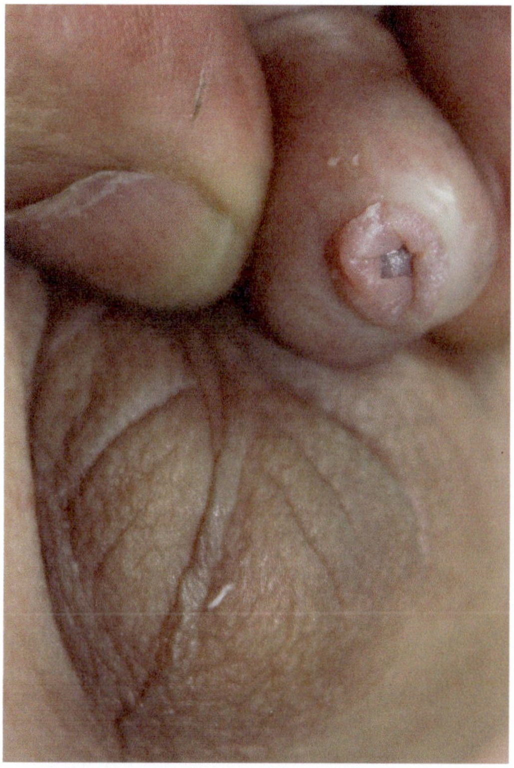

Fig. 5.17 Normally the one way valve preputial meatus prevent retraction of the prepuce at infancy

allow bacterial colonization both in the meatus itself and in the urethra, and result in urinary tract infection.

In children, the foreskin usually covers the glans completely but in adults it may not, in a study of 3000 young men from Germany there is only 49.6% of them had the glans fully covered by foreskin, 41.9% were partially covered and 8.5% were uncovered; around half of which (4%) had the foreskin atrophied spontaneously without previous surgery [11].

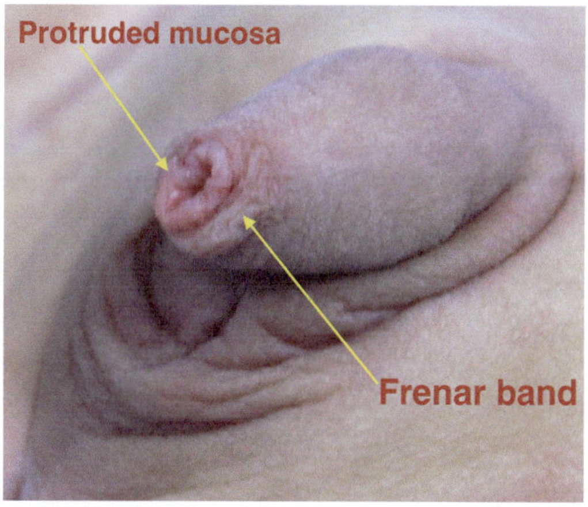

Fig. 5.18 Normally protruded mucous membrane from the preputial meatus

Preputial meatus, Frenar band and tip are totally absent in cases of hooded prepuce in hypospadias and in some isolated cases. The length of the prepuce in the human population varies from large problematic to a very small or absent prepuce i.e., aposthia. Radojicic and Perovic [12] found 6 various morphological forms of the prepuce associated with hypospadias, indicating its quantitative nature "monk's hood", "cobra eyes", "normal" (intact), "flat", "v-shaped" and "collar-scarf". This variation in shape and size of the prepuce in the population suggests that it may be a dominant quantitative trait [13].

The preputial meatus lies commonly central at the tip of the conically shaped prepuce, and in a direction plane perpendicular to he long axis of the glans penis, with a slight downward direction to guide the stream of urine properly downward and forward, any abnormal positioning or deviation of this direction will disturb the micturition process and annoying the person (Fig. 5.20).

The whole prepuce may be rotated -commonly to the left side- along the congenital anomaly of penile rotation, in such cases the meatus and subsequently the urine stream is deviated to one side.

Abnormally upward meatal direction is very rare, but there is a few reported cases (Fig. 5.21).

At the meantime the more dipping direction will results in a rare anomaly called igloo like prepuce and this will be discussed in Chap. 15.

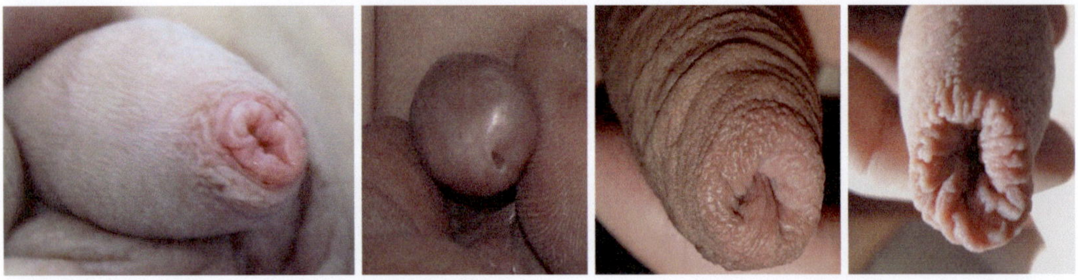

Fig. 5.19 Mucocutaneous junction obvious at the meatus at rest and on stretch in neonate and adult

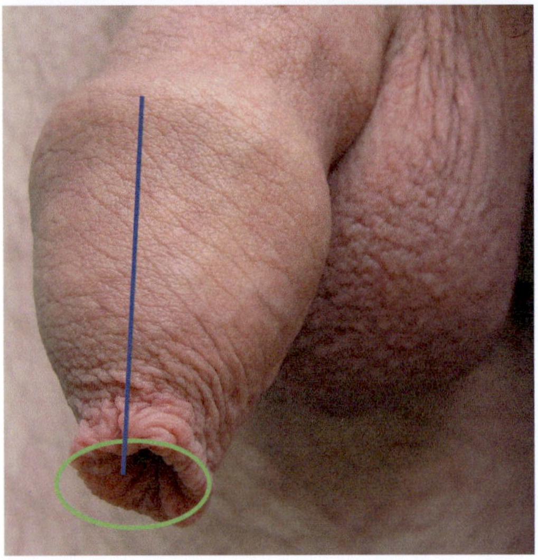

Fig. 5.20 Normal direction of the preputial meatus

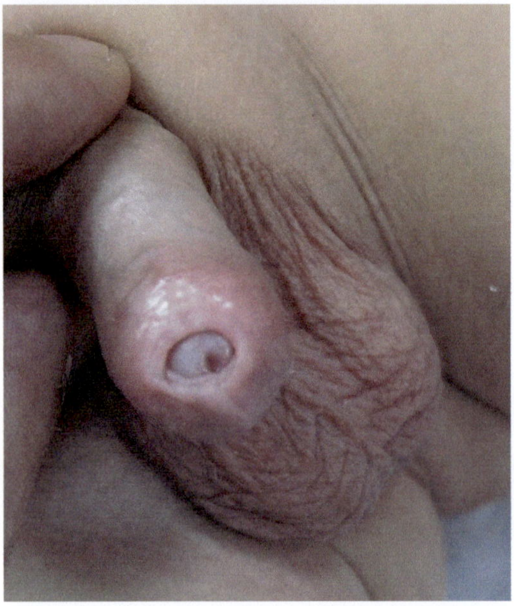

Fig. 5.21 Abnormal upward direction of the preputial meatus

Preputial Mucosa: (Internal Lamella)

When the prepuce retracted, its inner surface displays two distinct dermatological zones, ridged bands and smooth mucosa, as well the as the frenulum, the inner preputial mucosa is less pigmented than the outer skin of the prepuce, as it is not containing any melanocytes, but it have a plenty of Langerhan's cells and specialised nerve endings (Fig. 5.3).

The inner mucosal layer attached to the penile shaft at the coronal sulcus proximally, forming the mucocutaneous junction distally, and forming the preputial sac with the glans dorsally, but ventrally it forms a three structures; ridged band, ridged mucosa and the frenulum (Fig. 5.22). The male prepuce has looser collagen than the dense collagenous lamina propria of the glans penis.

The Ridged Mucosa (Ridged Band)

Ridged band is the name given by John R. Taylor at 1996 [14] to a unique part of the human male prepuce, it is also called "Cingulus rugosus", which is another anatomical Latin name suggested by Ken McGrath [15], but this term is not commonly in use. There is no other structure like it in the human body.

The ridged mucosa is a pleated band that start just proximal to the mucocutaneous junction, it contains 10–12 transverse ridges, whose collective width is 10–15 cm wide in adult, mainly in the ventral surface of the prepuce, but in the dorsal midline the ridged band lies above the level of the adjacent smooth mucosa and merges smoothly, the remainder of the preputial lining between the ridged band and the glans is smooth and lax, and commonly called smooth mucosa (Fig. 5.22).

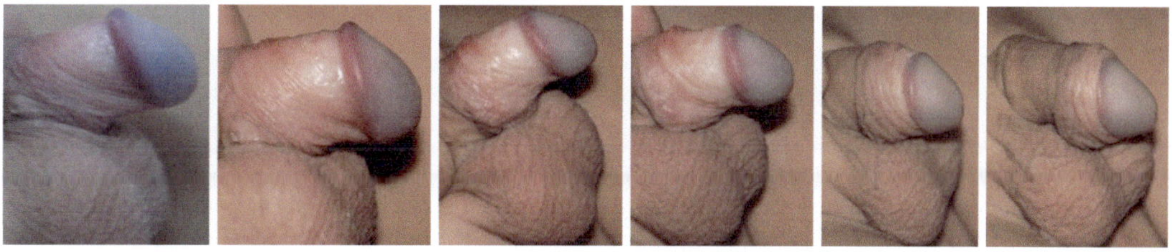

Fig. 5.22 Different structures of the inner mucosa at different degrees of retraction

Clusters of the tactile nerve endings of Meissner's corpuscles are found in abundance in the crests of these ridges, which are not present in the sulci (furrows) in between the ridges [16]. Meissner's corpuscles were more plentiful in some subjects than others but, perhaps significantly, they were only seen in the crests of the ridges, occasionally in small clumps that expanded the tips of corial papillae. Nerve endings were not seen in sulci between ridges. Special stains for nerve tissue showed the additional end-organs and myelinated nerve fibers in the ridges.

When the prepuce is retracted, the main part of the ridged band lies across the top and sides of the shaft of the penis (Fig. 5.23). On the underside of the penis, the ridged band merges into the frenulum. Stretching of the accordion-like ridged band triggers important sexual reflexes and erogenous sensation, and may also trigger and sustain erection.

Unretracted, the adult ridged band usually lies flat against the glans; retracted, the ridged band is everted on the shaft of the penis. There is considerable variation in the degree of ridging: older subjects showed less and younger men had more marked ridging, and it could be seen clearly at younger age; if the preputial retractability permits. In males with a short prepuce, the ridged band lies immediately inside the junctional rim at rest and against the glans in a variable position according to the preputial length.

Taylor and colleagues further noted that the ridged band is intensely vascularized, which is typical of components of the nervous system. The intense vascularity of the ridged band was best seen in transilluminated mucosa. When magnified, the ridged mucosa has a pebbled or coral-like appearance [17].

The tightly pleated concentric bands of the ridged band have been likened to the elastic bands at the top of a sock. These expandable pleats arise from the frenulum and encircle the inner lining of the foreskin. They allow the lips of the foreskin to open and roll back, exposing the glans. The ridged mucosa also gives the foreskin its characteristic taper [18].

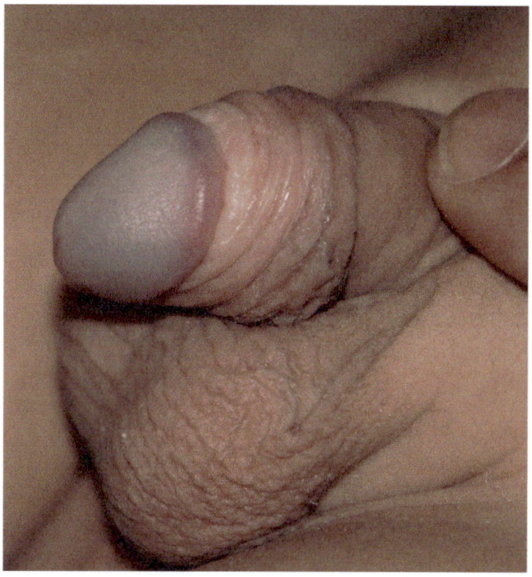

Fig. 5.23 Sloping configuration of the ridged bands with fanning from ventral to dorsal surface

Smooth Mucosa

It is also called "Cingulus levis"; this is an anatomical Latin name suggested by Ken McGrath for the zone or band of smooth mucosa on the inner foreskin [14].

The remainder of the preputial lining between the 'ridged band' and the glans is smooth and lax, histological examination of the smooth zone of the mucosa showed no ridging. In adult during erection the smooth mucosa incorporated to the skin covering the penis and it lies just proximal to the corona (Fig. 5.8).

Frenulum

The fusion of the prepuce on the ventral aspect of the glans creates the frenulum, which is a bridge-like structure that joins the ventral prepuce to the glans, the point of attachment of the prepuce is advanced towards the meatus; which usually assumes a longitudinal direction on the same line with the frenulum, which is continuous with the ridged band proximally.

It is similar to the labiogingival frenulum, which connects the upper lip to the upper gum and the lingual frenulum, which connects the tongue to the floor of the mouth, frenula tether movable structures to non-movable organs. The lingual frenulum, for example, not only prevents the tongue from being swallowed, but also restricts movement of the tongue in the distal direction. The preputial frenulum restricts proximal movement of the ridged bands, specially those in ventral surface, and assists in returning the prepuce back to its distal position over the glans. Plenty of Meissner's corpuscles were seen in the frenulum (Figs. 5.24 and 5.25).

The preputial mucosa of triangular shape distal to the ridged band in the ventral aspect having the frenulum at its point, and its sides defined by the ridged band is called *Frenular Delta* by McGrath [15]. It presents as the greater area of the mucosa ventrally and does not include the ridged band which is a zone in its own right. The median raphe runs longitudinally through its mid-line to become the frenulum and bisects the delta into two equal halves (Fig. 5.25).

The frenular delta in males with short prepuce does not extend beyond the lateral aspects. On the other hand, males with a long prepuce have their ridged band lying over the glans tip at rest. In this situation, the frenular delta base extends beyond the lateral aspects in a ribbon-like band as the extra dorsal strip of mucosa between the junctional rim and the ridged band. The frenular delta is noted by men as the most sensitive area of their penis, especially in the mid-line nearest the frenulum, and the frenulum itself [15].

Frenular anomalies will be discussed in Chap. 32.

Preputial Sac and Balanopreputial Membrane

Balanopreputial membrane is a common membrane binds the prepuce to the glans penis in the fetus and neonate. This is the same binding mechanism that fuses the eyelids of newborn kittens. This shared membrane inhibits the retraction of the prepuce and thereby it may protects the developing surface of the infantile glans and inner prepuce from the amniotic fluid intrauterine, and faecal contamination in neonates. The desquamation of this membrane, resulting in separation of the prepuce from the glans, which is gradual and variable from individual to other, and the preputial space is subsequently developed. The final separation often commences during puberty under male hormonal influences, but an incomplete separation process may occasionally occur in some indi-

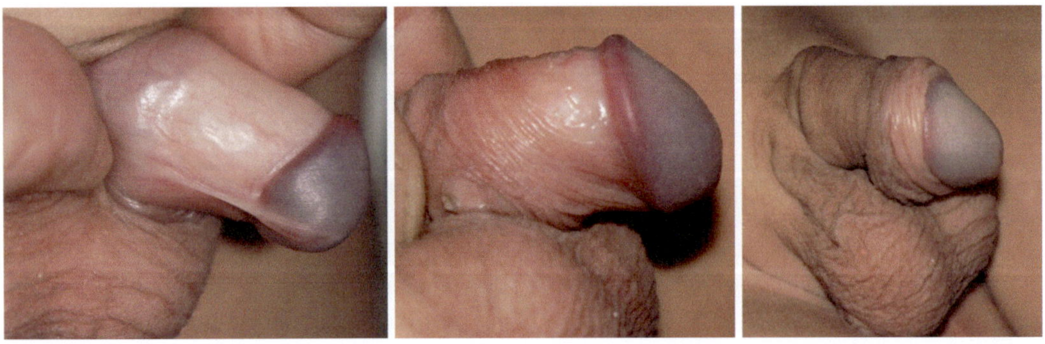

Fig. 5.24 Smooth mucosa and frenulum in stretched mucosa

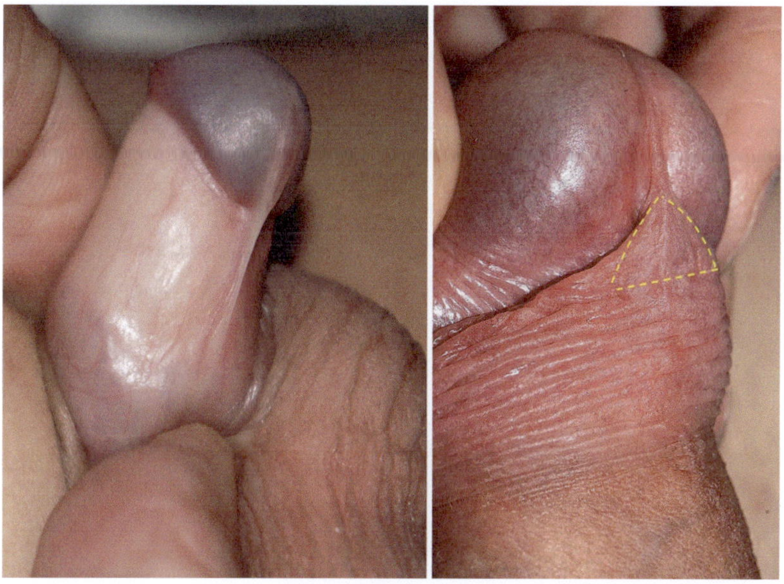

Fig. 5.25 Stretched smooth mucosa and frenulum in the ventral surface, dotted lines represent the frenular delta

viduals. Nutrition and birth weight of the infant is a definite factor in the advancement of this process. No degree of difference is apparent in the character and rate of separation in the white and negro races [19].

The separation of the prepuce in the human penis is essentially a process of keratinization of the intervening epithelium. It begins anteriorly and posteriorly at about the same time and proceeds toward the center. When confined on all sides the separation manifests itself as an epithelial pearl formation [20].

Whorls of cells form in the balanopreputial membrane and gradually die from the inside of the whorls out, creating hollows, over time these hollows coalesce to form the preputial space, which usually contain a variable smegma contents (smegma will be discussed in Chap. 17).

We have hundreds of neonates delivered with an already separated glans from the prepuce, and on the other hand many adolescents may had an adherent glans to the inner prepuce; either circumferentially or at some spots.

The practice of early separation of the prepuce from glans during neonatal circumcisions carries a lot of complications, and commonly there is a superficial abrasion of the glandular surface, which may be deep enough to form ulcers; also these bared area may be infected, disfigure the glans and latter on the glans may be adherent to the circumcised cut edge of the penile skin or mucosal cuff to form different forms of skin bridges, Figs. 5.26, 5.27, and 5.28 demonstrate the spectrum of such problem [21].

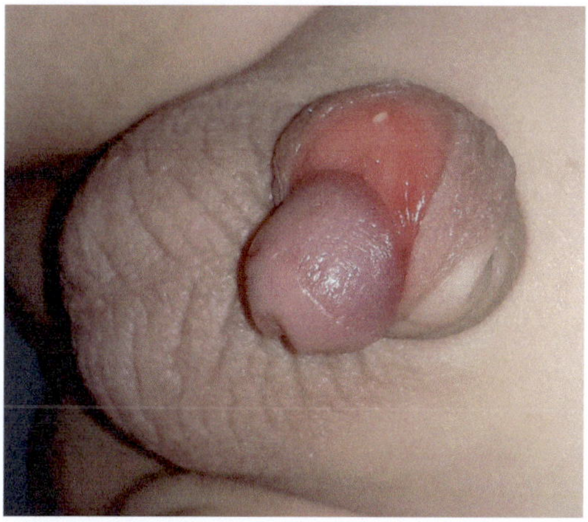

Fig. 5.26 Denuded glans surface in a neonate due to early forcible separation of balanopreputial membrane before commencing circumcision

In few cases a natural skin bridge may be formed between inner mucosa of the prepuce and the glans; this may be due to local failure of balanopreputial membrane separation, or due to a repeated attacks of balanoposthitis, this natural but pathological skin bridge is completely

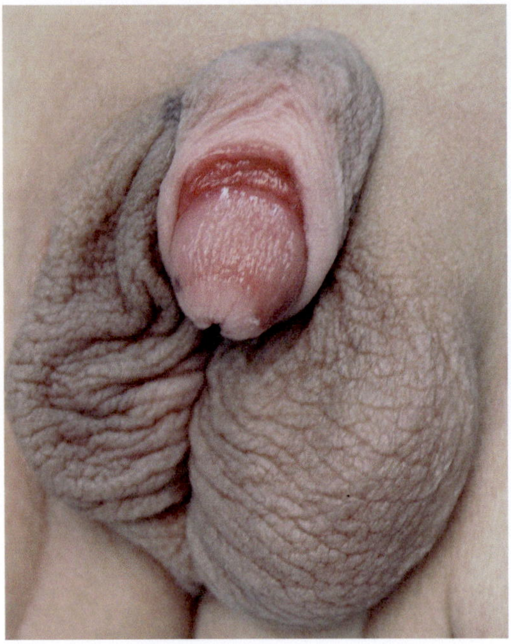

Fig. 5.27 Deepithelized glans surface due to forcible early retraction of the prepuce

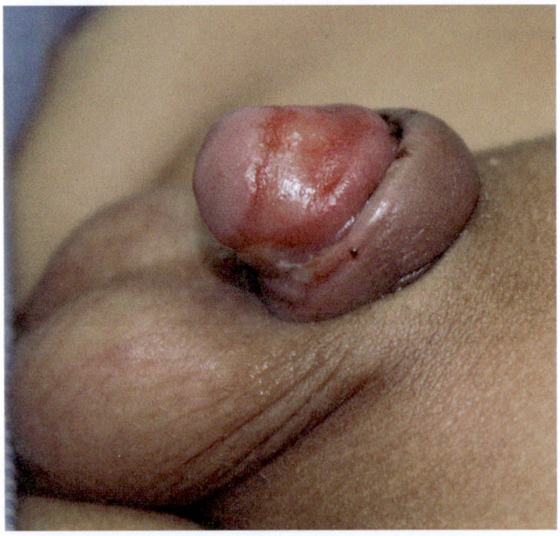

Fig. 5.28 Superficial ulceration and balanitis secondary to early separation of balanopreputial membrane

different from skin bridge which develops after circumcision secondary to the adhesions between denuded or deepithelized glans surface and penile skin edges (Fig. 5.29).

At the same time the natural or pathological adhesion of the inner prepuce to the glans penis attributed to failure of preputial retraction, which falsely diagnosed as phimosis (Chap. 18).

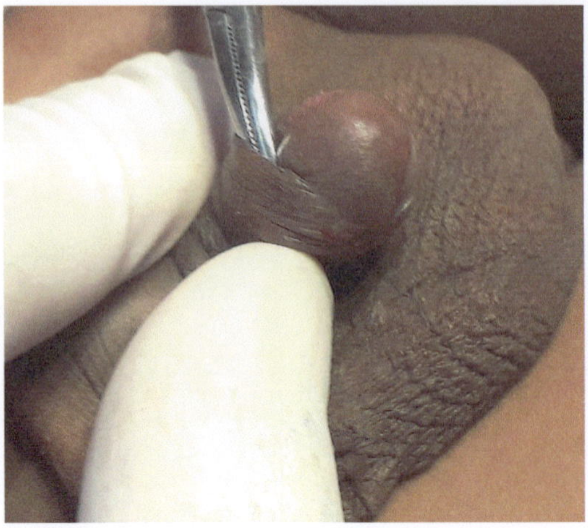

Fig. 5.29 Natural skin bridge between inner prepuce and the glans in uncircumcised child

The sub-preputial area is normally slightly moist in toddlers and adults, Taylor et al. [13] didn't find any sweat or sebaceous glands in prepuce, however, Fleiss et al. [22] reported apocrine glands that produce cathepsin B, lysozyme chymotrypsin, neutrophil elastase, cytokine, and pheromones such an androsterone. Prostatic, vesicular, and urethral secretions also contribute to the moisture of this area. Moisture may be exuded through the mucosa of the foreskin. Others reported that the sub-preputial moisture contains lytic material, which has an anti-bacterial and anti-viral action. The natural oils lubricate, moisturize, and protect the mucosal covering of the glans penis and inner foreskin [23].

Physiologically the preputial space behaves as an intertriginous zone, i.e., a body area where skin lies on contact with other skin surface, preputial space characterized as a warm, moist space with a higher degree of humidity, it had a tendency to have a more alkaline pH value, and with retained skin excretions such as corneocytes, sweat, and sebum with a different aggregations of smegma.

The normal microbial flora of the preputial space is not uniform and varies individually both qualitatively and quantitatively. Frequently, coagulase-negative staphylococci and propionibacterium acnes are present, and especially the very typical bacterium of the preputial space is the bacteroides melaninogenicus, the nosological significance of which is not entirely clear [23].

Preputial Musculatures (Fig. 5.30)

The penile dartos fascia is a loose areolar tissue devoid of fat that contains the superficial vessels and nerves of the penis. It is contiguous with Scarpa's fascia of the abdominal wall, and extends throughout the entire penile shaft between dermis and deep penile fascia (Buck's facia). At the shaft, the dartos fascia harbors the dartos muscle fibers which were arranged in a mosaic pattern, but form a circular sphincter-like configuration at the tip of the prepuce. Ventrally at the penile base, the superficial fascia fuses with the scrotal tunica dartos and further extends into the perineum to become continuous with the layers of the superficial perineal fascia "Colles fascia". Dartos facia and muscle lies one to two millimetres under the penile and preputial skin as a smooth muscle sheath. Preputial skin not containing any subcutaneous fat, which allow transmission of the dartos fascia contraction directly to the epidermis, and this is responsible for the corrugations of the prepuce specially at its distal part, which is similar to the architecture of scrotum. Different configurations of the attachment of dartos muscle fibers to the preputial skin is responsible for the highly variable patterns and shapes of the prepuce from one person to another (Figs. 5.9 and 5.14).

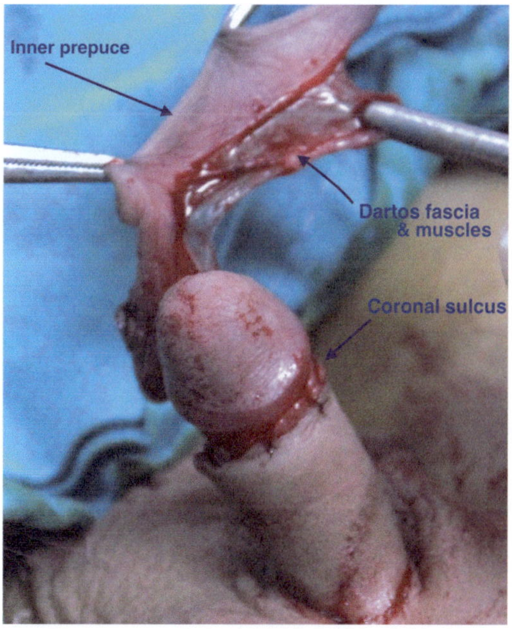

Fig. 5.30 Dartos muscle fibers embedded in dartos fascia deep to the preputial mucosa seen during circumcision by dissection

The sphincteric action of this muscle can inhibit inadvertent preputial retraction. This should be seen as normal physiology rather than a pathological condition. This sphincteric closing mechanism, beyond the urinary meatus, allows for the passage of urine while guarding against the entrance of foreign pathogens into the preputial space, also the muscle fibers keep the prepuce snug against the glans penis, and gives the prepuce a great elasticity, and allowing it to stretch.

Also the elasticity of the prepuce plays an important role in the erogenous and sexual functions of the prepuce [24].

Preputial Blood Supply

The blood supply of the penile skin is symmetrical, the superior and inferior external pudendal arteries arise from the femoral artery. They are attached to the Scarp's fascia, which extends to the base of the penis, at this point they divide into four branches as superficial penile arteries. Two enter the superficial penile fascia (Colles fascia) dorsolaterally and two enter it ventrolaterally. Numerous collaterals between these four arteries create a fine subcutaneous arterial plexus up to the preputial ring [25].

So these four arteries provide blood supply to the prepuce (Fig. 5.31). Beyond the preputial ring on the inner surface, the terminal branches become minute. At the level of the prepuce, certain branches are reflected to the anterior extremity towards the balanopreputial groove where they anastomose with the collaterals of the dorsal arteries. This is virtually the only point of anastomosis between the superficial and deep blood supply. However, an extensive network of collateral vessels across the midline forms a rich subdermal vascular plexus [25]. The foreskin is immensely vascularised and acts as a conduit for essential blood vessels within the penis, such as

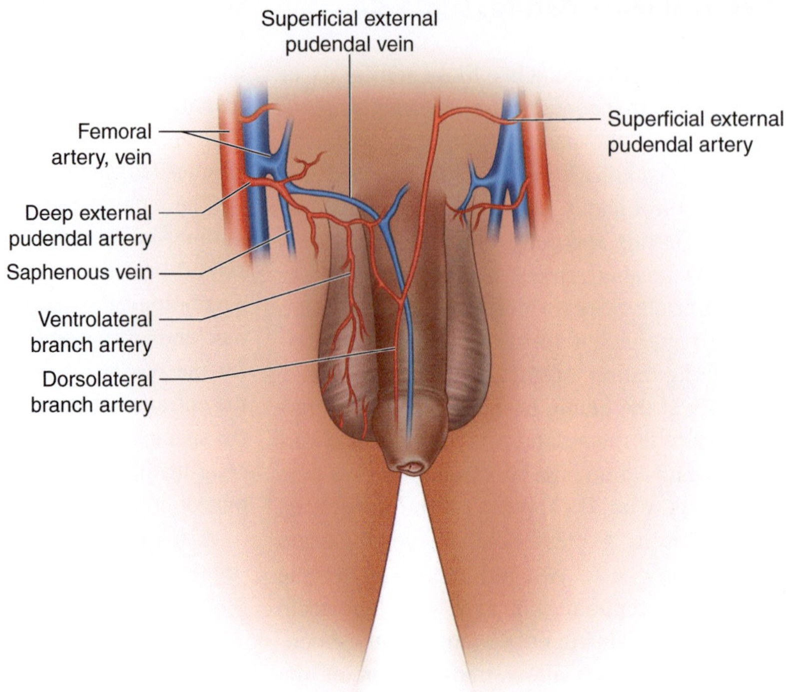

Fig. 5.31 Blood supply of the prepuce; arterial, venous

supplying the glans via the frenular arteries, which are symmetrical and arise from the dorsal penile artery, it branches at the level of the sulcus with small arteries that curve around each side of the distal shaft to enter the glans and the frenulum ventrally (Fig. 5.32).

On reaching the preputial ring the branches of the superficial penile arteries become tortuous and minute (Fig. 5.33), and the terminal branches were running circumferentially toward the coronal sulcus. Although the deep and superficial vascular systems anastomose at the level of the coronal sulcus, only some marginal blood supply of the prepuce was derived from the deep arterial system. The inner layer of the prepuce remains well vascularized because after the minute terminal and communicating branches are severed it still receives a blood supply from the glans.

The mean density of microvessels was significantly higher in the inner layer of the prepuce (31.8 ± 1.5/HPF). Microvessels are small size arterioles regularly arranged just underneath the epithelium of the inner prepuce. The outer prepuce shows scattered arterioles and capillaries of less microvessel density (14.7 ± 0.9/HPF). Microvessels density is high in the subepithelium of the inner prepuce in normal prepuce than the outer layer (31.8 ± 1.5 vs 140.8 ± 0.9/HPF) [26].

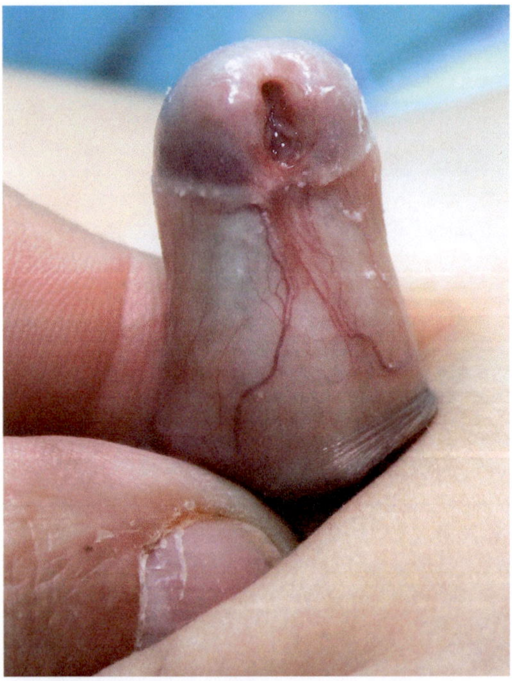

Fig. 5.32 Frenular arterial branches along the midline, (the urinary meatus is abnormally wide in this case)

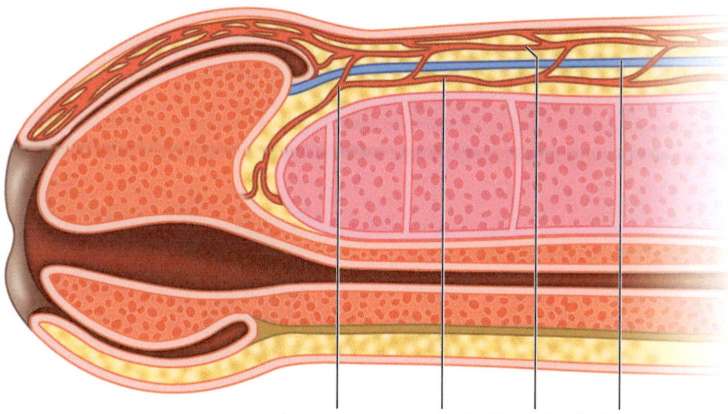

Fig. 5.33 Anastomosis between the dorsal penile artery and superficial arterial plexus of the prepuce proximal to the corona

Variations of the superficial penile arteries are possible with dominance of one side pair. The variations of the penile vascular anatomy have been reported previously. Marty et al. distinguished 3 main patterns of vascularization of the penile shaft skin. Both inferior external pudendal arteries supply the skin of the penile shaft but one is dominant [27].

Based on the transillumination technique, 4 types of preputial vascularization in normal boys were defined:- One artery predominant (41.67%), 2 arteries predominant (25%), H-type (12.5%) and net-like (no predominant artery) (20.83%) (Fig. 5.34).

Venous drainage of the prepuce is less well organized (Fig. 5.31). Multiple small veins in the prepuce without a particular orientation join the superficial dorsal veins and drain into the saphenous vein. Superficial venous drainage occurs through a number of veins that course in the dartos fascia along the dorsolateral, lateral, and/or ventrolateral aspect of the penis. These vessels unite at the base of the penis to form a superficial dorsal vein. Drainage of the latter is usually into the left saphenous vein, but communication with the deep dorsal vein of the penis may sometimes occur.

The penile lymphatics drain into the superficial inguinal and subinguinal lymph nodes.

The blood supply of the hypospadiac prepuce is crucial for successful hypospadias surgery. The hypospadiac prepuce could be used for neourethra reconstruction and penile body skin closure. Well vascularized flap is the main factor for a successful outcome of hypospadias surgery, although the severity of the hypospadias and macroscopic morphology of penis and prepuce generally determine the type of operative technique, recently many studies reported the anatomical variations of the blood supply of the hypospadiac prepuce from the normal one and its affect in surgery outcome [28] (Chap. 13).

Preputial Innervation (Fig. 5.35)

Many doctors or paramedical personals performing circumcision daily in dozens of children may not recognising that prepuce include any nerves at all. The first recorded reference about innervation of the prepuce is the notation by Bichat at 1801, Dogiel at 1893 is 1st one to describe Meissner corpuscles in the inner prepuce and the frenulum [29].

The foreskin contains 20,000–70,000 erogenous nerve endings, the majority of which are concentrated in the ridged band and the frenulum. The prepuce provides a large and important platform for several nerves and nerve endings. The innervation of the outer skin of the prepuce is impressive; its sensitivity to light touch and pain are similar to that of the skin of the penis as a whole [30]. The glans, by

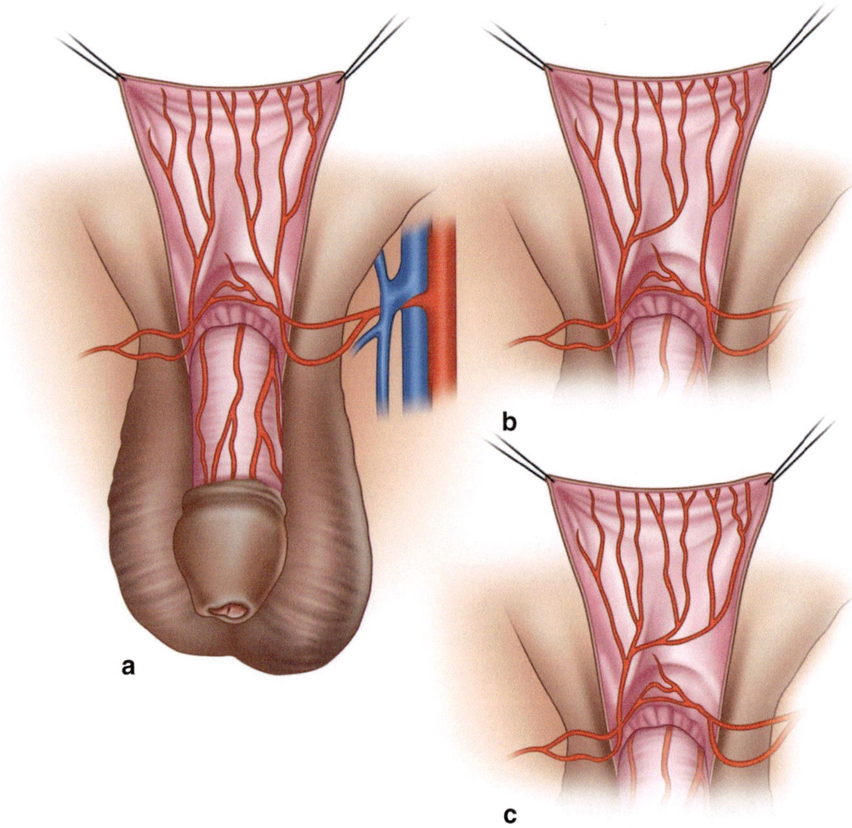

Fig. 5.34 Preputial end arteries variation: (**a**) normal blood supply, with equal distribution from both sides; (**b**) dominant right-sided distribution and (**c**) the whole blood supply from the right artery

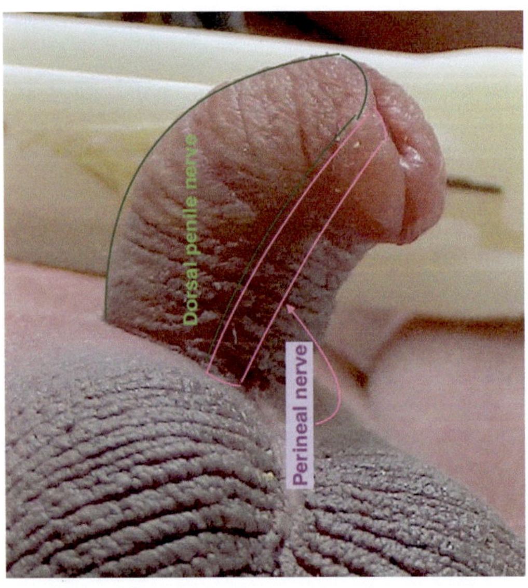

Fig. 5.35 The dorsal and lateral aspects of the prepuce innervated by the dorsal penile nerve, ventral prepuce and frenulum are innervated by the perineal nerve

contrast, is insensitive to light touch, heat, cold and, as far as to pin-prick. Le Gros Clark [31] noted that the glans penis is one of the few areas on the body that enjoys nothing beyond primitive sensory modalities. The glans penis is primarily innervated by free nerve endings and has primarily protopathic sensitivity. Protopathic sensitivity refers to cruder, poorly localized feelings (including pain, some temperature sensations and certain perceptions of mechanical contact). In the glans penis, encapsulated end-organs are sparse, and found mainly along the corona and the frenulum. The only portion of the body with less fine-touch discrimination than the glans penis is the heel of the foot. The innervation difference between the protopathic sensitivity of the glans penis and the corpuscular receptor-rich ridged band of the prepuce is part of the normal complement of penile erogenous tissue [32].

The foreskin has an erogenous function, due to its unique innervation. The Dorsal Nerve of the penis (DNP) and branches of the perineal nerve (including the posterior scrotal nerves) are responsible for the preputial somatosensory innervation.

The dorsal and lateral aspects of the prepuce are innervated by the dorsal penile nerve, but the ventral prepuce and frenulum are innervated by the perineal nerve (Fig. 5.35). The dorsal and perineal nerves are branches of the pudendal nerve, which derives from the second, third, and fourth sacral plexus.

Autonomic innervation is derived from the pelvic plexus, the parasympathetic visceral afferent and efferent fibers arise from sacral roots (S2–S4) and course adjacent to and through the walls of the membranous urethra, while sympathetic preganglionic and visceral afferent fibers arise from thoracolumbar nerve roots (T11–L2) (Fig. 5.36).

Sensory receptors can be classified as mechanoreceptors, e.g. Meissner's corpuscles, Vater-Pacinian corpuscles, Merkel cells and nociceptors (free nerve endings). Merkel cells mediate tactile sensations, and are found in glabrous skin; they have also been reported in the clitoris and can be identified in the male prepuce.

A multitude of names have been used to describe these encapsulated receptors, e.g. Krause, Dogiel, genital corpuscles, Endkalpsen and mucocutaneous end-organs [33].

The term corpuscular (encapsulated) receptors is usually used to include all of these mechanoreceptors. Most of the encapsulated receptors of the prepuce are Meissner corpuscles, as they contact the epithelial basement membrane [14].

Numerous specialised nerve endings have been identified in the prepuce, among them are:

- Pacinian corpuscles (responsible for pressure sensing)
- Ruffini's corpuscles (mechanical receptors)
- End-bulbs of Krause (most likely responsible for sensing cold)
- Free nerve endings (pain receptors)
- Meissner's corpuscles, which are sensitive to light touch, and perhaps are the most important in terms of erogenous sensation. It represent the majority of sensory receptors (genital corpuscles) that are found in prepuce. They are distributed throughout the skin, but concentrated in areas that are particularly sensitive, such as the fingertips, palms and soles, lips, tongue, face, and genitals.

It has been calculated that circumcision results in the loss of at least 10,000–20,000 specialized erotogenic nerve endings [31].

Although the sensory and autonomic innervation of the penis and clitoris are similar, but there is a remarkable difference in their encapsulated

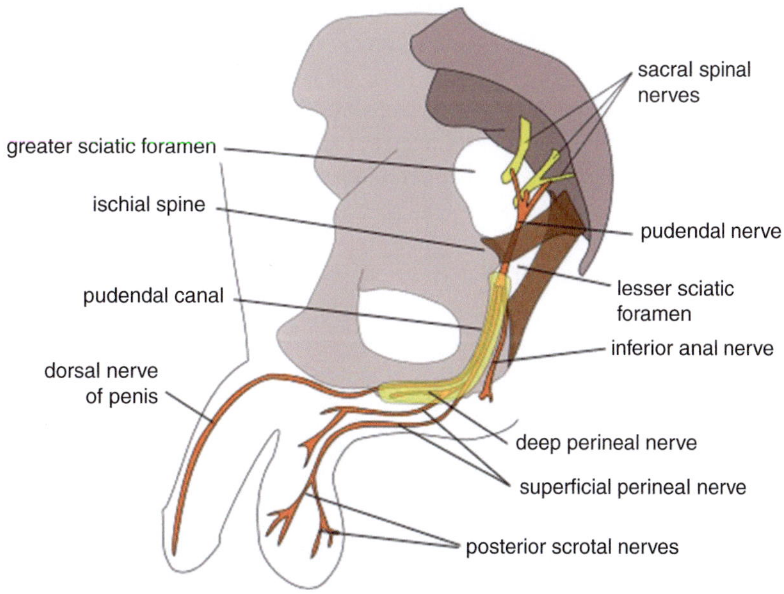

Fig. 5.36 Innervation of the prepuce

somatosensory receptors; in females, the glans clitoris and the inner plate of the prepuce have corpuscular receptors on their oppositional surfaces. The glans clitoris also has a much denser concentration of Vater-Pacinian corpuscles than either the glans penis or the male prepuce. Also the fused common epithelium of the clitoris and the inner plate of the prepuce are reported to have intraepithelial nerve endings.

Neonatal Innervation

There is an extensive network of nerves within the prepuce at birth, newborns appear to have a higher density of preputial nerves than adults [34]. The fused inner plate of the male prepuce/glans has also been reported to have intraepithelial nerves.

Studies of the complete human foetal penis with careful attention to this area will be required before the assertions of Dogiel and Ohmori for intraepithelial nerves of the male prepuce can be dismissed [29].

Preputial Development and Maturity in Adolescence

Adhesion and the common membrane attaching the inner mucosa of the prepuce and the glandular surface is a unique difference between neonatal and adult prepuces and this discussed with the balanopreputial space. The genital organs, specially the prepuce are in a very immature stage of development at birth. The growth and development continues through puberty and into adulthood. Neonatal prepuce is completely different from adult one (Fig. 5.6).

The tubular, tapered, and elongated prepuce of the young boy should not be seen as "hypertrophic" or "redundant" tissue that requires "trimming" (Fig. 5.14). As the corpora cavernosa develop in adolescence, the penis will enlarge to take up the slack. A prepuce that in childhood appears long, may, at maturity, fail to completely cover the glans. A study published in the Journal of Urology finds that by ages 8–10, 50% of boys will have a fully retractable prepuce [26].

In the infant, the muscle fibres are intertwined and arranged in a mosaic- like pattern, causing the distal prepuce to pucker and close like a one-way valve.

When comparing the dartos muscle layer of the prepuce in males before and after puberty, the ratio of muscle fibres to elastic fibres decreases. This may explain why on gross inspection the distal prepuce is puckered in the infant and appears more relaxed in the adult [35].

May be there is an ethnical developmental variability in the appearance of the normal foreskin throughout childhood and puberty, in Malaysia, New Guinea, Sri Lanka and southern India the foreskin is very long and ends in a narrow extension that acts like a muzzle. This is an impediment to sexual intercourse. A short prepuce that rarely covers the glans completely is seen in Whites of the northern Mediterranean and many Asians (Chinese and Japanese) [9].

A tight preputial orifice with normal histology is not pathological in young boys, but should be considered as a normal stage of penile development.

Normal Preputial Variations

Prepuce shows a great variabilities between individuals as regard its length, configurations, colour, its retractability, wideness of the meatus and extension of its frenulum (Fig. 5.37).

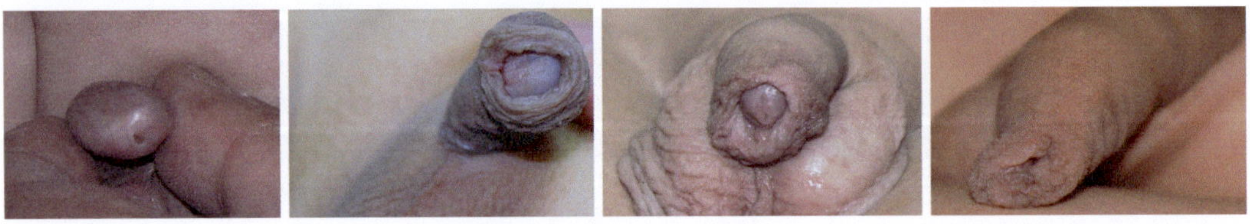

Fig. 5.37 Normal variation in the preputial length and preputial meatus

A recent study conducted in 30 preputial specimens obtained from 3 groups of boys undergoing ritual circumcision (<3 years, 3–5 and 5–7 years) showed that the number of vein clusters in the prepuce and the incidence of vessel wall fibrosis grow with age. The number of nerve, vessel, and collagen fibers also increased with age [36].

So far there have been a scanty knowledges analyzing the incidence of non-pathological lesions or normal variants on the male external genitalia in general, and nothing was written as regard the prepuce in particular. Subsequently, the number of patients consulted due to the presence of such lesions remains unknown. As most of the penile and preputial variants may be interpreted by the patients as a venereal or sexually transmitted diseases; so such variants may lead to apprehension, which recently known as "venerophobia" [37].

The most common normal variations were hyperpigmentation of the whole or the tip of the prepuce, followed by difference in preputial length and penile coverage.

Constitutive pigmentation variations are due to race, sun-induced facultative pigmentation is rarely relevant in the genital area, but postinflammatory hyperpigmentation is common. Linear hyperpigmentation of the ventral penile shaft, along the median raphe, is often seen.

Other common normal lesions are:

Pearly Penile Papules (PPP) (Fig. 5.38)

Synonyms: Papillae Coronae Glandis, Hirsuties papillaris penis, hirsutoid penis papilloma.

This is a manifestation without a disease significance at the proximal border of the glans, before its transition into the coronary sulcus, manifested as one or many fringed papillary, whitish-red, fine, very regularly sized excrescences, partly vascularized. These fine serrated papillae constitute a rare, normal finding and histologically it looks like acral angiofibromas [38].

PPP are common; they may be found in up to 50% of men. They present as flesh-coloured, pink, smooth, rounded, 1–3 mm papules, occurring predominantly around the coronal margin of the glans, rarely on the glans itself, in rows or rings, sometimes this tiny nodules extend to the undersurface of frenulum. Despite their benign nature, PPP are known to cause significant distress because of their resemblance to sexually transmitted infections such as condyloma acuminata. For patients who still desire treatment after counselling and reassurance, cryotherapy and laser therapy represent two reliable treatment options with low rates of recurrence [39].

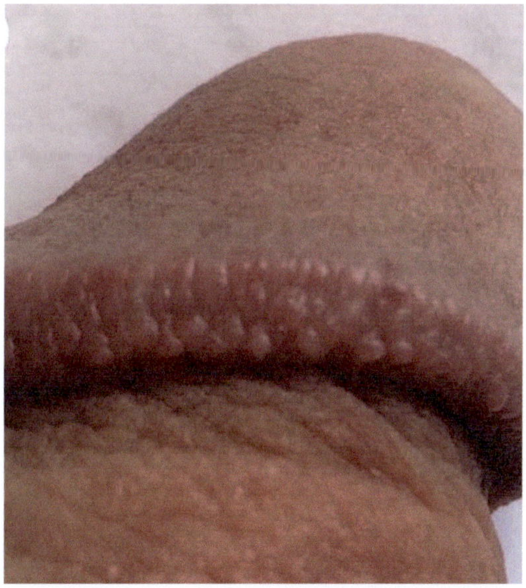

Fig. 5.38 Pearly penile papules at the coronal sulcus

Skin Tags

It is also termed acrochordons. According to Banik et al. [40] in a group of 750 males selected at random, skin tags were diagnosed in 46% cases. The most common sites of genital skin tags in male include groins, sometimes scrotum, penile shaft and the glans. Preputial tags are very rare. They occur as multiple dark or skin-colored, filiform or smooth-surfaced papules, approximately 2–3 mm in diameter. The stalk of skin tags is fibrous and consists of loose connective tissue with dilated capillaries. in Fig. 5.39 a child

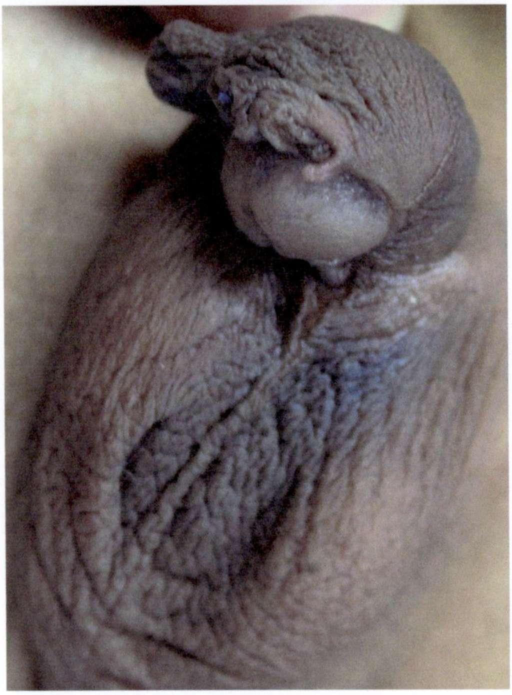

Fig. 5.39 Preputial skin tag in hypospadiac prepuce

have a hypospadias and a well demarcated skin tag at the top of the hooded prepuce. As a rule these lesions are asymptomatic, but in some cases, contact with the underwear may result in a painful bleeding or predispose to bacterial superinfection. Treatment involves removal of the skin tags by means of electro- or cryosurgery.

References

1. Scott S. The anatomy and physiology of the human prepuce. In: Denniston GC, et al., editors. Male and female circumcision. Boston: Springer; 1999. https://doi.org/10.1007/978-0-585-39937-9_2.
2. Blouin K, Richard C, Brochu G, et al. Androgen inactivation and steroid-converting enzyme expression in abdominal adipose tissue in men. J Endocrinol. 2006;191:637–49.
3. Werker PMN, Terng ASC, Kon M. The prepuce free flap: dissection feasibility study and clinical application of a super thin new flap. Plast Reconstr Surg. 1998;102(4):1075–82.
4. Fahmy MA. The spectrum of genital median raphe anomalies among infants undergoing ritual circumcision. J Pediatr Urol. 2013;9:872. http://www.sciencedirect.com/science/article/pii/S147751311200294X#FCANote
5. Fahmy MA. Penile median raphe anomalies as an indicator of megameatus intact prepuce anomaly in children undergoing routine circumcision. Urology. 2018;121:164–7.
6. Velazquez EF, Bock A, Soskin A, Codas R, Arbo M, Cubilla AL. Preputial variability and preferential association of long phimotic foreskins with penile cancer. Am J Surg Pathol. 2003;27(7):994–8.
7. Sorrells ML, Snyder JL, Reiss MD, Eden C, Milos MF, Wilcox N, Van Howe RS. Fine-touch pressure thresholds in the adult penis. BJU Int. 2007;99:864–9. https://doi.org/10.1111/j.1464-410X.2006.06685.x.
8. Gairdner D. The fate of the foreskin: a study of circumcision. BMJ. 1949;2:1433–7.
9. Kayaba H, Tamura H, Kitajima S, Fujiwara Y, Kato T, Kato T. Analysis of shape and retractability of the prepuce in 603 Japanese boys. J Urol. 1996;156:1813–5.
10. Hiraoka M, Tsukahara H, Ohshima Y, Mayumi M. Meatus tightly covered by the prepuce is associated with urinary infection. Pediatr Int. 2002;44:658–62.
11. Schöberlein W. Significance and incidence of phimosis and smegma. [Article in German]. Munch Med Wochenschr. 1967;108(7):373–7.
12. Radojicic ZI, Perovic SV. Classification of prepuce in hypospadias according to morphological abnormalities and their impact on hypospadias repair. J Urol. 2004;172:301–4.
13. Sadeghipour S, Esmailzadehha N. Aposthia: a case report. J Pediatr Surg. 2010;45(8):17–9.
14. Taylor JR, et al. The prepuce: specialised mucosa of the penis and its loss to circumcision. Br J Urol. 1996;77:291–5.
15. McGrath K. The frenular delta. In: Denniston GC, Hodges FM, Milos MF, editors. Understanding circumcision. Boston: Springer; 2001.
16. Hunter RH. Notes on the development of the prepuce. J Anat. 1935;70:68–75.
17. Snell RS. Atlas of clinical anatomy. Boston: Little, Brown and Company; 1978. p. 136.
18. Hodges FM. What your doctor may not tell you about circumcision. New York: Warner Books; 2002. p. 7.
19. Wells LJ, Lund CJ. Effects of steroid hormones upon the developmental separation of the prepuce from the glans penis. J Clin Endocrinol Metab. 1947;7:192–200.
20. Deibert GA. The separation of the prepuce in the human penis. Anat Rec. 1933;57(4):387.
21. Fahmy MA. Complications in male circumcision. St. Louis: Elsevier; 2019. https://doi.org/10.1016/C2018-0-03679-8.
22. Fleiss PM, Hodges FM. What your doctor may not tell you about circumcision. New York: Warner Books; 2002. p. 7.
23. Günsar C, Kurutepe S, Alparslan O, et al. The effect of circumcision status on periurethral and glandular bacterial flora. Urol Int. 2004;72:212–5.
24. Aldahan AS, Brah TK, Nouri K. Diagnosis and management of pearly penile papules. Am J Mens Health. 2018;12(3):624–7. https://doi.org/10.1177/1557988316654138.

25. Sonnex C, Dockerty WG. Pearly penile papules: a common cause of concern. Int J STD AIDS. 1999;10:726–7.
26. Lakshmanan S, Prakash S. Human prepuce: some aspects of structure and function. Indian J Surg. 1980;44:134–7. http://www.cirp.org/library/anatomy/lakshmanan/.
27. Juskiewenski S. A study of the arterial blood supply to the penis. Anat Clin. 1982;4:101–7.
28. Schwartz O. Langerhans cells lap up HIV-1. Nat Med. 2007;13:245–6.
29. Winkelmann RK. The cutaneous innervation of the human newborn prepuce. J Invest Dermatol. 1956;26:53–67.
30. Marty B, Perruchoud C, Wicky S, Guillou L, Von Segesser LK. Atheroembolization: a harmful complication of therapeutic internal iliac artery occlusion. J Vasc Surg. 2002;36:1062–5.
31. Le Gros Clark WE. The tissues of the body. 5th ed. Oxford: Clarendon Press; 1965. p. 329.
32. Yucel S, Guntekin E, Kukul E, et al. Comparison of hypospadiac and normal preputial vascular anatomy. J Urol. 2004;172:1973–6. https://doi.org/10.1097/01.ju.0000142131.37693.05.
33. Modwing R, Valderrama E. Immunohistochemical analysis of nerve distribution patterns within preputial tissues. J Urol. 1989;141(Suppl 1):489A.
34. Winkelmann RK. The mucocutaneous end-organ. Arch Dermatol. 1957;76:225–35.
35. Ohmori D. Uber die entwicklung der innervation der genital apparatus als peripheren aufnahme-apparat der genitalen reflex. Ztschrj Jges Anat U Entw. 1924;70:347–410.
36. Dossanova A, Lozovoy V, Manekenova K, Lozovaya Y, Seidakhmetov M, Dossanov B, Omarov T, Botabaeva A, Shakeeva A, Baubekov Z. Histological and morphological characteristics of the prepuce of penis skin structure in different age groups. J Pediatr Urol. 2018;14:280.e1–6. https://doi.org/10.1016/j.jpurol.2018.02.022.
37. Michajłowski I, Sobjanek M, Michajłowski J, Włodarkiewicz A, Matuszewski M. Normal variants in patients consulted in the dermatology clinic for lesions of the male external genitalia. Cent European J Urol. 2012;65(1):17–20. https://doi.org/10.5173/ceju.2012.01.art5.
38. Dogiel AS. Die nervenendigunngen in der schleimhaut der aussen genitalorgane des menschen. Arch F Mikr Anat. 1893;41:585–612.
39. Tanagho EA. Anatomy of the lower urinary tract. In: Walsh PC, Retik AB, Stamey TA, Vaughan ED, editors. Campbell's urology, vol. 1. 6th ed. Philadelphia: W. B. Saunders; 1992. p. 61.
40. Banik R, Lubach D. Skin tags localization and frequencies according to sex and age. Dermatologica. 1987;174:180–3.

Histology of the Prepuce

6

Skin of the Prepuce (Fig. 6.1)

The skin (outer) layer of the prepuce shows typical characteristics of a thin, true skin. However, there are distinctive features that characterize the prepuce histologically from other parts of the body:-

- The papillary dermis is rich in nerves and lymphoid cells.
- Dense capillary networks can be observed in both the upper and lower dermal zones.
- Lacks of the dense collagenous zone, both in density and thickness, which usually seen in most areas of the body
- Scant in lanugo hair follicles, sweat and sebaceous glands.
- Although limited in number, melanocytes can be observed.
- There are scattered smooth muscle bundles located in the lower reticular dermal zone.
- Elastin fibers and bundles are very abundant and dense.

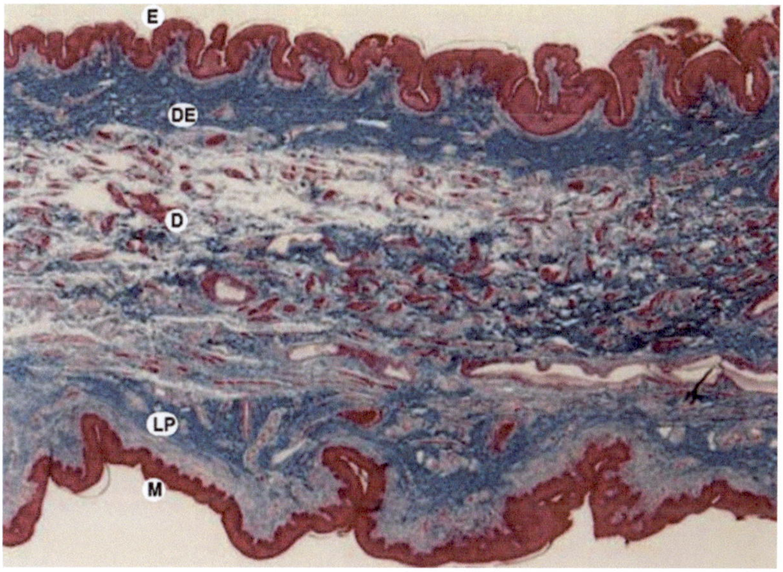

Fig. 6.1 Male prepuce: Mucosa (M), lamina propria (LP), dartos muscle (D), dermis (DE) and glabrous outer epithelium (E). Note there are more black elastic fibres in the dermis than in the mucosal lamina propria. Elastin trichrome ×25 [17]

M. A. B. Fahmy, *Normal and Abnormal Prepuce*, https://doi.org/10.1007/978-3-030-37621-5_6

The outer epithelium of the prepuce consists of stratified squamous cells that are keratinized, Melanocytes are present in the basal layers. Langerhans cells and Merkel cells are also detectable, which are a specialized neuroendocrine cells that mediate tactile sensations and stain positively with cytokeratin [1].

Generally the Merkel cells of glabrous skin contain characteristic membrane-bound dense core granules and are sometimes associated with unmyelinated neurites, it may express VIP, neurone-specific enolase, chromogranin A and cytokeratin [2]. The function and concentration of Merkel cells within the external genitalia has not been extensively studied.

Preputial Sweat Glans

There is debate about whether humans have a functional homologues to preputial glands, which were first noted by Edward Tyson and in 1694 and fully described by William Cowper who named them Tyson's glands [3]. They are described as a modified sebaceous glands located around the corona and inner surface of the prepuce of the human penis. They are believed to be most frequently found in the balanopreputial sulcus, also they thought that its secretion may be one of the components of smegma, but latter on, other authors disputed their existence [4].

The existence of these Tyson's glands being rejected by many European investigators as far back as 1884. The problem has arisen because one of the findings of Tyson's paper of 1699 on the orangutan was interpreted as applying to humans, which it does not [5]. No actual description of them in humans exists and a number of modem investigations have failed to find any glands in the inner prepuce or sulcus [6]. In conclusion; human preputial skin containing few sebaceous and sweat glands, but it is devoid of any other specific glands which was described in animals.

Dermis of the Prepuce

The dermis of the prepuce consists of connective tissue, blood vessels, nerve trunks, Meissner corpuscles within the papillae, and occasionally scattered sebaceous and sweat glands. The dermis of the male prepuce appears to have more elastic fibres than the lamina propria. The difference between the elastic fibres in the lamina propria and dermis may also help form the 'muzzle' configuration around the glans penis. The elastic tissue of the prepuce dermis, along with the dartos muscle and frenulum, tether the prepuce and help return it to its anatomically correct position after deployment during erection or after manual retraction. The clitoral prepuce has only a dermal component with fewer elastic fibres than the male prepuce (Fig. 6.2).

Nerve fibres of the dermis are arranged into a deeper and a more superficial network. These

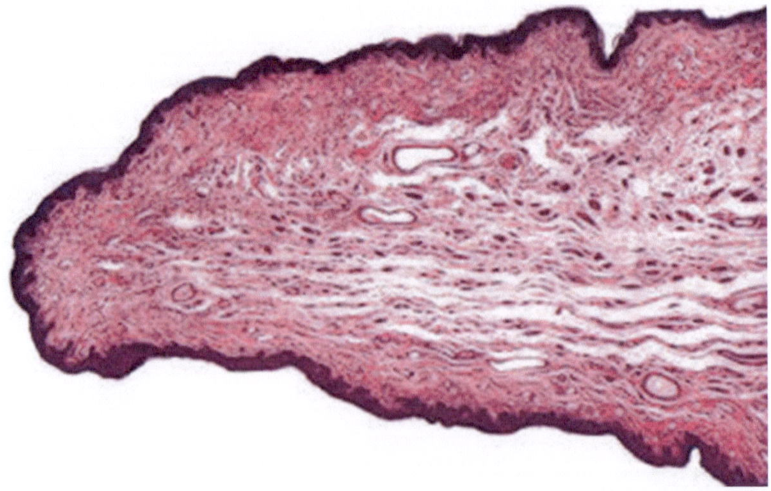

Fig. 6.2 Full thickness of preputial edge shows all five layers: keratinized stratified squamous epithelium, dermis with sebaceous glands, dartos, submucosa and squamous mucosa. H&E

networks constitute the chief form of innervation of human prepuce. The deeper net is oriented with the rete of arterioles in the reticular layer and may be considered limited to this portion of the dermis [7].

Dartos Muscle

The dartos smooth muscle is specific to the male external genitalia and the vast majority of the penile dartos muscle is contained within the prepuce. The dartos muscle consists of smooth muscle cells invested with elastic fibres. From the prepuce, the delicate, attenuated penile dartos muscle surrounds the shaft of the penis and is continuous with the scrotal dartos muscle. The penile dartos muscle is temperature-dependent and allows for the volume changes required for erection [8] (Fig. 6.3).

In the infant, the muscle fibres are intertwined and arranged in a mosaic- like pattern, causing the distal prepuce to pucker and close like a one-way valve.

When comparing the dartos muscle layer of the prepuce in males before and after puberty, the ratio of muscle fibres to elastic fibres decreases. This may explain why on gross inspection the distal prepuce is puckered in the infant and appears more relaxed in the adult [9]. The increase in elastic fibres may be necessary for the uncomplicated eversion of the glans in the adult. While the aetiology of this transformation is unknown, steroid hormones may have an influence, as their topical application can accelerate the retractability of the prepuce in prepubescent boys. Nerve bundles of the prepuce run alongside the dartos muscle (Fig. 6.4).

Lamina Propria of Preputial Mucosa

The lamina propria of the male and female prepuce is very vascular, but the male prepuce has looser collagen than the dense collagenous lamina propria of the glans penis. The ridged bands of the prepuce lie near the mucocutaneous tip of the male prepuce and, in the unretracted prepuce, it usually lie against the glans penis. The mucosal lamina propria (corion) is devoid of lanugo hair follicles, sweat and sebaceous glands.

Mucosal Epithelium (Inner Plate of the Prepuce)

The mucosal epithelium of the male prepuce is the same as the squamous mucosal epithelium that covers the glans penis. The glans penis and the inner prepuce share a common, fused mucosal

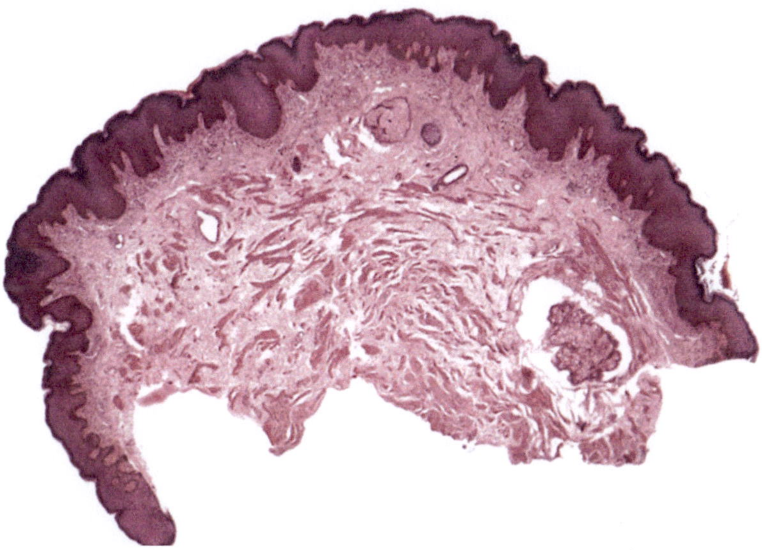

Fig. 6.3 Muscle bundles of the dartos are seen beneath the keratinized squamous epithelium

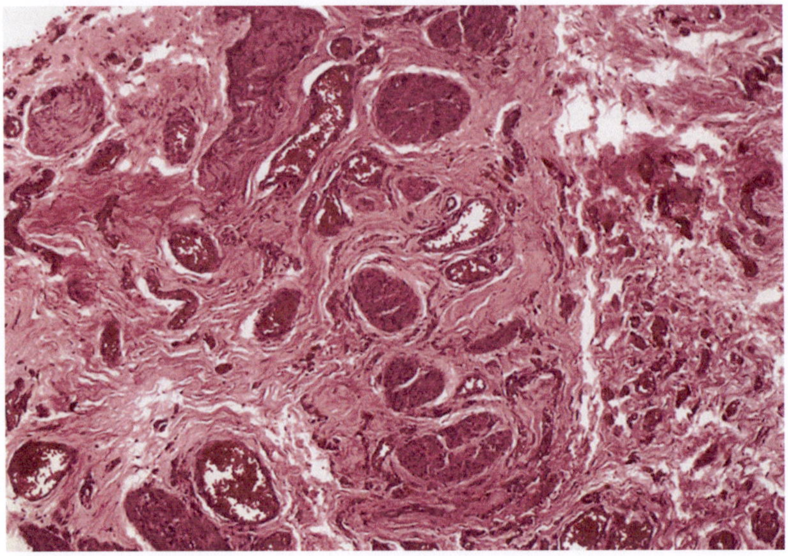

Fig. 6.4 Thick bundles of conspicuous smooth muscle in the deep reticular dermis

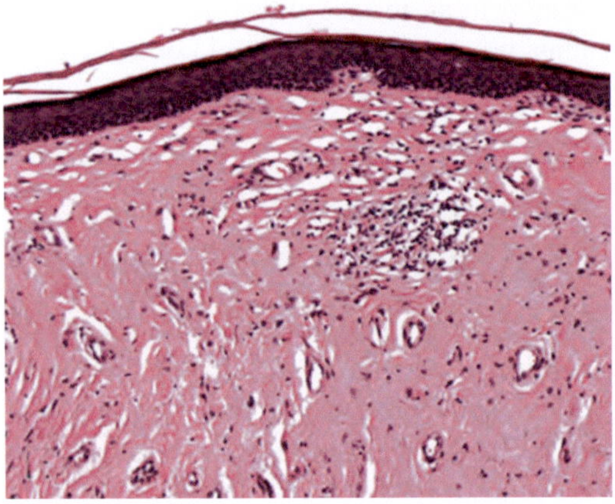

Fig. 6.5 The foreskin inner mucosa is formed by a nonkeratinized squamous epithelium similar to that covering the glans and the coronal sulcus. Note the almost flat epithelial base and the absence of pigmented keratinocytes

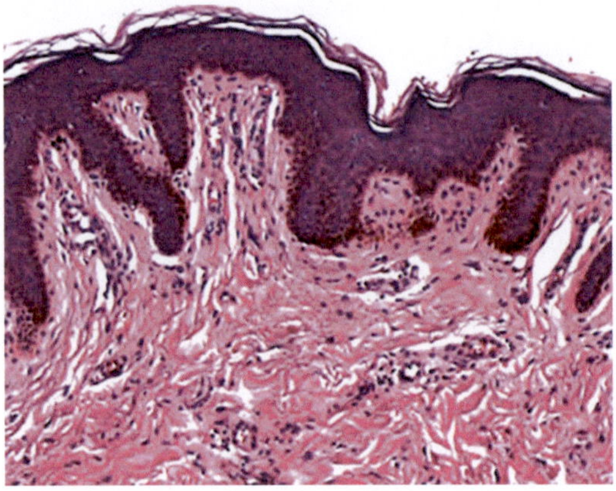

Fig. 6.6 The foreskin outer surface is covered by a slightly keratinized squamous epithelium. Note the irregular rete ridges of the basal epithelium and the easily recognized pigmentation of the basal cells

epithelium at birth. Regardless of the embryological explanation, this common epithelium does not separate until the proper hormonal and growth factors are present. The fused inner plate of the male prepuce/glans has also been reported to have intraepithelial nerves, but many researchers disputed existence of any nerve endings in the balanopreputial membrane [10] (Fig. 6.5).

The inner surface of the prepuce is lined by variably keratinized squamous epithelium similar to frictional mucosa of the mouth, vagina and oesophagus. The epithelium is papillated by stromal or 'corial' tissue and is rich in nerves, Schwann cells, lymphoid cells and capillaries. Papillae are continuous with a highly vascular, loose-knit tissue layer that resembles the corium of oral mucosa. Preputial mucosa also lacks the dense collagenous zone seen in most areas of true (skin) dermis and, again unlike true skin of the penile shaft and outer surface of the prepuce, the mucosal surface of the prepuce is completely free of lanugo hair follicles, sweat and sebaceous glands, and it is also devoid of melanocytes (Figs. 6.6 and 6.7).

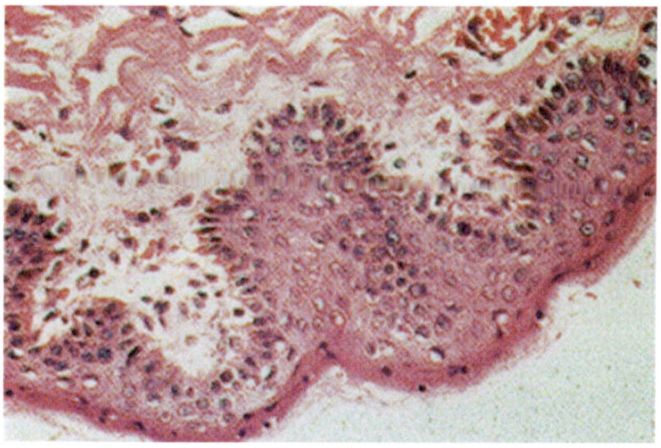

Fig. 6.7 Meissner's corpuscles appear as large oval or elongated bodies attached to the basement membranes of corial papillae of the ridged band Haematoxylin and eosin × 100

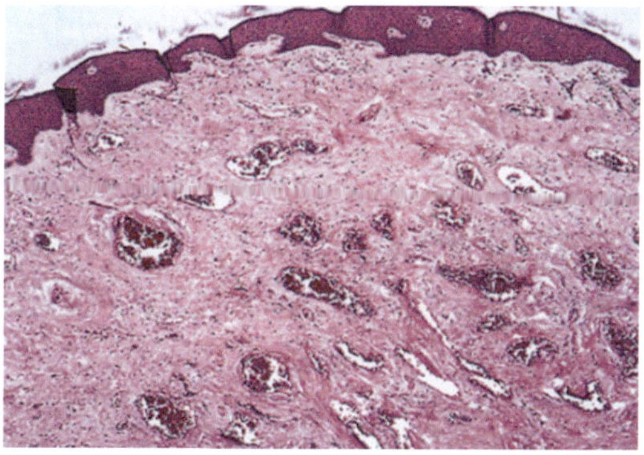

Fig. 6.8 Normal histology of the glans penis, with three layers are noted: nonkeratinized stratified mucosa, lamina propria and corpus spongiosum. H&E

Dense capillary networks can be observed in both upper and lower dermal zones. Papillae resemble the corium of oral mucosa. The absence of the dense collagenous zone, both in density and thickness, compared with most areas of true (skin) reticular dermis is obvious. Smooth muscle bundles can be observed in the lower reticular dermal zone. Elastin fibers and bundles are more abundant and dense than the preputial skin.

Histological cross-sections of the 'ridged band' showed focal, spiky or more rounded, broader and flatter ridges interspersed with sulci. Meissner's corpuscles were more plentiful in some subjects than in others but perhaps significantly, they were only seen in the crests of ridges, occasionally in small clumps that expanded the tips of corial papillae (Fig. 6.8).

S100 staining of the preputial mucosa (Fig. 6.9) showed additional end-organs and myelinated nerve fibres within papillae and confirmed the richly innervated nature of the 'ridged band'. The distribution of Meissner's corpuscles in the mucosal ridges was best seen in tangential sections through the epithelium and tips of corial papillae of some but not all persons. Sections of 'smooth mucosa' showed no ridging of the mucosal surface, slightly shallower corial papillae and few Meissner's corpuscles [11].

Histologically, no clear demarcation line can be drawn between true skin of the penile shaft and the 'ridged band' at the precise tip of the prepuce.

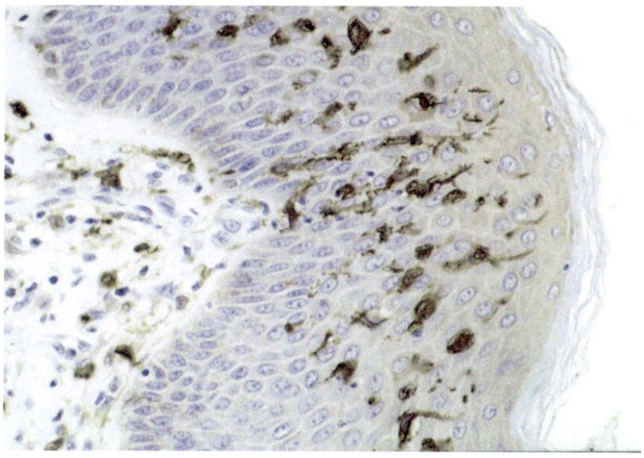

Fig. 6.9 Section of skin showing large numbers of dendritic (Langerhans) cells in the epidermis. S100 immunoperoxidase stain (Public Domain photo)

There are four clinically obvious distinctions between the preputial skin and mucosa were reported:

1. Early graft edema, especially in mucosal grafts, that resolves spontaneously after 48 h.
2. Better "take" of mucosal grafts.
3. Hyperpigmentation in both graft types, with the skin being darker.
4. Less secondary contraction in mucosal grafts.

Electron Microscopic Studies of the Prepuce

The reticular dermal layer of the skin, especially the lower zone, displays a loose appearance among collagen bundles, almost similar to the characteristics of loose areolar tissue. Collagen bundles are oriented in both the longitudinal and horizontal directions. The epidermal layer is very thin with scant keratinization. The abundance of active fibroblasts and mast cells is clearly obvious. Schwann cells, and myelinated and nonmyelinated nerve fibers emphasize the good sensation of the prepuce [12]. The reticular dermal layer of the mucosa has a loose appearance that is more intensive than preputial skin. The epidermal layer is very thin and almost lacks keratinization. The abundance of active fibroblasts, mast cells, myelinated and nonmyelinated nerve fibers, and Schwann cells is clearly obvious.

Preputial Immunology

The prepuce covers and protects the glans penis and urinary meatus. In most males, the prepuce protects the sterile urinary tract environment in infancy and maintains the moistness of the mucosal surface of the glans penis throughout life. Fleiss et al. [13] have identified several immunological functions of the prepuce that help to protect the body from pathogens:

- Sphincter action of the preputial orifice functions like a one-way valve, allowing urine to flow out but preventing the entry of infectious contaminants;
- Apocrine glands of the inner prepuce, which secrete lysozyme, which helps on break down of the cell walls of pathogens (and also acts against HIV).
- Sub-preputial moisture that lubricates and protects the mucosa of the glans penis.
- High vascularity to bring phagocytes to fight infection.

The mucosal surface of the foreskin produces plasma cells, part of the body's defence system, they secrete antibodies and antibacterial and antiviral proteins, including lysozyme.

Langerhans cells are dendritic cells (antigen-presenting immune cells) of the skin and some mucous membranes, and contain organelles called Birbeck granules. They are present in all layers of the epidermis and are most prominent in the stratum spinosum. They also occur in the papillary dermis, particularly around blood vessels (Fig. 6.9).

Epithelial Langerhans cells (ELCs), is a component of the immune system, help the body recognise and process antigens, directing them to lymphocytes or macrophages, it migrate to the regional lymph nodes and convert into mature dendritic cells capable of priming naive T cells.

ELCs have been demonstrated in skin by electron microscopy at 14 weeks gestation. Immunohistochemical techniques have detected ELCs in foetal skin as early as 43 days. Weiss et al. noted an abundance of ELCs in the outer surface of the neonatal prepuce comparable with the general density found in adult skin. ELCs secrete cytokines, hormone-like low molecular-weight proteins, which regulate the intensity and duration of immune responses [14].

de Witte and colleagues [15] reported that the (ELCs) of the prepuce produce *langerin*, a substance that provides a barrier to HIV infection.

Specialized immunological properties should be noted by the presence of Langerhans cells and other lytic materials, which defend against common microbes, and there is robust evidence supporting HIV protection [16].

On the other hand Langerhan's cells can be found in both the mucosal epithelium of the prepuce and in the outer keratinized epithelium. Since superficial Langerhans' cells on the inner aspect of the foreskin, frenulum, and urethral meatus are poorly protected by keratin, they could act as potential virus target cells and play an important role in primary HIV infection in males [17].

These findings may thus provide a possible anatomical explanation for the epidemiologically observed protective effect of male circumcision against HIV and other sexually transmitted infections (STIs).

An increased level of ELCs in the prepuce may be the result of continuous stimulation of bacteria found in the periurethral area, and expressions of CD4 and CD8 in the prepuce and normal skin may help the colonization of uropathic bacteria under the foreskin [18].

Immune inactivation of the ELCs render the mammal in a perilous and vulnerable state. The removal of the prepuce leads to the permanent loss of 673,547 ELCs in the outer layer and 30,968 cells in the inner layer, with a total loss of 704,515 ELCs (The tissue loss from circumcision was calculated using the formula of Ritter and Denniston) [19].

References

1. Barreto J, Caballero C, Cubilla A. Penis. In: Sternberg SS, editor. Histology for pathologists. 2nd ed. New York: Raven Press; 1997. p. 1043–4.
2. Gould VE, Moll R, Moll I, et al. Neuroendocrine (Merkel) cells of the skin: hyperplasia, dysplasia, and neoplasms. Lab Invest. 1985;52:334–53.
3. Parkash S, Jeyakumar K, Subramanya K, Chaudhuri S. Human subpreputial collection: its nature and formation. J Urol. 1973;110(2):211–2.
4. Batistatou A, Panelos J, Zioga A, Charalabopoulos KA. Ectopic modified sebaceous glands in human penis. Int J Surg Pathol. 2006;14(4):355–6. https://doi.org/10.1177/1066896906291779.
5. Dickinson RL. Human sex anatomy: a topographical hand atlas, vol. 82. Baltimore: Williams & Wilkins; 1949.
6. Barreto J, Caballero C, Cubilla A. Penis. In: Sternberg S, editor. Histology for pathologists. New York: Raven Press; 1992. p. 725.
7. Winkelmann RK. The cutaneous innervation of human newborn prepuce. J Investig Dermatol. 1956;26(1):53–67.
8. Jefferson G. The peripenic muscle: some observations on the anatomy of phimosis. Surg Gynecol Obstetr. 1916;23:177–81.
9. Van Howe RS. Coste Cective: treatment of phimosis. Pediatrics. 1998;102:E43.
10. Dogiel AS. Die nervenendigunngen in der schleimhaut der aussen genitalorgane des menschen. Arch F Mikr Anat. 1893;41:585–612.
11. Taylor JR, Lockwood AP, Taylor AJ. The prepuce: specialized mucosa of the penis and its loss to circumcision. Br J Urol. 1996;77:291–5.
12. Tuncali D, Bingul F, Talim B, et al. Histologic characteristics of the human prepuce pertaining to its clinical behaviour as a dual graft. Ann Plast Surg. 2005;54(2):191–5. https://doi.org/10.1097/01.sap.0000141939.42990.70.
13. Fleiss P, Hodges F, Van Howe RS. Immunological functions of the human prepuce. Sex Transm Infect. 1998;74(5):364–7. http://www.cirp.org/library/disease/STD/fleiss3/
14. Weiss GN, Sanders SM, Westbrook KC. The distribution and density of langerhans cells in the human prepuce: site of a diminished immune response? Isr J Med Sci. 1993;29:42–3.
15. de Witte L, Nabatov A, Pion M, et al. Langerin is a natural barrier to HIV-1 transmission by Langerhans cells. Nat Med. 2007;13:367–71. Abstract available at http://www.nature.com/nm/journal/v13/n3/abs/nm1541.html
16. Parkash S, Raghuram R, Venkatesan K, et al. Subpreputial wetness—its nature. Ann Nat Med Sci. 1982;18:109–12.
17. Anderson D, Politch JA, Pudney J. HIV infection and immune defence of the penis. Am J Reprod Immunol. 2011;65:220–9.
18. Ganor Y, Bomsel M. HIV-1 transmission in the male genital tract. Am J Reprod Immunol. 2011;65:284–91.
19. Ritter RJ, Denniston GC. Say no to circumcision. 2nd ed. Aptos: Hourglass Book Publishing; 1996.

7 Functions of the Prepuce

Human prepuce is a highly specialized junctional mucocutaneous tissue which plays an integral part in the global aspect of external male genitalia and has many underestimated features [1].

Principal functions associated with the prepuce could be considered (1) protective, (2) immunological, (3) erogenous, (4) mechanical.

Particularly, the prepuce comprises:

- A double layer of epithelium which covers the glans and the urinary meatus, safeguarding them from abrasion and friction and contributing to its protective function (see Chap. 5);
- Specialized immune cells, thousands of lymphatic vessels and exocrine glands secreting lytic material, contributing to its immunological function (see Chap. 6);
- The frenulum, where most of the erotogenic nerves end on the penis and thousands of coiled fine-touch receptors and pheromone producing apocrine glands, contributing to its erogenous function (see Chap. 6);
- Approximately half of the smooth muscle sheath of the penis, called the dartos fascia, which elongates and accommodates the entire penis during erection, contributing to its mechanical function [2] (see Chap. 5).

Understanding the global functions of male prepuce can throw new light on the ongoing circumcision debate, with proponents supporting it for health issues and opponents arguing about its detrimental outcomes.

With approximately one third of the world's male population being circumcised for non-therapeutic reasons, in fact, prophylactic circumcision is perhaps the world's most commonly performed, and debated, paediatric surgical procedure.

Albeit the ancient roots of male circumcision and its worldwide spread over centuries, the persistence of prepuce in primates for at least 65 million years raises questions about whether it is only a vestigial tissue devoid of function (see Chap. 2).

Protective Function

The more intuitive function of the foreskin is to protect the glans and the urinary meatus from abrasion and drying, decreasing external irritation and keeping it protected from contamination by dirt (see Chap. 9).

This primary task is ascribed to the peripenic muscle, a layer of smooth muscle cells intertwined with elastic fibres, direct prolongation of the scrotal dartos within the prepuce (see Chap. 6).

In the first months of life, the sphincter action of these muscle fibres causes the distal prepuce to pucker and close like a one-way valve, preventing the entry of contaminants while allowing the passage of urine [2].

During the stage when the baby is incontinent the prepuce completely covers the glans to protect it and to avoid permanent contact with

M. A. B. Fahmy, *Normal and Abnormal Prepuce*, https://doi.org/10.1007/978-3-030-37621-5_7

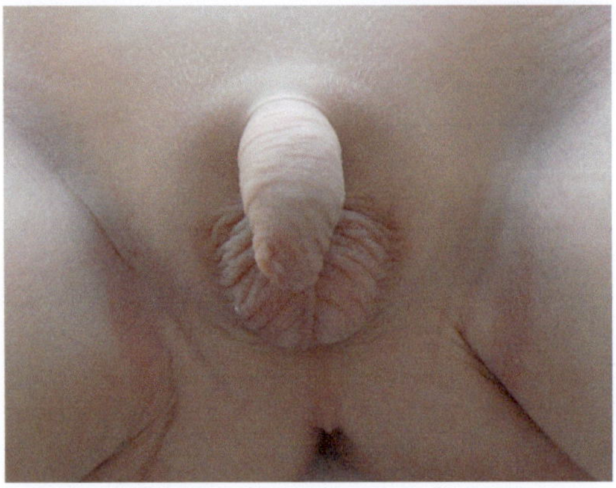

Fig. 7.1 Normal prepuce in a 2 years old boy

ammonia and other irritants contained in the urine (Fig. 7.1).

The loss of this protective layer exposes the glans and the urinary meatus to direct friction and abrasion. Consequently, the glans mucosa keratinizes abnormally and the chronically irritated urinary meatus can lose its elliptical shape into a rounded one.

Several observational studies, systematic reviews and meta-analyses, in fact, have demonstrated higher prevalence of meatal stenosis in the circumcised male, underlining the importance of the male prepuce in protecting the external urethral orifice against continuous trauma [3, 4].

These results are not clinically meaningless since even asymptomatic meatal stenosis may lead to potentially serious obstructive urological conditions in a significant percentage of cases.

Urinary stream deflection, pain at the initiation of micturition, dysuria, haematuria, urinary frequency, enuresis and incontinence are the most common symptoms of meatal stenosis, the occurrence of which is, mostly, prevented by male prepuce.

Immunological Function

Both the mucosa of the inner plate and the squamous epithelium of the outer plate of the human prepuce, containing Langerhans cells, contribute to its immunological function [5] (see Chap. 6).

These cells play an essential role in the cutaneous mucosal immune system as they are the first line of the body's immune defence system. They help the body to recognise and process antigens, directing them to lymphocytes and macrophages, through thousands of lymphatic vessels contained within the prepuce layers.

In addition, the preputial sac is colonized by benign commensal organisms, such as Corynebacterium, Gram-negative anaerobes (especially Bacteroides melaninogenicus), Enterococci, Enterobacteria, coagulase-positive Staphylococci, mycobacterial contaminants from soil and water (such as *M. gordonae*) and *M. smegmatis*, their relative composition being age dependent [2]. Whether the biodiversity of subpreputial flora contributes to prevent infections is still not fully proven.

The preputial cavity also contains desquamated squamous epithelial cells and a white creamy material produced by the ectopic sebaceous glands concentrated near the frenulum called smegma praeputii. The smegma praeputii comprise squalene, beta-cholestanol, sterols and long-chain fatty acids, which may exert protective function, as elsewhere on the skin [2].

The apocrine glands concentrated in the inner layer secrete cathepsin B, lysozyme, chymotrypsin, neutrophil elastase and cytokine, that have the function to destroy bacterial cell walls [5].

Although, after circumcision, all these immunoprotective structures are irreversibly lost and the unprotected glans is constantly exposed to dirt, several studies reported a lower incidence of Urinary Tract Infections (UTIs) [6] and Sexually Transmitted Infections (STIs) [7–13] in circumcised men.

In a systematic review and meta-analysis, Singh-Grewal et al. [6] proved that the benefit of circumcision in preventing UTIs outweighed its surgical risk but only in children with recurrent infections or with high grade vesicoureteric reflux. However, the authors admitted that observational studies of variable quality dominated the meta-analysis while the only randomised controlled trial had a small sample size and failed to achieve independent statistical significance.

Regarding STIs, three African randomised controlled trials reported a reduction in the risk of heterosexual Human Immunodeficiency Virus (HIV) transmission after circumcision in high-risk developing countries with a low baseline circumcision rate [7–9].

Similarly, other randomized controlled trials found that adult circumcision decreases the incidence of Herpes Simplex Virus type-2 (HSV-2) infection and the prevalence of Human Papilloma Virus (HPV) infection [11, 13], well-known risk factors for penile and cervical cancer.

A lower incidence of genital ulceration, Trichomonas and bacterial vaginosis in female partners of circumcised men was also reported by randomized controlled trials performed in Uganda [12].

An hypothesis to explain why male circumcision could reduce the risk of STIs is to consider that removing the foreskin decreases the surface area of the penile skin particularly rich in Langerhans' cells, dendritic cells, CD4+ T cells and macrophages, all possible targets of viral and bacterial infection [7–9]. To validate this hypothesis a randomized trial looked at the incidence of HIV in relation to foreskin surface area. The study, published by Kigozi et al. [14], reported that the risk of male HIV acquisition was increased among Ugandan men with larger foreskin surface areas.

Another possible biological mechanism by which the presence of the prepuce could lead to a greater risk of infection may include poor hygiene [8] and a longer interaction between the vaginal fluids and the wet subpreputial cavity, which could provide a favourable environment for pathogens survival and replication [15].

Furthermore, uncircumcised men may be at increased risk of STIs as the result of pathogens entry through the lightly keratinised and highly vascularized inner mucosa of the prepuce, particularly at the frenulum. Micro-abrasions of the foreskin and frenulum, occurring during intercourse, may also increase its vulnerability to infection [15, 16].

Although the results of these studies were scientifically valid, they are appropriate in the context of developing countries while their extrapolation to other populations and societies has not been confirmed [17, 18].

Erogenous Function

Sexual arousal relies on anatomical, neural, psychological, hormonal and genetic factors but it is also highly influenced by the cultural environment.

Although it is well-known that erogenous penile sensation is based on sophisticated somatosensory information coming from the glans and the male urethra, the relative function of the prepuce is still widely debated.

Anatomical studies demonstrated that the somatosensory innervation of the prepuce is provided by the dorsal penile nerve and branches of the perineal nerve (including the posterior scrotal nerves), while its autonomic innervation is from the pelvic plexus (the parasympathetic fibres arise from the sacral centre and the sympathetic fibres arise from the thoracolumbar centre) [2] (see Chap. 5).

Histological studies showed that the prepuce has more spreading nerve networks than the rest of the penile skin, in particular, the presence of various sensory receptor types, resembling typical Pacinian and Meissner corpuscles has been proven [19] (see Chap. 6).

The highest concentration of Meissner's corpuscles, which are non-capsulated mechanoreceptors involved in fine-touch sensitivity is found at the ridged band at the mucocutaneous junction, merging smoothly with the frenulum [19].

This dense concentration of sensory corpuscles, which are also sensitive to motion, touch, temperature and erogenous stimulation, highly contrasts with the protopathic sensibility of the glans [20]. This is composed of free nerves responsible only to deep pressure and pain.

However, for normal copulatory behaviour, the corpuscular receptor-rich ridged band of the male prepuce should interact with the protopathic sensitivity of the corpuscular receptor-deficient glans.

Taylor et al. hypothesized that the stretching of the peripenic muscle fibers of the prepuce during coitus activates Meissner's corpuscle endings, triggering the penilo-cavernosus reflex responsible for deep erogenous sensation and ejaculation [21].

This observation was confirmed by Podnar, who found more difficult to clinically elicit the penilo-cavernosus reflex in circumcised men [22].

A more recent neurophysiological study performed by Senol et al. also showed that both mean pudendal evoked potential (PEP) and ejaculatory latency times became significantly longer after circumcision [23].

These results were validated by Senkul et al. in a prospective clinical trial including 42 patients who experienced a significantly increased mean ejaculatory latency time after circumcision [24].

Understanding the correlation between the sensory receptors located in the foreskin and the overall penile sensitivity could be useful to better understand the impact of a circumcision in sexual performance and satisfaction.

Unfortunately, however, only few published studies have thoroughly investigated the effects of circumcision on penile sensitivity and the reported results are contradictory.

Long-term implications on adult sensation and sexual pleasure following circumcision, therefore, still remain controversial.

Masters and Johnson's pioneering work on sexual physiology failed to identify any difference in sensitivity of the ventral and dorsal surfaces of the glans between 35 circumcised and 35 uncircumcised men, while other studies report different (sometimes opposite) outcomes [25].

Sorrells et al. in an objective quantitative study provided the first extensive map of the fine-touch static pressure thresholds of the penis [26]. They found that the most sensitive location on the circumcised penis corresponded to the ventral scar of the glans and, interestingly, that the five most sensitive locations on the uncircumcised penis were all more sensitive than the analogue sites on the circumcised penis.

Bronselaer et al. proved that the stimulation of the foreskin elicited sexual pleasure in uncircumcised men and that the glans sensitivity was significantly reduced in circumcised individuals [27].

Studies have also demonstrated that, as a consequence of the loss of preputial primary sensory endings associated with the desensitization of the sensory nerve receptors of the glans and the keratinization of the exposed glans epithelium, circumcised penises require a more vigorous and prolonged stimuli to trigger orgasm [27].

In another study that compared penile sensitivity in men who had been circumcised in the neonatal period with uncircumcised ones, it was found that the foreskin was, amongst the genital sites tested, the most sensitive to tactile sensation and more sensitive to warmth detection than the glans [28]. In the same study, however, authors failed to find any significant difference in overall penile sensitivity for punctate tactile and pain thresholds or for warmth detection and heat pain thresholds.

Their findings suggested that, although neonatal circumcision seems not to be associated with impaired sexual functioning or decreased penile sensitivity in adulthood, some minimal long-term implications to penile sensitivity could be expected.

In order to explore how sexual arousal affected sensation, Payne et al. compared penile touch and pain sensations between uncircumcised and circumcised men [29]. They found that, although no difference in genital sensation was reported, participants in the uncircumcised group had lower baseline penile temperature and a greater increase in penile temperature after arousal.

The real effects of circumcision on penile sensitivity, however, remains debated due to a number of methodologically questionable reports and controversial results.

In their systematic reviews, Cox et al. failed to correlate the histological features of the prepuce with penile sexual sensation [30] while Morris at al stated that the absence of the prepuce does not affect sexual function, sensitivity and satisfaction [4].

A meta-analysis published by Tian et al. did not find any correlation between circumcision and impaired sexual function and sensitivity; however, the authors admitted that the quality of the reviewed literature was very low with great heterogeneity across the various studies [31].

A robust analysis of a national health survey in Denmark of more than 5000 people (2573 men and 2979 women), showed that circumcision was three times more likely associated with orgasm difficulties in men and with a wide range of women's sexual function impairment, notably orgasm difficulties, frequent episodes of dyspareunia and a sense of incomplete sexual needs fulfilment [32].

Moreover, an article published in 2007 by Solinis et al. reported that 35% of men and 46% of female partners experienced a worsened sex life after circumcision [33].

To provide more evidence of the effects of circumcision on male sexual function, however, further research, including high-quality study designs, randomized controlled trials and physiological tests performed in a standardized setting, is required.

Mechanical Function

The double layers of the prepuce provide the necessary tissue to cover the penis also during erection and allows the underlying corpora cavernosa and corpus spongiosum to glide easily over the glans during intercourse [2].

The dartos layer is exclusive to the external male genitalia and consists of smooth muscle cells intertwined with elastic fibres which, from the apex of the prepuce, continue to the scrotum (Fig. 7.2).

Interestingly, the vast majority of the penile dartos muscle is contained within the prepuce (see Chap. 6). It is temperature-sensitive and its texture allows for the volume changes required for erection. This is demonstrated by the fact that the organization pattern and the relative ratio of its elastic fibres change with puberty: in adulthood, in fact, an increase is required to achieve an uncomplicated eversion of the glans during erection.

Another function of the prepuce is to facilitate the penetration and the smooth movements between the glans and the vaginal mucosa during intercourse. Indeed, the prepuce allows the glans to move into the vaginal cavity without friction as the foreskin unfolds inside its own self-lubricating layers.

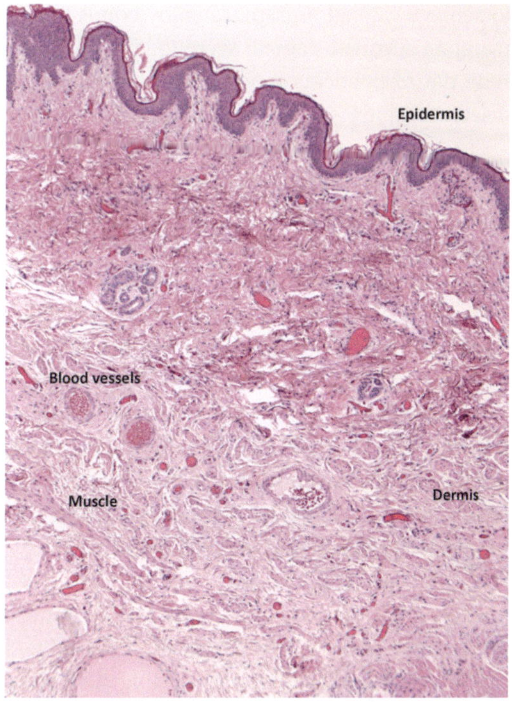

Fig. 7.2 Histology of a normal foreskin. We can recognize two layers (epidermis and dermis) with presence of blood vessels and muscle

In an experimental study, Taves et al. proved that an unretracted foreskin reduces the force required to penetrate by tenfold [34].

In addition, the foreskin helps to maintain the sub-preputial space in a wet status, thanks to the accumulation of prostatic, vesicular and urethral secretions produced by the urethral glands of Littré [2]. This natural emollient protects and lubricates the glans and the inner layer of the prepuce, contributing to and facilitating erection, glans eversion and an atraumatic vaginal intercourse.

Conversely, the skin of a circumcised penis rubs into the vaginal cavity with increased friction and attrition, leading to an unnatural dryness and possible painful coitus for female partners [27].

Confirming the above findings a large survey that included 139 women who had sexual experience with both circumcised and uncircumcised partners, reported that sex with circumcised partners was associated with reduced woman's ability to achieve vaginal orgasm, to enjoy coitus and to maintain adequate vaginal secretions; at the same time the respondents reported increased vaginal discomfort [35].

To reinforce the contentious attitude towards the foreskin and its function, in parallel with the growing popular custom of practising circumcision, historically, there has also been a demand for restoring the foreskin.

Initially, this was not for health or sexual reasons, but rather, for fear of religious persecution. This practice has been well described and analysed by Dr. Dirk Schultheiss, a German urologist who in 1998 published an article in which, among other findings, he reported that the first evidence of demand for restoration of the prepuce after circumcision is mentioned in the Bible [36].

In the last few decades, instead, there has been a growing movements against circumcision as many people who, for sexual reasons and emotional distress caused by feeling they were victims of genital mutilation, has led them to request a foreskin restoration in order to achieve emotional wholeness, and improve their satisfaction [37].

References

1. Gairdner D. The fate of the foreskin, a study of circumcision. Br Med J. 1949;2(4642):1433–7, illust.
2. Cold CJ, Taylor JR. The prepuce. BJU Int. 1999;83(Suppl 1):34–44.
3. Frisch M, Simonsen J. Cultural background, non-therapeutic circumcision and the risk of meatal stenosis and other urethral stricture disease: two nationwide register-based cohort studies in Denmark 1977-2013. Surgeon. 2018;16(2):107–18.
4. Morris BJ, Krieger JN. Does circumcision increase meatal stenosis risk?-A systematic review and meta-analysis. Urology. 2017;110:16–26.
5. Fleiss PM, Hodges FM, Van Howe RS. Immunological functions of the human prepuce. Sex Transm Infect. 1998;74(5):364–7.
6. Singh-Grewal D, Macdessi J, Craig J. Circumcision for the prevention of urinary tract infection in boys: a systematic review of randomised trials and observational studies. Arch Dis Child. 2005;90(8):853–8.
7. Gray RH, Kigozi G, Serwadda D, Makumbi F, Watya S, Nalugoda F, et al. Male circumcision for HIV prevention in men in Rakai, Uganda: a randomised trial. Lancet. 2007;369(9562):657–66.
8. Bailey RC, Moses S, Parker CB, Agot K, Maclean I, Krieger JN, et al. Male circumcision for HIV prevention in young men in Kisumu, Kenya: a randomised controlled trial. Lancet. 2007;369(9562):643–56.
9. Auvert B, Taljaard D, Lagarde E, Sobngwi-Tambekou J, Sitta R, Puren A. Randomized, controlled intervention trial of male circumcision for reduction of HIV infection risk: the ANRS 1265 trial. PLoS Med. 2005;2(11):e298.
10. Weiss HA, Thomas SL, Munabi SK, Hayes RJ. Male circumcision and risk of syphilis, chancroid, and genital herpes: a systematic review and meta-analysis. Sex Transm Infect. 2006;82(2):101–9; discussion 10.
11. Tobian AA, Serwadda D, Quinn TC, Kigozi G, Gravitt PE, Laeyendecker O, et al. Male circumcision for the prevention of HSV-2 and HPV infections and syphilis. N Engl J Med. 2009;360(13):1298–309.
12. Gray RH, Kigozi G, Serwadda D, Makumbi F, Nalugoda F, Watya S, et al. The effects of male circumcision on female partners' genital tract symptoms and vaginal infections in a randomized trial in Rakai, Uganda. Am J Obstet Gynecol. 2009;200(1):42.e1–7.
13. Auvert B, Sobngwi-Tambekou J, Cutler E, Nieuwoudt M, Lissouba P, Puren A, et al. Effect of male circumcision on the prevalence of high-risk human papillomavirus in young men: results of a randomized controlled trial conducted in Orange Farm, South Africa. J Infect Dis. 2009;199(1):14–9.
14. Kigozi G, Wawer M, Ssettuba A, Kagaayi J, Nalugoda F, Watya S, et al. Foreskin surface area and HIV acquisition in Rakai, Uganda (size matters). AIDS. 2009;23(16):2209–13.
15. Szabo R, Short RV. How does male circumcision protect against HIV infection? BMJ. 2000;320(7249):1592–4.
16. Bailey RC, Plummer FA, Moses S. Male circumcision and HIV prevention: current knowledge and future research directions. Lancet Infect Dis. 2001;1(4):223–31.
17. Frisch M, Earp BD. Circumcision of male infants and children as a public health measure in developed countries: a critical assessment of recent evidence. Glob Public Health. 2018;13(5):626–41.
18. Mazor J. The child's interests and the case for the permissibility of male infant circumcision. J Med Ethics. 2013;39:421–8.
19. Martín-Alguacil N, Cooper RS, Aardsma N, Mayoglou L, Pfaff D, Schober J. Terminal innervation of the male genitalia, cutaneous sensory receptors of the male foreskin. Clin Anat. 2015;28(3):385–91.
20. Halata Z, Munger BL. The neuroanatomical basis for the protopathic sensibility of the human glans penis. Brain Res. 1986;371(2):205–30.
21. Taylor JR, Lockwood AP, Taylor AJ. The prepuce: specialized mucosa of the penis and its loss to circumcision. Br J Urol. 1996;77(2):291–5.
22. Podnar S. RE: clinical elicitation of the penilo-cavernosus reflex in circumcised men. BJU Int. 2012;110(5):E161.

23. Senol MG, Sen B, Karademir K, Sen H, Saraçoğlu M. The effect of male circumcision on pudendal evoked potentials and sexual satisfaction. Acta Neurol Belg. 2008;108(3):90–3.
24. Şenkul T, İşerİ C, Karademİr K, Saraçoğlu F, Erden D. Circumcision in adults: effect on sexual function. Urology. 2004;63(1):155–8.
25. Master MD, Johnson VE. Human sexual response. Boston: Little Brown; 1966.
26. Sorrells ML, Snyder JL, Reiss MD, Eden C, Milos MF, Wilcox N, et al. Fine-touch pressure thresholds in the adult penis. BJU Int. 2007;99(4):864–9.
27. Bronselaer GA, Schober JM, Meyer-Bahlburg HF, T'Sjoen G, Vlietinck R, Hoebeke PB. Male circumcision decreases penile sensitivity as measured in a large cohort. BJU Int. 2013;111(5):820–7.
28. Bossio JA, Pukall CF, Steele SS. Examining penile sensitivity in neonatally circumcised and intact men using quantitative sensory testing. J Urol. 2016;195(6):1848–53.
29. Payne K, Thaler L, Kukkonen T, Carrier S, Binik Y. Sensation and sexual arousal in circumcised and uncircumcised men. J Sex Med. 2007;4(3):667–74.
30. Cox G, Krieger JN, Morris BJ. Histological correlates of penile sexual sensation: does circumcision make a difference? Sex Med. 2015;3(2):76–85.
31. Tian Y, Liu W, Wang JZ, Wazir R, Yue X, Wang KJ. Effects of circumcision on male sexual functions: a systematic review and meta-analysis. Asian J Androl. 2013;15(5):662–6.
32. Frisch M, Lindholm M, Grønbæk M. Male circumcision and sexual function in men and women: a survey-based, cross-sectional study in Denmark. Int J Epidemiol. 2011;40(5):1367–81.
33. Solinis I, Yiannaki A. Does circumcision improve couple's sex life? J Mens Health Gend. 2007;4(3):361.
34. Taves D. The intromission function of the foreskin. Med Hypotheses. 2002;59(2):180–2.
35. O'Hara K, O'Hara J. The effect of male circumcision on the sexual enjoyment of the female partner. BJU Int. 1999;83(Suppl 1):79–84.
36. Schultheiss D, Truss MC, Stief CG, Jonas U. Uncircumcision: a historical review of preputial restoration. Plast Reconstr Surg. 1998;101(7):1990–8.
37. Collier R. Whole again: the practice of foreskin restoration. CMAJ. 2011;183(18):2092–3.

Medical and Surgical Uses of the Prepuce

8

Aside from a number of functions described previously, an intact prepuce can be extremely useful for both medical and surgical purposes.

The main field where the foreskin is used is for reconstructive surgery in patients affected by hypospadias [1], but it can also be used as a source of cutaneous grafts or flaps, for example for creation of a neo-scrotum in case of congenital scrotal agenesis [2], for burn wound coverage [3], scar contractures [4, 5], eye reconstruction [6, 7], syndactyly repair [8, 9], reconstruction of foot injuries [10] anal repair [11, 12].

In addition, more recently, the prepuce has been considered as a potential source of immunotherapeutic Mesenchymal Stromal Cells (MSCs) [13, 14] and human Dermis-Isolated Adult Stem cells (hDIAS) [15]. Moreover, fibroblasts obtained from the foreskin have been used to generate induced Pluripotent Stem Cell line (hiPSCs) [16].

Foreskin for Hypospadias Repair

Hypospadias is the second most common congenital anomaly of male genitalia with an incidence of one in 300 male births [1]. It is due to an arrest of the normal development of the penile structures occurring during embryogenesis, which leads to a triad of defects, including proximal displacement of the urethral opening, ventral penile curvature and deficient hooded foreskin [1].

Although several classifications have been proposed, the position of the native urethral meatus remains the most commonly preferred criterion to judge the severity. According to this, roughly 70% of hypospadias is either glanular or distal penile, 10% is mid-penile and 20% is proximal [1]. In regard to the surgical repair, it is also important to consider the presence and the degree of any penile curvature, the development of the groove of the urethral plate and the global appearance of the glans.

The aim of the surgical repair is to obtain a good functional and cosmetic reconstruction with the lowest complication rate. In particular, the reconstruction should achieve the creation of a straight penis, an adequate urethral calibre and a natural-shaped meatus located at the apex of the glans.

In the majority of patients, a single procedure is sufficient but in the most severe cases or when a re-do operation is required a two-stage approach is preferred.

The one-stage repair is performed in distal cases when the urethral plate is adequate in width and depth to be safely tubularized.

In some patients however, if the urethral plate is not adequate in width and depth to be directly tubularized, it could be either released by a midline deep dorsal incision [17] or

M. A. B. Fahmy, *Normal and Abnormal Prepuce*, https://doi.org/10.1007/978-3-030-37621-5_8

augmented through an "inlay graft" [18] or an "onlay flap" [19].

Instead, the two-stage repair is the most reliable solution in those cases in which the severity of the hypospadias and/or the associated penile curvature require the transection of the urethral plate and a urethral plate substitution [1].

The Tubularized Incised Plate (TIP) urethroplasty procedure has become increasingly popular in the last few years due to its simplicity and its favourable cosmetic and functional outcomes and it now represents for the majority of surgeons the gold standard technique for less severe type of hypospadias. However, if the urethral plate is narrow and inelastic, a dorsal releasing incision may not be enough to guarantee a safe tubularization and a urethral plate augmentation is recommended. In this case, a vascularized flap or a free graft are used to widen the existing urethral plate: flaps are obtained from tissues moved from the proximity of the penis via vascularized pedicles, or free grafts are harvested from more distant sites [20]. The inner preputial layer is the preferred source while parameatal tissues, the tunica vaginalis or the scrotal skin have been used as alternative vascularized flaps [20]. As popularized by Duckett [19], the onlay preputial island flap involves the anterior rotation of the inner foreskin and its ventral displacement to form the roof of the neourethra. The preputial vascular peduncle is preserved and the neourethra is covered interposing a dartos fascia between the urethra and the skin. This solution has the advantage of preserving the native urethral plate and relying on a proper vascular pedicle.

More recently, a "Snodgraft repair" has been proposed as an alternative technique for urethral plate augmentation [18]. As the traditional TIP procedure, which has been proposed and popularised by Snodgrass, it involves a midline incision of the urethral plate. However, in this technique, the dorsal defect is covered by a free graft quilted into the urethral plate to promote an effective re-epithelialization and to prevent scar formations (Fig. 8.1).

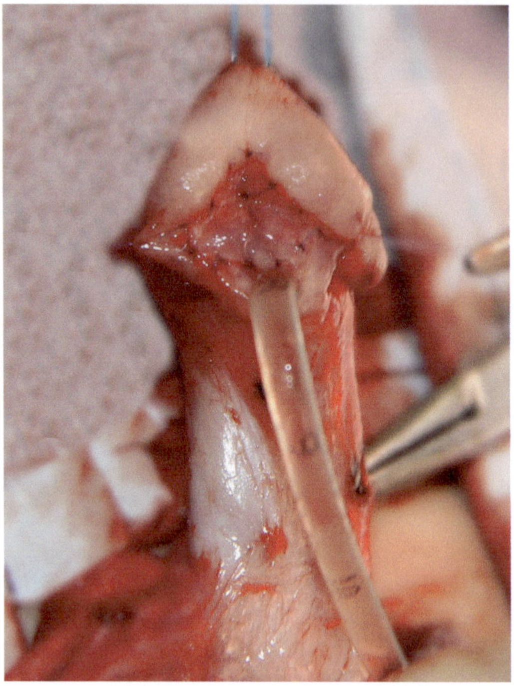

Fig. 8.1 "Snodgraft repair" with the insertion of a foreskin graft for urethral plate augmentation

The donor site for free grafts is usually the internal prepuce layer or, less commonly, the buccal mucosa. Although they share many advantages, such as anti-infection properties, a high vascularisation and a long survival rates, the inner prepuce layer has the unique advantage of being directly accessible without adding any risk of donor site morbidity. Shuzhu et al. [21] have shown that, compared to the TIP, the inlay buccal mucosa graft and the inlay internal preputial graft are both reliable techniques in terms of surgical outcomes. Long-term follow up studies have confirmed that the neourethra created from free preputial grafts or vascularized preputial flaps grows well, while few data are available regarding the long-term outcome of tissues with less androgen-sensitivity, such as buccal mucosa.

In the case of proximal hypospadias associated with severe ventral curvature, the transection of urethral plate is necessary in order to release the significant ventral chordees. In these cases, a substitution urethroplasty becomes necessary [22].

During the initial first-stage surgery the aim is to create a new and adequate urethral plate: the existing narrow and poorly developed plate is excised, the glans is clefted, the chordee are

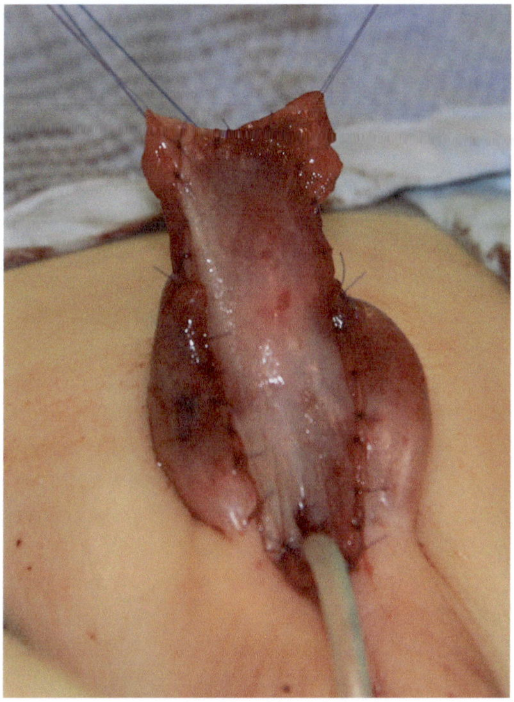

Fig. 8.2 First-stage surgery for the correction of proximal hypospadias. The urethral plate is substituted with a graft from the inner layer of the prepuce

released and the resulting defect is covered with a graft which is usually taken from the inner layer of the prepuce (Fig. 8.2).

During the second stage (performed about 6–9 months later) the new urethral plate is tubularized to form the neourethra.

Besides its use as a flap (in the onlay island procedure) or as a free graft (in a single or two stage repair), a different use of the foreskin has been described in techniques that create a preputial tubularized island flap [23].

Where there are postoperative complications, the steps of salvage surgeries are similar to those previously described for the primary repair, however, the challenge is the presence of scarred, less vascular and deficient tissues. In those cases, dorsal inlay grafts are generally preferred to the island onlay flaps because the ventral tissues are usually less vascularized and offer a loose mechanical support for the flaps, which are therefore more prone to further complications (such as fistula formation or abnormal urethral dilatations) [20].

During primary hypospadias surgery, the foreskin can also be reconstructed; since foreskin reconstruction at the time of the single-stage hypospadias repair does not increase the number of complications nor the need for reoperation in the long-term follow-up [24], in some cases a planned surgical strategy could include foreskin preservation and reconstruction not only to provide a normal cosmetic aspect of the penis but also to maintain a precious potential graft donor in the event of postoperative complications.

Foreskin as Skin Graft and Flap

The prepuce could be used as an autologous source of full-thickness skin graft and flap.

Wound management depends on the underlying cause and the scale, the extension and the position of the primary lesion. Although superficial tissue losses affecting small areas could be simply treated by debridement, application of topical antibiotics and proper wound dressing, deeper wounds affecting larger areas may need a more aggressive approach.

In these more severe cases, skin grafts may be required to cover the tissue defect. Cutaneous grafts are useful to protect denuded areas from further traumas, to prevent infections and to shorten the healing time, by the so-called 'healing by tertiary intention'. In addition, skin grafts can be used successfully to prevent or to treat scar contractures—possible causes of movement limitation of the affected area. When a fasciotomy is required, skin grafts can also be used to cover the tissue defect produced by the surgical procedure performed to release the tension occurring after a severe soft tissue contusion of the extremities.

Several body sites may be used as a source of skin autografts, such as the buttock, the anterior side of the thighs, the groin, the cubital or the post-auricular area. However, in these cases, hypo-pigmented areas or scars in the donor sites inevitably develop.

Since 1937 the prepuce has been described as a widely available full-thickness skin graft to cover denuded areas in boys [25]. Several advantages of skin grafting using the foreskin have been reported. First of all, the donor site is hidden, the loss of tissue is minimal and the circumcised penis is considered as a normal variant rather than an abnormality. Moreover, compared to other body sites, the penis has less tendency to form keloid or hypertrophic scars. Histopathological studies have revealed that the prepuce inner mucosa has a considerable vascular supply (see Chap. 5) and epithelial proprieties like those of the mouth, vaginal and esophageal mucosa [4]. In particular, its keratinocytes have a high division capacity leading to heal wounds in a very short time. In addition, using the prepuce, has resulted in fewer secondary graft contractures and more elastic and pliable tissues have been achieved. This is particularly important for areas exposed to frequent movements, such as joints. The absence of hair follicles and a large graft size are two other important pros of the foreskin, which can be harvested in a simple surgical procedure with low morbidity and with almost no need for donor site care. However, its availability is limited to the male population and a slight hyperpigmentation in the recipient area is usually noted, which restricts its usage in the face and neck area.

Once the surgical indication of skin grafting using the foreskin is established, the recipient area is measured, the prepuce size is evaluated and the circumcision is performed. The foreskin is then unfolded so that the two layers become a larger piece for grafting. It is worth noting that, thanks to its natural elasticity, about 20% more than the actual measured foreskin could be obtained removing the subcutaneous tissue from the skin. Moreover, when the donor size is not sufficient to cover the affected area, meshing or multiple relaxing incisions can be made to enlarge the donor graft.

In their study, Chittmittrapap et al. [26] reported good surgical outcomes of 42 boys (aged from 2 to 14 years) undergoing full thickness autografting using their own prepuce to cover different types of skin lesions or congenital defects. In particular, 11 patients were treated for scar contractures, eight for syndactyly and for skin necrosis, six for traumatic skin loss of the extremities, three required grafting of the defect after fasciotomy, three had burn granulated wounds, while three others had a large granulated tissue area where grafting was used to shorten the healing time. They reported that more than 90% of the grafts had taken after 7 days.

In several other conditions, the prepuce has been used as a good autologous full-thickness skin graft with very low tendency to contract and a good recipient adaptation.

D'Alessio et al. [27] reported the use of the foreskin to cover a large cutaneous defect made by the surgical excision of a congenital nevus occupying the plantar surface of the foot of a 4-year-old boy. Izzuddin et al. [28] used the preputial skin as a full-thickness skin graft to cover an 18-month-old boy's cutaneous defect produced by the excision of a verrucous hemangioma of the thumb.

Zaroo et al. [29] reported the use of prepuce for post-burn contractures of digits in 12 children.

Scar and contracture formations are common sequelae of severe burns, which can lead to important limitation of the range of movement, especially around joints. Further reconstructive surgeries are therefore required to release the contractures and to restore the complete range of motion.

No graft loss was reported with wounds that had healed within 2 weeks without complications.

The foreskin has been used as a free skin graft for a number of other indications, including excision of large melanoma (Fig. 8.3), eyelid reconstruction [6], replacement of conjunctiva [7], correction of ectropion [7], creation of an anal canal [11, 12], reconstruction of extravasation injury to the foot [10], syndactyly repair [8, 9] and to resurface the first web space of a child with a burn to the palmar aspect of his hand [30].

In addition, a well-vascularized preputial flap provided an excellent source of tissue for creation of a neo-scrotum in the series of three congenital scrotal agenesis reported by Benson et al. [2]. The prepuce was harvested on a pedicle of dartos and rotated to the perineum to create a neo-scrotal pouch. No complications were

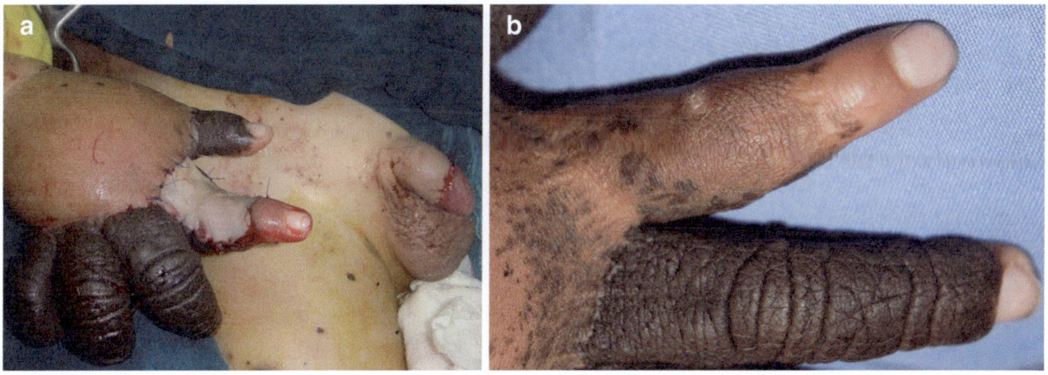

Fig. 8.3 A case of the use of foreskin as skin graft for a large melanoma. (**a**) At the time of procedure (**b**) 5 years follow up (kindly provided by Prof M. Fahmy)

reported and both testes were accommodated in a capacious scrotal sac 12–14 weeks after the initial procedure.

Immunotherapeutic and Tissue Engineering Potential of Foreskin-Derived Regenerative Cells

The foreskin is considered a reservoir of regenerative cells with therapeutically relevant functions.

In particular, it is a stable source of immunotherapeutic Mesenchymal Stromal Cells (MSCs) [14].

Originally isolated from the bone marrow, MSCs are multipotent fibroblast-like cells that have been more recently identified in many other tissues, including the adipose tissue and Wharton's jelly of the umbilical cord [14]. MSCs display well-characterized properties related to their multi-lineage differentiation potential and their ability to support haematopoiesis and to modulate the immune response.

Such properties make them ideal candidates for use in tissue engineering and in cellular immunotherapies.

Although the MSCs, isolated from the prepuce, demonstrate inconsistent stemness, they have high clonogenic and proliferative capacities. They exhibit a tri-lineage potential and can differentiate into adipogenic, osteogenic and chondrogenic cells [31]. This multi-lineage differentiation potential represents an attractive quality for several therapeutic applications in the field of regenerative medicine. For example, skin-derived MSCs have been used to promote innovative bone tissue renewal [14].

In addition, neonatal prepuce harbours skin stromal cells which can differentiate to the endothelial lineage and thus represent a new source for vascular tissue regeneration [14, 31].

Beside their proliferative abilities and their possible use in regenerative medicine, MSCs also have some promising immunomodulatory proprieties which could be valuable tools in the field of immunotherapy.

Although structurally MSCs display a well-characterized immunological profile, they are non-immunogenic and therefore they do not elicit any immune response. For this reason, they could have safe and efficient therapeutic applications also in allogeneic settings.

MSCs are extremely sensitive to environmental signals and are able to adapt their biological functions to the surrounding milieu and translate these messages into immunomodulatory responses [14]. In particular, by expressing and modulating an array of Toll-like receptors (TLR), they are able to recognize microbial pathogens and thus sense signs of infection [31].

Additionally, in response to the surrounding environment, they can regulate the innate and the adaptive immune cells. As other non-lymphoid cells, MSCs play a fundamental suppressive role in the maintenance of immune system tolerance by secreting regulatory mediators, such as cytokines and other biologically active substances [14]. Indeed, their actions are usually mediated by the release of soluble factors or extracellular vesicles that stimulate or inhibit the surrounding target cells. Moreover they demonstrate a specific pattern of cell adhesion molecules, which allow a close interaction with immune cells, especially with T-cells [32]. Thus MSCs can inhibit lymphocyte activation and proliferation in a cell dose-dependent way.

For all these reasons, they are very promising cell populations for the development of cell therapies aimed to treat a range of systemic inflammatory and autoimmune diseases, particularly of the skin.

Compared to other classical sources of MSCs, the foreskin offers several advantages: it is easily collected after male circumcision and its use raises fewer ethical concerns.

To sum up, the multi-lineage differentiation and the self-renewal abilities make MSCs a promising tool in the field of regenerative medicine while their different immune-regulatory functions could be wisely used to manage inflammatory or immunological disorders.

Moreover, the foreskin holds promise as a potential cell source of human Dermis-Isolated Adult Stem (hDIAS) cells [15]. They provide a number of possible tissue engineering applications without the ethical concerns carried by pluripotent embryonic stem cells.

Foreskin hDIAS cells are attractive because they are easily accessible, abundant and also small tissue can potentially yield large cell numbers after expansion.

Kwon et al. showed that foreskin hDIAS have multi-lineage differentiation potential. In particular, they exhibited osteogenic and chondrogenic differentiation but limited adipogenic capabilities. In vivo, they were able to form spheres and self-assembly into constructs which disclose stability, integrity and no adverse reactions in host animals. All these proprieties make foreskin hDIAS a potential cell source for tissue-engineered cartilage.

Fibroblasts from the foreskin have also been used to generate induced Pluripotent Stem Cell lines (hiPSCs) which open them up to a wider potential usage.

In the field of the tissue engineering, a recent report has also demonstrated that foreskin can be utilised to obtain a decellularized extracellular scaffold with potential to be used in a regenerative approach in the reconstruction of the human foreskin [33].

In conclusion, the foreskin, usually considered as a biological waste material, should instead be considered a reservoir of cells with self-renewal capacity, multilineage potential and immunomodulatory properties, which make it a very attractive tool for cell-based immunotherapy and a wide range of tissue-engineering applications.

References

1. Manzoni G, Bracka A, Palminteri E, Marrocco G. Hypospadias surgery: when, what and by whom? BJU Int. 2004;94(8):1188–95.
2. Benson M, Hanna MK. A novel technique to construct a neo-scrotum out of preputial skin for agenesis and underdeveloped scrotum. J Pediatr Urol. 2018;14(5):449.e1–4.
3. Yildirim S, Akan M, Aköz T, Tanoğlu B. The preputium: an overlooked skin graft donor site. Ann Plast Surg. 2001;46(6):630–4.
4. Aslan G, Sarifakioglu N, Tuncali D, Terzioglu A, Bingul F. The prepuce and circumcision: dual application as a graft. Ann Plast Surg. 2004;52(2):199–203.
5. Mak AS, Poon AM, Tung MK. Use of preputial skin for the release of burn contractures in children. Burns. 1995;21(4):301–2.
6. Grabosch A, Weyer F, Gruhl L, Bruck JC. Repair of the upper eyelid by means of the prepuce after severe burns. Ann Plast Surg. 1991;26(5):427–30.
7. Parkash S. The use of preputial skin to replace conjunctiva and to correct ectropion. Br J Plast Surg. 1982;35(2):206–8.
8. Oates SD, Gosain AK. Syndactyly repair performed simultaneously with circumcision: use of foreskin as a skin-graft donor site. J Pediatr Surg. 1997;32(10):1482–4.
9. Levin LAR. The use of spare parts in surgery of the hand. Atlas Hand Clin. 1998;3:235.
10. Schäfer T, Kukies S, Stokes TH, Levin LS, Donatucci CF, Erdmann D. The prepuce as a donor site for reconstruction of an extravasation injury to the foot in a newborn. Ann Plast Surg. 2005;54(6):664–6.
11. Fucini C, Caminati F, Basiricò F, Bartolini N, Mirasolo VM. Free graft foreskin anoplasty. Color Dis. 2012;14(8):e506–7.

12. Freeman NV. The foreskin anoplasty. Dis Colon Rectum. 1984;27(5):309–13.
13. Najar M, Crompot E, van Grunsven LA, Dollé L, Lagneaux L. Foreskin-derived mesenchymal stromal cells with aldehyde dehydrogenase activity: isolation and gene profiling. BMC Cell Biol. 2018;19(1):4.
14. Najar M, Lagneaux L. Foreskin as a source of immunotherapeutic mesenchymal stromal cells. Immunotherapy. 2017;9(2):207–17.
15. Kwon H, Haudenschild AK, Brown WE, Vapniarsky N, Paschos NK, Arzi B, et al. Tissue engineering potential of human dermis-isolated adult stem cells from multiple anatomical locations. PLoS One. 2017;12(8):e0182531.
16. Skrzypczyk A, Giri S, Bader A. Generation of induced pluripotent stem cell line from foreskin fibroblasts. Stem Cell Res. 2016;17(3):572–5.
17. Snodgrass W. Tubularized, incised plate urethroplasty for distal hypospadias. J Urol. 1994;151:464–5.
18. Kolon TF, Gonzales ET. The dorsal inlay graft for hypospadias repair. J Urol. 2000;163(6):1941–3.
19. Hollowell JG, Keating MA, Snyder HM, Duckett JW. Preservation of the urethral plate in hypospadias repair: extended applications and further experience with the onlay island flap urethroplasty. J Urol. 1990;143(1):98–100; discussion 100–1.
20. Wallis MC, Braga L, Khoury A. The role of flaps and grafts in modern hypospadiology. Indian J Urol. 2008;24(2):200–5.
21. Shuzhu C, Min W, Yidong L, Weijing Y. Selecting the right method for hypospadias repair to achieve optimal results for the primary situation. Springerplus. 2016;5(1):1624.
22. Bracka A. Hypospadias repair: the two-stage alternative. Br J Urol. 1995;76(Suppl 3):31–41.
23. Duckett JW. The island flap technique for hypospadias repair. Urol Clin North Am. 1981;8(3):503–11.
24. Manuele R, Senni C, Patil K, Taghizadeh A, Garriboli M. Foreskin reconstruction at the time of single-stage hypospadias repair: is it a safe procedure? Int Urol Nephrol. 2019;51(2):187–91.
25. Ashley F. Foreskin as skin grafts. Ann Surg. 1937;106(2):252–6.
26. Chittmittrapap S, Vejchapipat P. Foreskin for skin grafting: an unthinkable positive aspect. Asian Biomed. 2009;3:675–80.
27. D'Alessio A, Piro E, Brugnoni M, Abati L. Use of preputial skin as cutaneous graft after nevus excision. Int J Pediatr. 2010;2010:951270.
28. Izzuddin MB, Normala BB. Use of preputial skin as cutaneous graft in post excision of a verrucous hemangioma of the thumb. J Surg Med. 2018;2:170–3.
29. Zaroo MI, Sheikh BA, Wani AH, Darzi MA, Mir M, Dar H, et al. Use of preputial skin for coverage of post-burn contractures of fingers in children. Indian J Plast Surg. 2011;44(1):68–71.
30. Emory RE, Chester CH. Prepuce pollicization: a reminder of an alternate donor. Plast Reconstr Surg. 2000;105(6):2100–1.
31. Najar M, Raicevic G, André T, Fayyad-Kazan H, Pieters K, Bron D, et al. Mesenchymal stromal cells from the foreskin: tissue isolation, cell characterization and immunobiological properties. Cytotherapy. 2016;18(3):320–35.
32. Najar M, Raicevic G, Fayyad-Kazan H, Kazan HF, De Bruyn C, Bron D, et al. Immune-related antigens, surface molecules and regulatory factors in human-derived mesenchymal stromal cells: the expression and impact of inflammatory priming. Stem Cell Rev. 2012;8(4):1188–98.
33. Purpura V, Bondioli E, Cunningham EJ, De Luca G, Capirossi D, Nigrisoli E, et al. The development of a decellularized extracellular matrix-based biomaterial scaffold derived from human foreskin for the purpose of foreskin reconstruction in circumcised males. J Tissue Eng. 2018;9:2041731418812613.

Part II

Congenital Preputial Anomalies

9 Aposthia

Preputial Diseases

Diseases affecting the prepuce could be addressed as a congenital anomalies and deformities; like aposthia, akroposthia, rotation and rare anomalies like igloo prepuce, acquired diseases like; phimosis, balanitis xerotica obliterans, balanitis, paraphimosis, neoplastic lesions and lastly focal lesions like cysts, nevi and vascular lesions. Most of these anomalies have no or minimal influence on urinary function, but had a great impaction in the psychological status and sexual life, usually these anomalies can be detected on clinical examination, but some specific investigations may be required to diagnose uncommon pathologies. Spontaneous improvement is possible in some cases. Majority of cases may need to undergo surgery, the potential psychological implications of genital malformation on patient development are the main reason for treatment, and the age generally recommended for surgery is after 12 months of age.

This review provides the paediatrician and general surgeons with a handy tool to identify the most common and also the rare preputial anomalies to make a sensible and adequately parents and patients assurance, and to plan the strategy of management.

Introduction

Soft tissues are rarely preserved in the fossil record, so we can expect little help from that quarter regarding the origin of foreskin. Nobody knows if the human beings created (or evolved) with a bared glans and the prepuce is just an acquired penile sheath, or the prepuce is a genuine organ?, also researches failed to detect the actual length of this double layered sheath, and if it is progressive or regressive along mankind history? So there is no clear answer if the prepuce is an acquired protection sheath, or it is a vestigial appendage. However, it is now settled in the conscience that prepuce is a common anatomical covering of the glans penis and clitoris of all human and non-human primates, Martin [1] reported, only based on its commonality as an anatomical feature in mammals, that prepuce not only has been present in primates for at least 65 million years, and is likely to be over 100 million years old, but also the reproductive advantages provided by the prepuce during the last 65 million years should not be taken lightly. The results of this study demonstrate that the human prepuce is not "vestigial" but it is an evolutionary advancement over the prepuce of other primates. This is most clearly seen in the evolutionary increase in corpuscular innervation of the human prepuce and the concomitant decrease in corpuscular receptors of the human glans relative to the innervation of the prepuce and glans of lower primate (Fig. 9.1).

From time to times, detection of babies delivered with a deficient prepuce arouse the confusion about the preputial origin.

M. A. B. Fahmy, *Normal and Abnormal Prepuce*, https://doi.org/10.1007/978-3-030-37621-5_9

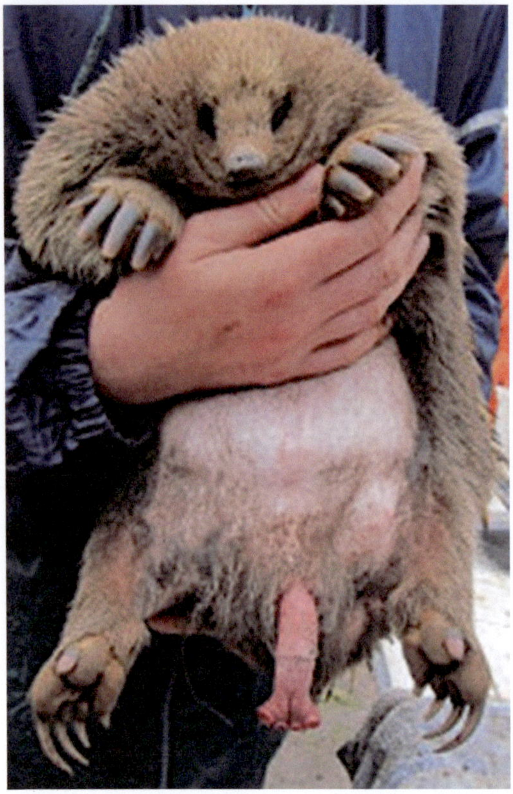

Fig. 9.1 Echidna-penis without any preputial covering

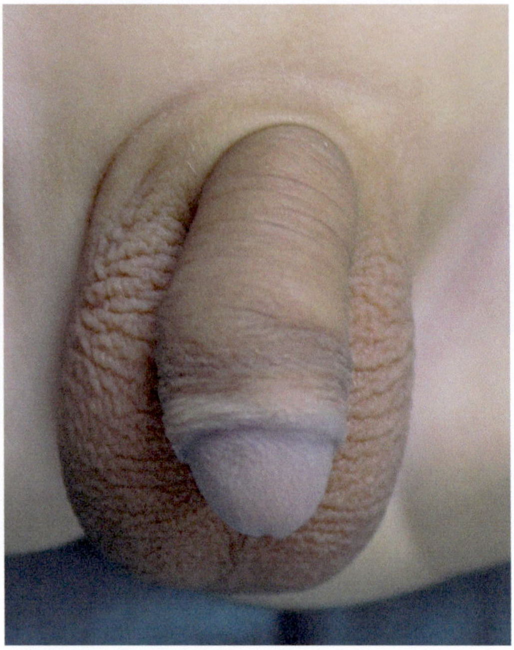

Fig. 9.2 Completely deficient prepuce in a 3 years old boy, with a normal penis and urethra

Definition

Aposthia is a rare congenital condition in humans, in which the foreskin of the penis is completely missing in a normally developed penis and urethra (Fig. 9.2).

Kim et al. [2] widened the spectrum of aposthia and described it as any male having relatively short prepuce but not phimotic, having prepuce fully retractable during erection, having a penis that looks more or less like a circumcised penis even when not erect, but this definition is not universally accepted.

In this textbook we consider aposthia only in male who had a completely deficient prepuce without any other anomalies in the urethra, or the urinary meatus, and without any previous history of trauma, and we will use the term "Microposthia" for cases with deficient prepuce not completely covering the glans penis.

Nomenclature

Natural circumcision, foreskinless, Preputial agenesis, Auto-amputation of the preputium. Congenital absence of foreskin.

Historical Background

Religious literature from various sources reflects the history of aposthia; as this condition was first referenced in Jewish law of 1567 CE, in relation to a child born circumcised.

Toward the end of the nineteenth century, E. S. Talbot [3] claimed in Medicine that aposthia among Jews was evidence for the now-discredited Lamarckian theory of evolution. It is likely that the cases he described were actually hypospadias. The Midrash of Ki Tetzei mentioned that Moses was born aposthic. Other sources tell us that Jacob and David were also born aposthic. Jewish law requires males born without a foreskin or who lost their foreskin through means other than a formal circumcision ceremony to have a drop of blood let from the penis at the point where the foreskin would have been attached. Later on, the Prophet Muhammad was said to have been born with "natural circumcision" (in Ibn Sad Tabaqatul-Kubara) [4].

Incidence

It is a very rare congenital anomaly; without any reported figure about incidence of aposthia among population, however in the last few years, various cases had been reported. Amin et al. [4] reported aposthia inheritance as a normal quantitative recessive human genetic trait in three strictly endogamous families, and aposthia reported as a sporadic and familiar cases.

In South Korea in 1999, Kim et al. [2] found 69% "naturally circumcised" among uncircumcised males during a survey, but their definition of aposthia is not accurate, it was most likely they describing hypospadias cases rather than a true aposthia.

So aposthia may be prevalent in certain ancient healthy and comparatively developed inbred population isolates; this condition has not been shown to have a higher frequency in Jews or Muslims [5]. If the hypospadias surgeons are fully aware about this condition, a cumulative number of cases will be reported either in association with other genital anomalies or as an entire pathology.

It is reported that there is no cases of aposthia in females have been described in the literature [6], but this not true in my opinion, as the clitoral hood varies in the size, shape, thickness, and other aesthetic aspects from female to female, some women have large clitoral hoods that completely cover the clitoral glans, which usually retractable, others have a smaller hoods that do not cover the full length of the clitoral glans, leaving it exposed all the time (Chap. 33).

I noticed a sort of aposthia in association with most cases of adrenogenital hyperplasia; actually in such cases there is no deficient hood, but the clitoris proportionally larger to exceed the preputial coverage (Fig. 9.3). Other cases of female aposthia are associated with an ill developed labia or bifid clitoris as in some cases of bladder exstrophy.

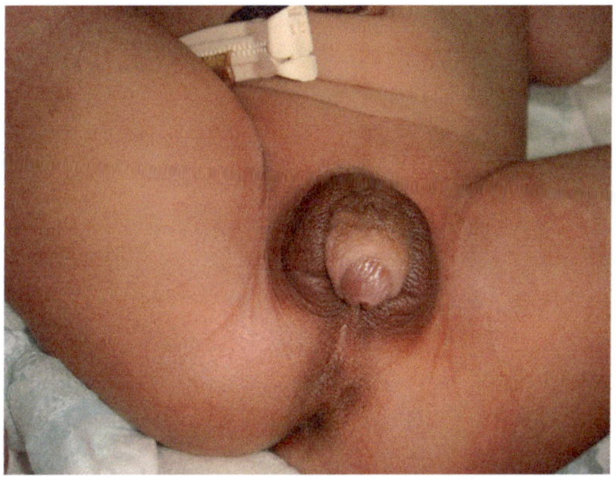

Fig. 9.3 A female child with adrenogenital hyperplasia, her clitorial glans completely exposed; secondary to a clitoromegaly, it looks like aposthia

Etiology

With the recent studies about preputial development, it is clear that aposthia represents a failure of the normal developmental progression of the prepuce, which start normally at the 12th intrauterine week from the coronal sulcus as a dorsal-ventral expansion of the preputial lamina, dorsal portion growing at a more rapid rate than the ventral component, prior to 11th weeks of gestation there is no evidence of preputial traces (Fig. 9.4).

The closure of the ventral portion of the prepuce is completed by the fifth month of gestation after closure of the glanular urethra, prepuce eventually develops an outer epidermal surface and an inner surface lined by a stratified epithelium. Preputial development is in someway linked to urethral development within the glans since in hypospadias, preputial tissue is absent ventrally, and excessive dorsally [7].

Amin et al. [4] reported that aposthia is inherited as normal quantitative recessive human genetic trait in three strictly endogamous families, and aposthia reported as a sporadic and familiar cases; in sporadic cases, all of cases had a hypospadias associated and the familiar case had a normal development of the urethra. Both groups had a history of consanguineous marriage and the study suggested that certain linked modifier loci as well as a number of autosomal recessive genes are required to express natural circumcision or aposthia. I think this not conclusive as there is no molecular or cytogenetic studies in the surveyed families, also we had an identical twins; one of them is aposthic and the other is completely normal, we exhausted all lab and chromosomal investigations without detection of any underlying abnormalities (Fig. 9.5).

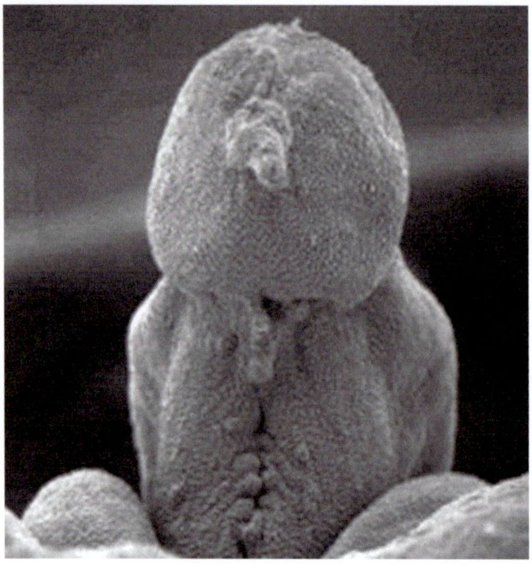

Fig. 9.4 Intrauterine male genitalia of 65 mm embryo, with the glans uncovered by prepuce, which start to creep from the coronal sulcus

It seems that aposthia is a congenital local field defect, which interfere and hinder proper preputial development, without any underling chromosomal or hormonal defect, it could be simply due to arrest of normal preputial development (Fig. 9.6).

Defective preputial development may be associated with defective urethral development; as in cases of hooded prepuce associating hypospadias, but cases of intact prepuce associating megameatus and epispadias disputes the relation between urethral and preputial developments.

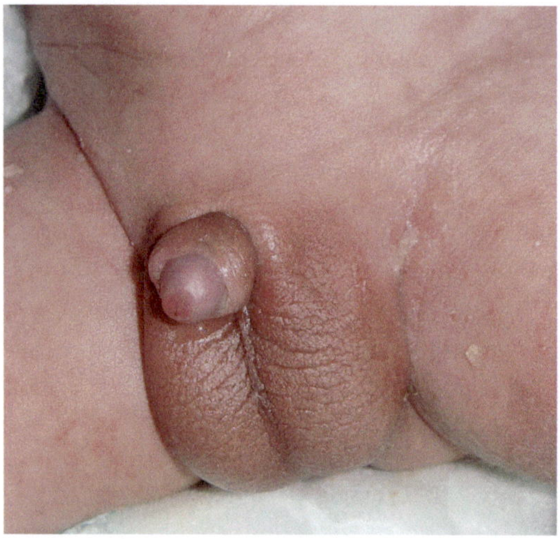

Fig. 9.6 Aposthia in neonate with completely normal glans and urethra

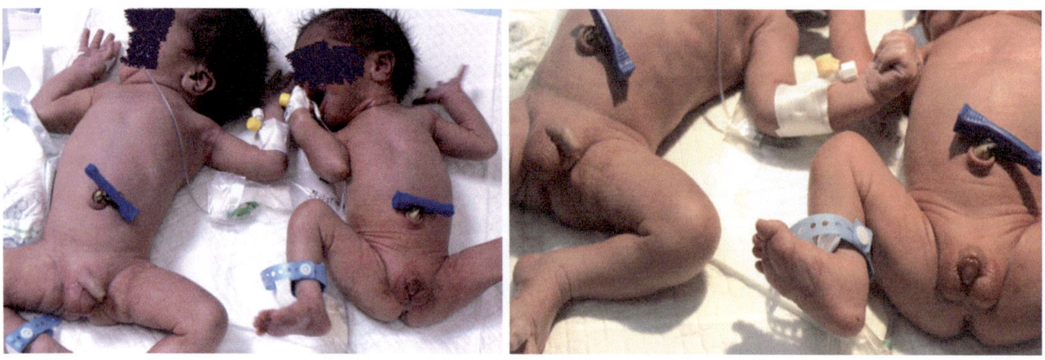

Fig. 9.5 An identical twins; one of them had a completely normal genitalia, other has an aposthia

Associated Anomalies

Ventral penile curvature with or without chordee is a common association in our collection of cases of aposthia (Fig. 9.7), cases of epispadias usually associated with a dorsal preputial defect, but complete aposthia with epispadias is not reported before, in Fig. 9.8 aposthia is recognisable in 1 year old child with an isolated epispadias.

Children with different spectrum of the androgen insensitivity syndrome, may had a variant grades of deficient prepuce, but a complete aposthia is a very rare associate; aposthia in such cases could be expected along the defective development of the glans penis [8]. Of course the defective preputial development in cases of androgen insensitivity syndrome is different from cases of hooded prepuce associating hypospadias; as in the earlier cases the prepuce is completely and circumferential absent (Figs. 9.9 and 9.10).

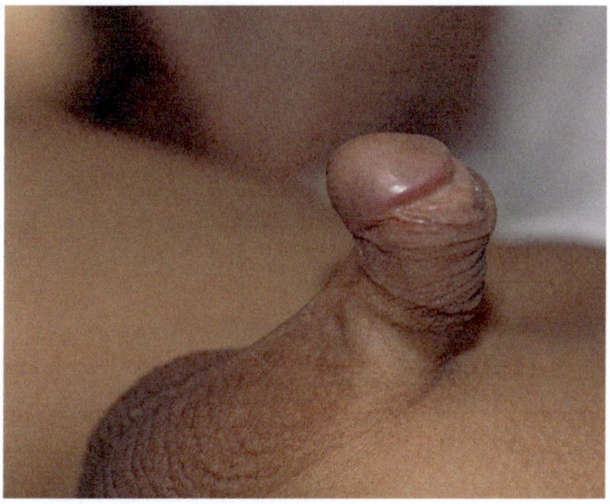

Fig. 9.7 Aposthia associated with a significant chordee and ventral penile curvature

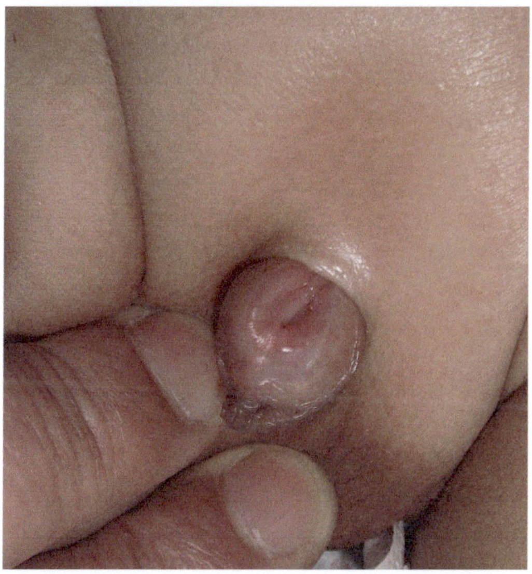

Fig. 9.8 An infant with epispadias and a completely deficient prepuce

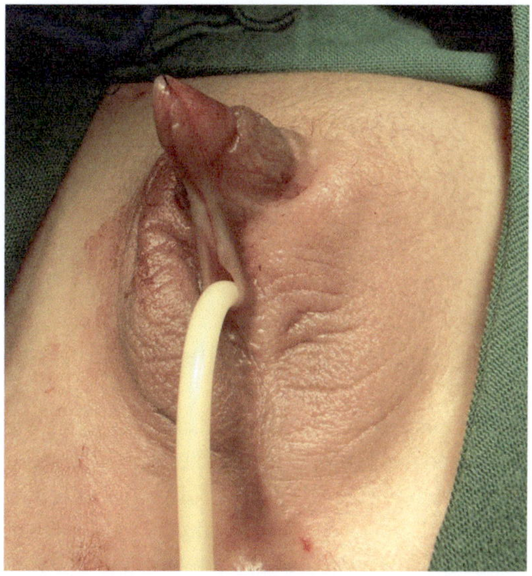

Fig. 9.9 A case of Androgen Insensitivity Syndrome with a completely deficient prepuce

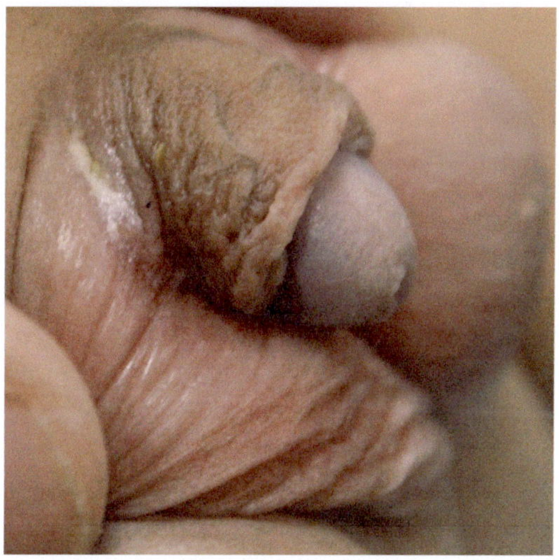

Fig. 9.10 A child with a mild form of androgen insensitivity syndrome with aposthia

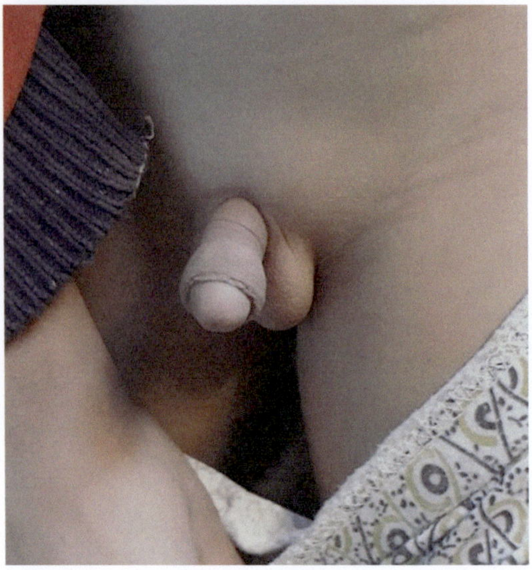

Fig. 9.11 An adolescent with aposthia with a normally developed penis and testicles

Diagnosis and Differential Diagnosis

It is distinctive in cases of aposthia diagnosed at adulthood to see a well formed penis, scrotum and even a frenulum, such cases should be investigated to detect any disease or syndrome which may associate this anomaly and affected the child at birth (Fig. 9.11).

Inspite of the obvious clinical findings, which can diagnose all cases of aposthia clinically, a through investigations should be carried on to detect any associated genitourinary anomalies or defective sex hormones, also cases of aposthia theoretically should be differentiated from other similar cases of microposthia or hyposthia (Chap. 10).

Significance and Management of Aposthia

Absent prepuce in a child is not an actual surgical problem, which usually needs no intervention; exclusion of any other associated anomalies and family reassurance may be enough in certain communities where circumcision is a routine or an acceptable practice, but preputial reconstruction and restoration may be considered in societies which considering an exposed glans without a preputial covering is a socially unacceptable condition, also many adults with aposthia may ask for preputial restoration. Many procedures had been described to develop a neo-prepuce, either by non-surgical foreskin restoration, which accomplished through traction, tissue expansion, or with a circular fasciocutaneous penile flap or other different grafts, which typically taken from the scrotum [9]. Several commercial retaining devices are available to hold the remaining skin. Tissue expansion cannot restore the specialized structures, and it is unclear whether the process promotes any nerve regeneration. Nonsurgical tissue expansion methods are state of the art, as they produce a pseudo-foreskin with much higher cosmetic appearance and functionality than that produced by surgical methods; also they are far less expensive; and do not have an associated risks as surgical methods.

Surgical preputial reconstruction methods include the following:

1. Skin graft from the thigh or buttocks: A free skin graft is sutured into a circumferential cut made around the penile shaft at the circumcision scar. The transplanted tissue usually has a very different condition and texture and is quite inflexible and smooth.
2. Scrotal implant flap: A scrotal implant graft is a multiple-stage reconstruction, involving circumferentially cutting the shaft tissue at the circumcision scar. A tunnel is created in the front side of the scrotum between two incisions and then the penile shaft is threaded through the tunnel and stitched at both ends. After about 3–6 months, when healed, the penis is surgically removed with the new scrotal tissue cut on either side and wrapped around the shaft and sewn on the ventral side. There is then another healing period. At that point, it is typically necessary to reduce the 'overhang' and to enlarge the orifice of the new foreskin.
3. Z-plasty or Y-V plasty: It is used to lengthen the distal penile skin to cover the glans partially.

References

1. Martin RD. Primate origins and evolution: a phylogenetic reconstruction. Princeton: Princeton University Press; 1990. p. 42–3.
2. Kim DS, Lee JY, Pang MG. Male circumcision: a Korean perspective. BJU Int. 1999;83(1):28–33.
3. Talbot ES. Inheritance of circumcision effects. Medicine. 1898;4:473–5.
4. Amin Ud Din M, Salam A, Rafiq MA, Khaliq I, Ansar M, Ahmad W. Aposthia: a birth defect or normal quantitative recessive human genetic trait? East Mediterr Health J. 2007;13(2):280–6.
5. Parkash S, Jeyakumar K, Subramanya K, Chaudhuri S. Human subpreputial collection: its nature and formation. J Urol. 1973;110(2):211–2.
6. Garcia-Palacios M, et al. Congenital absence of preputial foreskin: an extremely uncommon anomaly. J Pediatr Surg. 2013;48:E13–5. https://doi.org/10.1016/j.jpedsurg.2012.10.072.
7. Liu X, Liu G, Shen J, Yue A, Isaacson D, Sinclair A, Cao M, Liaw A, Cunha GR, Baskin L. Human glans and preputial development. Differentiation. 2018;103:86–99. https://doi.org/10.1016/j.diff.2018.08.002.
8. Gleniste TW. A consideration of the processes involved in the development of the prepuce in man. Br J Urol. 1956;28:243–9.
9. Fahmy MA. Chapter 15: Reconstructive surgery for circumcision complications. In: Complications in male circumcision. St. Louis: Elsevier; 2019. https://doi.org/10.1016/C2018-0-03679-8.

10 Microposthia

Abbreviation

MIP Megameatus intact prepuce

Historical Background

Recently there is a scanty reports about the congenitally deficient prepuce, but a pathological deformity called lipodermus, a condition in which the foreskin was not long enough to cover fully the glans penis was described long time ago by Galen, Soronus, Pedanius Dioscorides, Antyllus and others [1], all published descriptions of lipodermus made recommendations for its correction, most of which involve the application of unguents and stretching [2]. The only pathological condition of the foreskin that Gabriele Fallopius (1523–1562) considered worthy of discussion was a shortness or absence of the foreskin, passing the unfavourable verdict that a penis with an exposed glans resembled a "horse's rump" Fallopius made various recommendations for repairing this defect. Needless to say, the concept of a foreskin being too long or too tight is nowhere to be found [3].

Epispasm is an operation that described early to correct a circumcised penis. Some might call it circumcision in reverse. Epispasm on a circumcised penis required a somewhat more difficult technique. Some Jews probably submitted to epispasm because they shared the common Greek and Roman revulsion toward circumcision [4].

For Greek art portrays the foreskin, often drawn in meticulous detail, as an emblem of male beauty; and children with congenitally short foreskins were sometimes subjected to a treatment, known as epispasm, that was aimed at elongation [5].

Nomenclature

Microposthia, Hypoposthia, Peeper penis, which is a term refers to the penis whose foreskin is short enough to expose some of the glans when flaccid. The term microposthia is our preference [6].

Incidence

In a sample of 3000 young men examined; W. Schöberlein found a lack of, or spontaneous atrophy of the foreskin among approximately 4% [7].

Definition

It is a condition of having a very small foreskin not covering the whole penis in a flaccid status; microposthia diagnosed if the glans penis could be seen partially in a flaccid penis (Fig. 10.1).

M. A. B. Fahmy, *Normal and Abnormal Prepuce*, https://doi.org/10.1007/978-3-030-37621-5_10

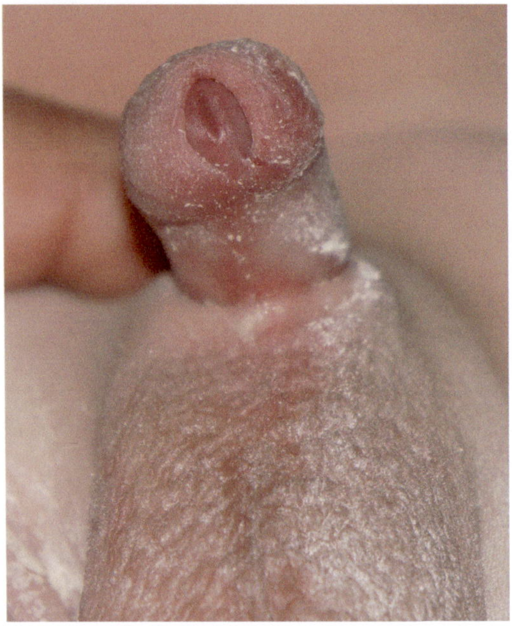

Fig. 10.1 A minimal degree of microposthia

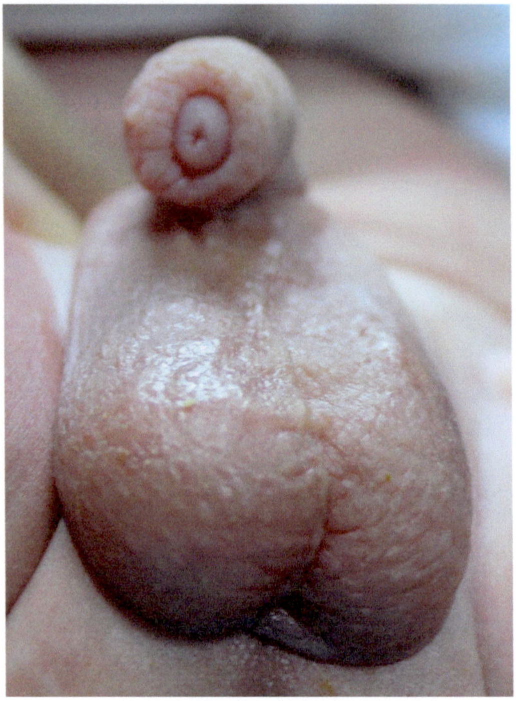

Fig. 10.2 A case of microposthia giving a typical example of the term peeper penis

It is not a rare condition, and it could be considered as a normal variation, where the prepuce looks shorter to give the chance for the glans or the urinary meatus to be visible in a neonate without foreskin retraction (Fig. 10.2). In all cases of microposthia the frenulum is absent or deficient and penile raphe end at the coronal sulcus (Fig. 10.3). Usually the foreskin is defective at the ventral aspect of the penis in hypospadias cases and in cases of hooded foreskin without hypospadias (Chap. 12) but in microposthia the prepuce is deficient all around the glans with a different grades (Fig. 10.4).

The preputial remnants with microposthia is a smooth skin with an exposed inner mucosal layer, but very rarely the prepuce had a disfigured serrated preputial remnants covering partially the dorsal surface of the glans as in Fig. 10.5.

Microposthia have to be differentiated from cases of aposthia (Chap. 9), where is the prepuce is completely deficient and the coronal sulcus clearly seen in a flaccid penis, but in microposthia the preputial remnants covering the sulcus but not reaching to tip of the penis.

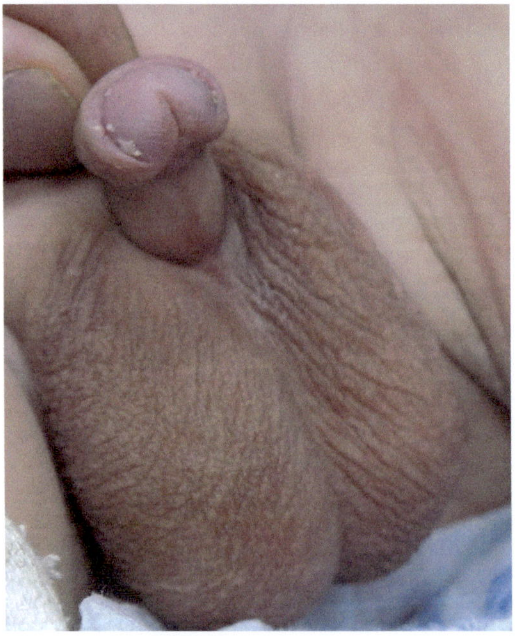

Fig. 10.3 A microposthia with a deficient prepuce, the preputial edges inserted directly to the glans

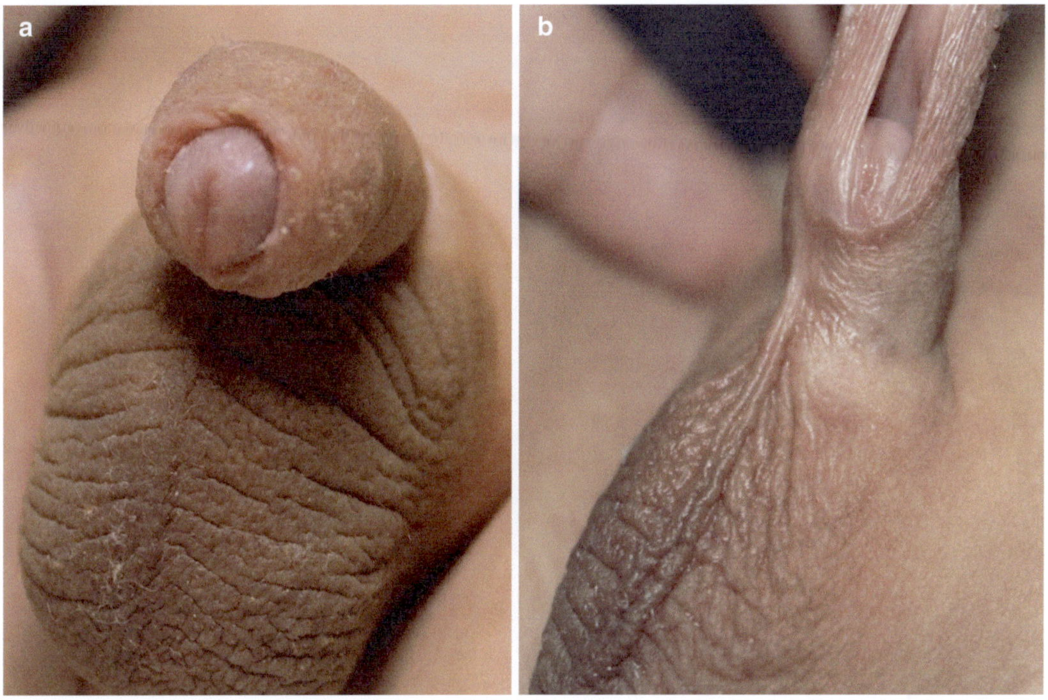

Fig. 10.4 Difference between microposthia with all around deficiency of the prepuce (**a**) and hooded prepuce with only ventral preputial deficiency, with normal urethra (**b**)

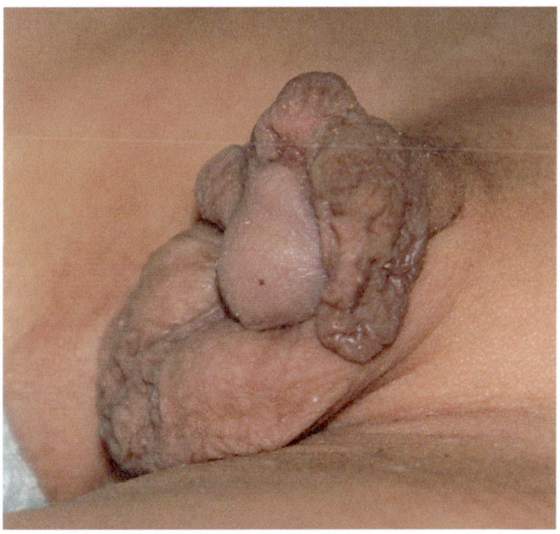

Fig. 10.5 Irregular serrated deficient prepuce

Significance of Microposthia

Failure of development of urethral groove; results in hypospadias and subsequently associated with ventrally deficient prepuce (hooded Prepuce). In female the urethral groove persist; so preputial hood is a normal finding which covers the clitoris partially, and it is extremely rare to have a complete prepuce ensheathing entirely the clitoris, but till now, there is no conventional explanation why there is some boys had a completely formed prepuce with hypospadias as in Megameatus Intact Prepuce (MIP) anomaly, and in contrary there are other cases with a deficient prepuce but with a normally formed urethra (Microposthia)?

So cases of microposthia may present as an arrest of the normal preputial development secondary to failure of complete folding process of the preputial lamella around the glans penis.

Generally there are only a few data in the literature on anatomical characteristics of the prepuce, also the course of embryonal development and the exact etiology of hypospadias still remain unknown. The difference in the shape and the development of the prepuce presumably depends on the potency of the causal agent and the moment when it disrupts penile development [8]. However, sometimes there is no correlation between the severity of hypospadias and the degree of vascularity and morphological underdevelopment of the prepuce [9].

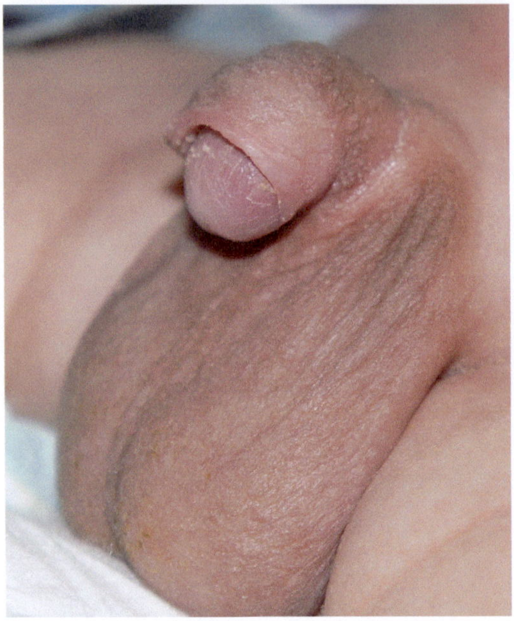

Fig. 10.6 Microposthia with penile chordee, but with a normal urethra

Differential Diagnosis

Cases of microposthia should be differentiated from aposthia (Chap. 9), hooded prepuce (Chap. 12), and cases of exposed glans with a normally long prepuce. Grade 1X of Kayaba et al. classification of the normal prepuces could't be considered as a degree of microposthia, as microposthia is a deficient prepuce which manifests as an exposed glans and not related to the degree of retractability of the foreskin [10].

Associated Anomalies

Microposthia itself is not a serious anomaly and could not be considered as a disease, but its importance came from the possibility of association with other congenital genitourinary anomalies, where the deficient foreskin is an indicator for a defective genital development, as the normal development of prepuce is an androgen dependent process; so many other genital anomalies could associated microposthia, and the most common association is hypospadias; as one of the cardinal signs of hypospadias is the ventrally deficient prepuce, and it is not rare to have a deficient prepuce with a chordee, but with normal urethra and meatus (Fig. 10.6). It is postulated that a disturbance in the development of the prepuce may leave the ventral penis with inadequate skin coverage, resulting in borrowing of scrotal tissue, and results in different grades of webbing or bending of the penis [11].

Microposthia may associate a wide range of penile, genital and other congenital anomalies:

1. Penile anomalies associating microposthia include:
   - Penile rotation: We reported many cases of different grades of an isolated penile rotation, mainly to the left side, in association with microposthia (Fig. 10.7).
   - Angulation of the glans penis, a different degrees of penile bending at the coronal sulcus are common with microposthia (Fig. 10.8).

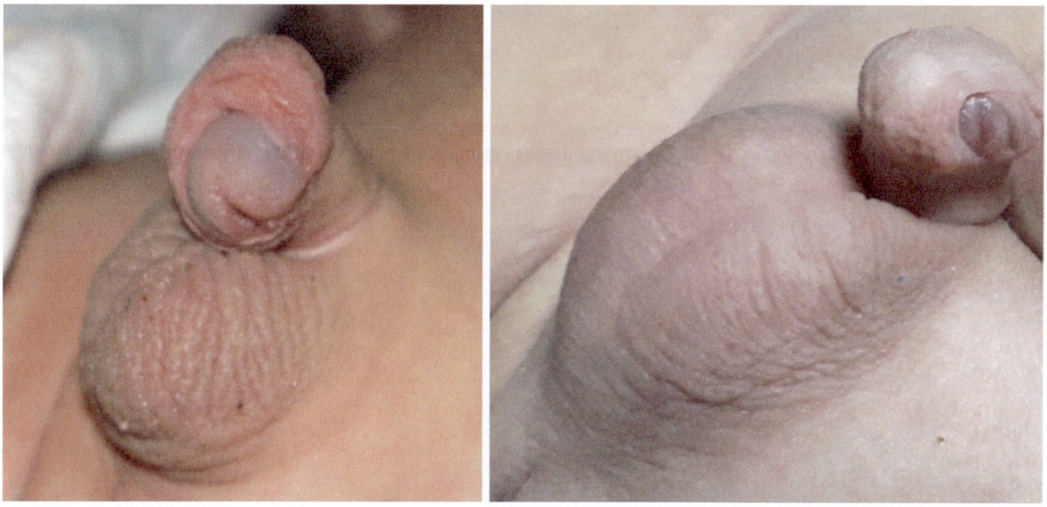

Fig. 10.7 Left sided penile rotation associated with microposthia

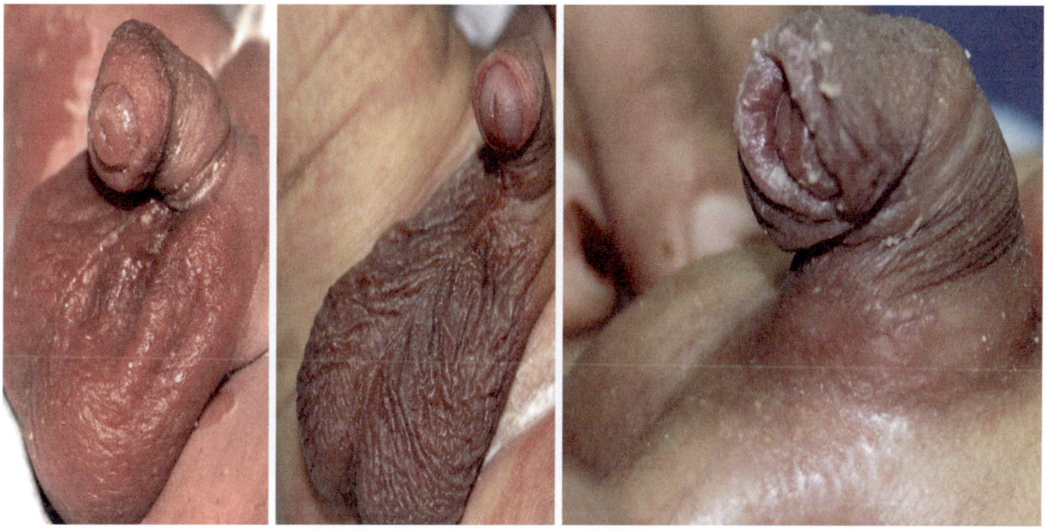

Fig. 10.8 Different grades of glandular angulation with the long axis of the penis in association with microposthia

- Penile chordee with a normal urethra is common with cases of hyposthia (Fig. 10.9).
- Abnormally wide meatus (Fig. 10.10).
- Absent frenulum (Fig. 10.11).
- Median raphe deviation (Fig. 10.12).
- Notched prepuce (Fig. 10.13).

2. Non penile genital anomalies:

   Undescended testicle (Fig. 10.14).

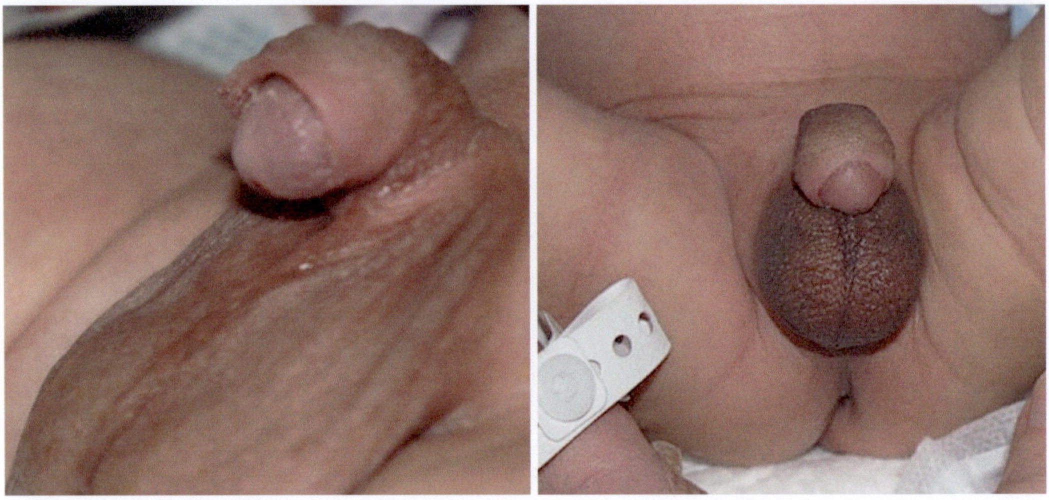

Fig. 10.9 Penile chordee with hyposthia

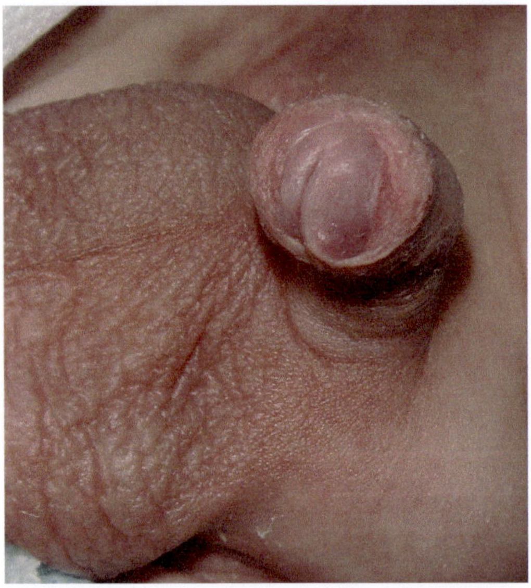

Fig. 10.10 Microposthia with a longitudinal wide urinary meatus, a degree of penile rotation is also noticeable

3. *Other congenital anomalies*: Imperforate anus (Fig. 10.15)

   Complications: Revision of the case series of microposthia revealed the importance of an intact prepuce for the neonates and infants, and this may justifying the concept of postponing neonatal circumcision, for those who are insisted to it, they have to wait till the baby could be taken out of napkins. The exposed

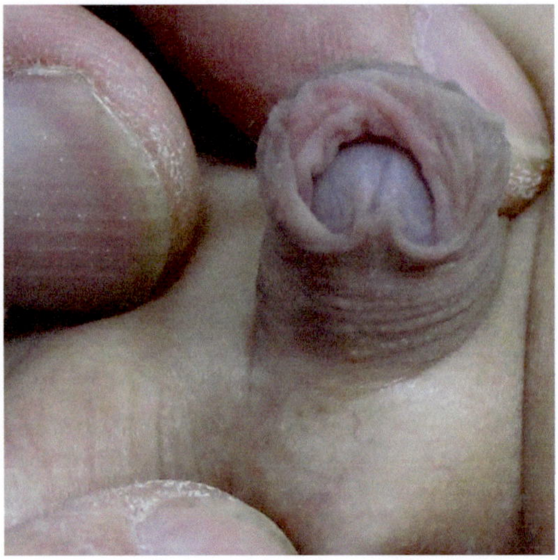

Fig. 10.11 Microposthia with an absent frenulum

deficient prepuce may be itself subjected to infection and results in posthitis (Fig. 10.16), smegma may aggregate under the adherent part of the microposthic prepuce and may end with balanitis (Fig. 10.17), also the exposed meatus without preputial protection from the napkins and its concentrated urinary contents, may be subjected to meatitis with a subsequent meatal stenosis (Fig. 10.18).

Management: A microposthic child may deserve a meticulous circumcision to make his

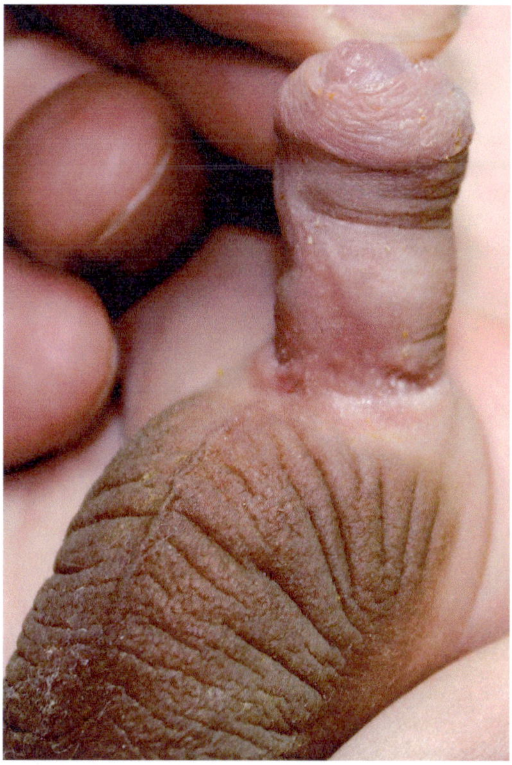

Fig. 10.12 Median raphe deviation with microposthia

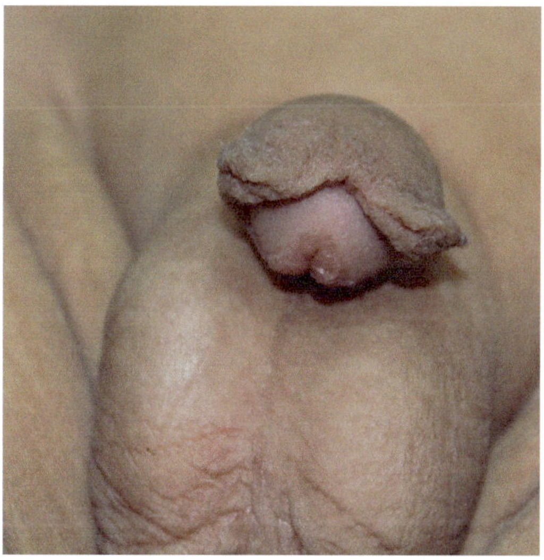

Fig. 10.13 A midline notched prepuce incompletely covering the glans, meatitis is obvious

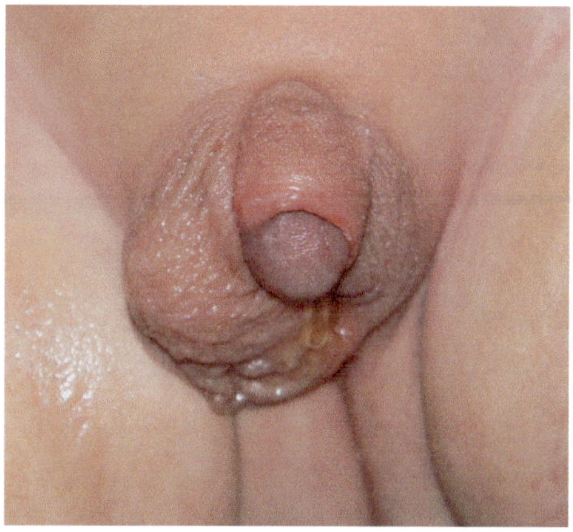

Fig. 10.14 Microposthia with left undescended testicle

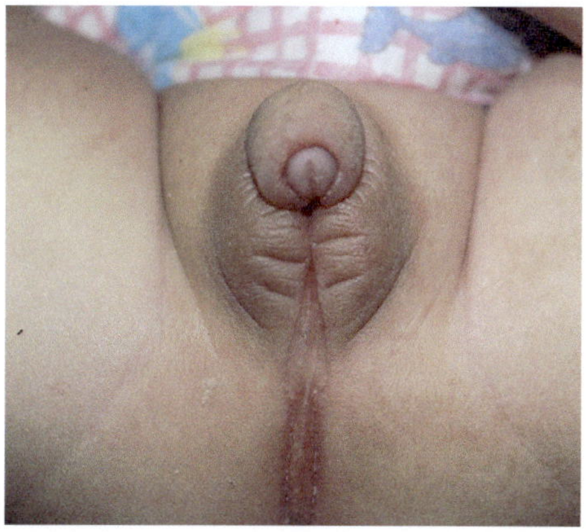

Fig. 10.15 A case of imperforate anus, wide median raphe and microposthia

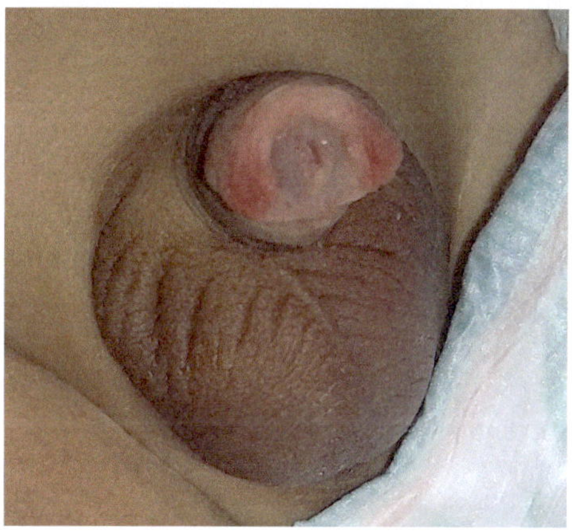

Fig. 10.16 (Posthitis) an inflammation of the deficient prepuce

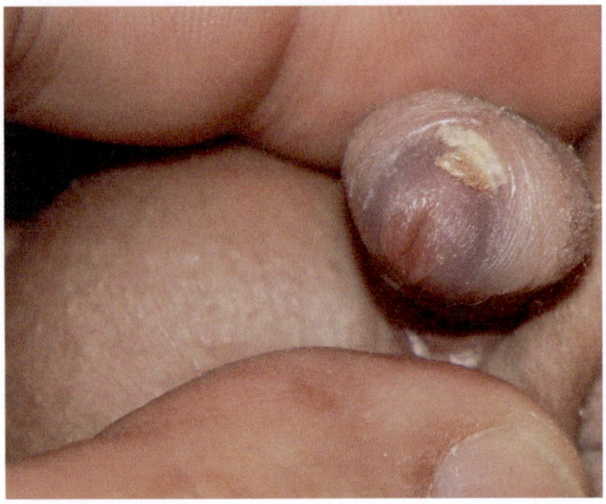

Fig. 10.17 Smegma collection and an early balanitis with microposthia

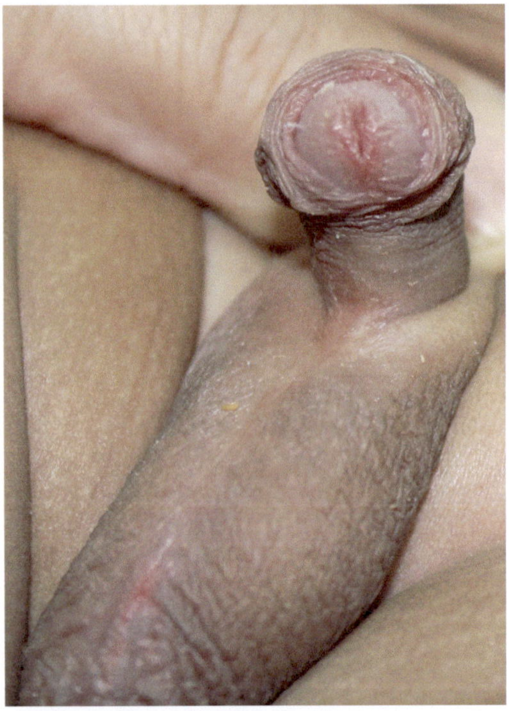

Fig. 10.18 Meatitis associating posthitis

penis looks like the normally circumcised one if the family wish, or the decision could be kept till the time when the child can decide about himself later on. In some occasions preputial reconstruction may be indicated for microposthia to restore the normally looking prepuce (preputioplasty), and this could be achieved without grafting in minor cases by preputial edges refreshment, midline closure and creation of a properly constricted tip distal to the glans in minor cases, but in cases with severe preputial deficiency, preputial restoration could be accomplished through non-surgical foreskin restoration techniques (developed to help circumcised men ‘regrow’ a skin covering for the glans by different modalities of tissue expansion) to lengthen the natural foreskin. In cases with marked preputial deficiency, foreskin restoration for those who are looking for a normal intact prepuce can be achieved by a circular fasciocutaneous penile flap or other different grafts which typically taken from the scrotum.

References

1. Cameron M. The sources of medical knowledge in Anglo-Saxon England. Anglo-Saxon England. 1982;11:135–55. https://doi.org/10.1017/S0263675100002593.
2. Hodges FM. The history of phimosis from antiquity to the present. In: Denniston GC, Hodges FM, Milos MF, editors. Male and female circumcision: medical, legal and ethical considerations in pediatric practice. New York: Kluwer Academic/Plenum Publishers; 1999.
3. *Gabrielis Falloppi Mutinensis MedicEi xcellentissimi Opuscula.* De Decoratione. De Praeputii Brevitate corrigenda Cap. XVIII. Padua: Lucam Bertellum. 156648-9.
4. Celsus AC. De Medicina 7.25.1. W.G. Spencer’s translation, Loeb Classical Library. Cambridge, MA: Harvard University Press/London: Heinemann; 1938.
5. Jacob Neusner, Approaches to ancient Judaism, new series: religious and theological studies (1993), p. 149, Scholars Press, Atlanta.
6. Fahmy MAB. Prepuce. In: Rare congenital genitourinary anomalies. Berlin: Springer; 2015. p. 33–41.
7. Schöberlein W. The significance and frequency of phimosis and smegma. Munch Med Wochenschr. 1966;108:373–7.
8. Baskin LS. Hypospadias and ureteral development. J Urol. 2000;163:951–6.
9. Radojicic ZI, Perovic SV. Classification of prepuce in hypospadias according to morphological abnormalities and their impact on hypospadias repair. J Urol. 2004;172:301–4. https://doi.org/10.1097/01.ju.0000129008.31212.3d.
10. Kayaba H, Tamura H, Kitajima S, Fujiwara Y, Kato T, Kato T. Analysis of shape and retractability of the prepuce in 603 Japanese boys. J Urol. 1996;156:1813–5.
11. Perlmutter AD, Chamberlain JW. Webbed penis without chordee. J Urol. 1972;107(2):320–1.

Macroposthia 11

Abbreviations

CMP	Congenital megaprepuce
CP/CPPS	Chronic Prostatitis/Chronic Pelvic Pain Syndrome
IMC	Infant male circumcision
MIP	Megameatus Intact prepuce
PE	Premature ejaculation

Definition and Nomenclatures

Macroposthia

We prefer this term as it generally means a congenitally long or excessive long prepuce, and this anomaly affects the whole layers of the prepuce and mainly confined to excessively long preputial tip; but till now there is no definite specific length matched with age for this anomaly. Macroposthia is not a synonymous to the term akroposthia, acroposthia or acroposthion; as these names describe a normally redundant longer part of the prepuce, which extend distal to the glans. Sometimes the penis which is affected by macroposthia is termed "Volcano penis" (Fig. 11.1).

The term: acroposthion literally means: "foreskin tip". This term found in Hippocratic aphorism that states: "When a bone, cartilage, sinew, the slender part of the jaw, or the acroposthion is severed, the part neither grows nor unites".

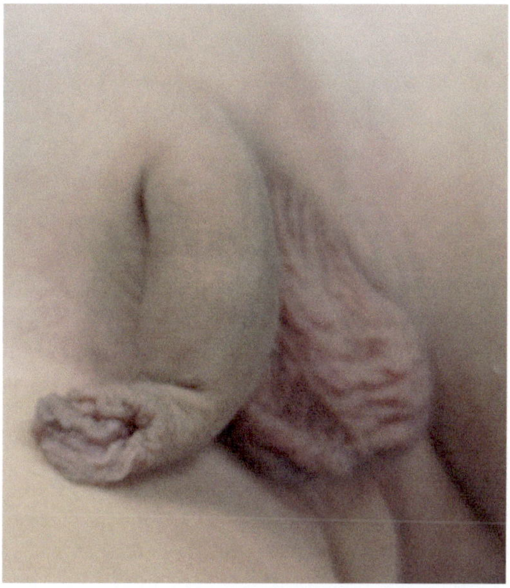

Fig. 11.1 A long macroposthitic prepuce, the prepuce length exceeding the penile length

Acroposthion is a Greek word, which designates the visually defining, tapered, fleshy, nipple-like portion of the foreskin that advances beyond the terminus of the underlying glans penis. The acroposthion, especially in early youth, can run to impressive lengths. Distinguished from the acroposthion is the posthe, which is the portion of the foreskin that merely enfolds the glans penis, beginning at the coronal sulcus. While it is not possible to make a definitive interpretation of the

M. A. B. Fahmy, *Normal and Abnormal Prepuce*, https://doi.org/10.1007/978-3-030-37621-5_11

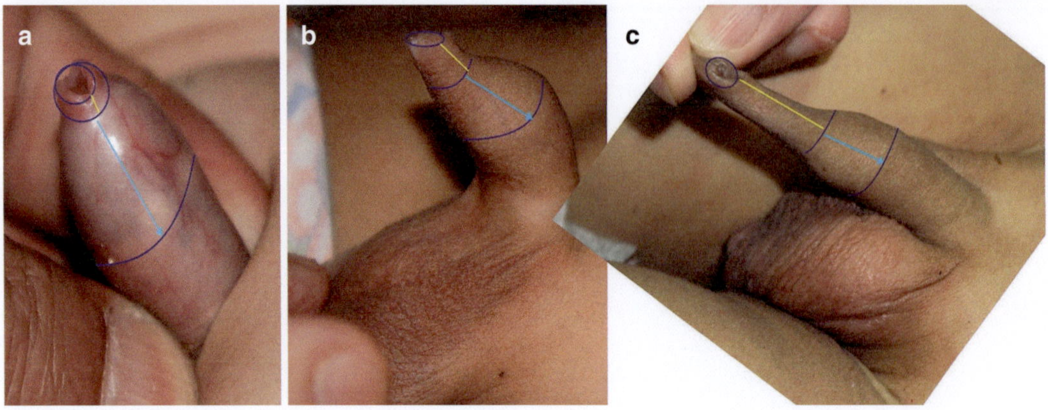

Fig. 11.2 Different grades of long preputial tip: (**a**) normal small tip, just distal to urinary meatus, (**b**) long preputial tip, and (**c**) a long tip could be considered as macroposthia, but with a smooth tapered tip

term. The acroposthion is the loose "snout" that hangs beyond the meatus of the penis. It may be tubelike, or resemble a spigot (Fig. 11.2).

In some argument about the merits of IMC (infant male circumcision), some authors claim that it is this acroposthion that was removed in ancient times, while the posthe was usually left, but modern "medical" IMC removes both [1].

The nomenclature, terminology and definition of the macroposthia is confusing in literature; as we can see in the International Classification of Diseases, 11th Revision (ICD-11), which gave a code: GB05.0 for redundant prepuce, with a short description: "A condition of the foreskin, caused by determinants arising during the antenatal period, this condition is characterized by the presence of excess foreskin tissue". https://icd.who.int/browse11/l-m/en#/http://id.who.int/icd/entity/1720564326

Another confusion came from merging between akroposthia and phimosis as in: "ICD 605" which gave a code for both; redundant prepuce and phimosis.

Akroposthia

Dictionaries usually give two definitions of this adjective: (1) abundant, copious, excessive; and (2) spare, surplus, turning to advantage. It was suggested that the justification used by surgeons is from the first; i.e., "excessive," or hypertrophic, and that is borne out by the writings of the nineteenth and early twentieth centuries [2].

We could counter with the questions: (1) how is this judged in respect of what may be considered normal? and (2) how can it be judged in light of the growth changes that will occur in the penis with puberty? The diagnosis is essentially a presumption; some authors claim that all boys have an acroposthion at birth, others considered the normal length of the prepuce of an adult is 6.4 cm (range 4.8–9.2 cm) [3].

Historical Background

The longer prepuce often serves as the object of erotic interest and as a signifier of the sexually attractive male along the history, the Greeks valued the longer over the shorter prepuce in relation to the length of the entire penis, and the smaller over the larger penis as a whole. The evolution of Greek and Roman medical conceptualizations of preputial aesthetics, utilizing evidence found in classical medical texts as well as clues from literature, legal sources, and art. A conclusive picture emerges that the Greeks valued the longer prepuce and pathologized the penis characterized by a deficient prepuce—especially one that had been surgically ablated—under the disease concept of lipodermos (Microposthia). The medical conceptualization of lipodermos is also placed in the historical context of the legal efforts to abolish ritual circumcision throughout the Seleucid and Roman empires [4, 5].

Significance and Presentation of Macroposthia

Diagnosis of macroposthia is essentially a presumption; there is no follow up for cases diagnosed early at childhood to know if macroposthia is retained into adulthood, or just it provides an extra skin for later penile growth.

Foreskin types were classified according to its length as:

- Long (with the preputial orifice located beyond glans meatus and entirely covering the glans)
- Medium (with the preputial orifice located between meatus and glans corona),
- Short (with the preputial orifice located between corona and coronal sulcus).

  From Fig. 11.2; we can appreciate the wide normal variation in the length of the preputial tip (The part of the prepuce extended from the preputial ring proximally to the level of urinary meatus) (Chap. 5).

  Of course cases considered to be an abnormal "macroposthetic" will had a longer and usually disfigured preputial tip, but usually they had a prow glans and high or long frenulum with more extensive frenular delta (Fig. 11.3).

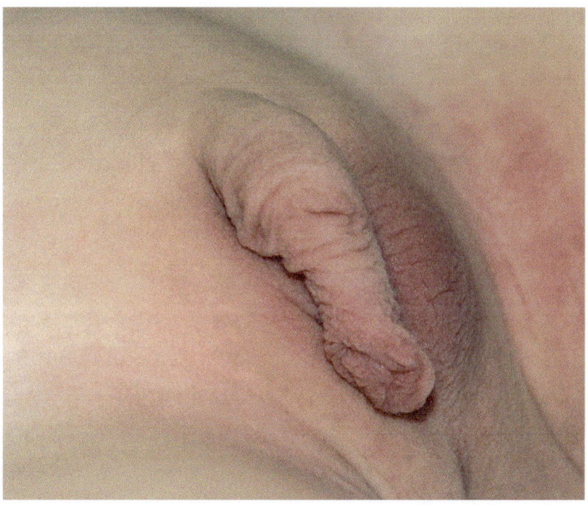

Fig. 11.3 Long disfigured macroposthia

In a rare occasions the prepuce in macroposthia is extensively puckered, corrugated, with many furrows and hyperpigmented (Fig. 11.4).

We didn't encounter any high incidence of phimosis associating macroposthia, instead; the long redundant preputial tip may acquire a normally wide preputial ring (Fig. 11.5).

But the long redundant foreskin during infancy in macroposthia is more liable to

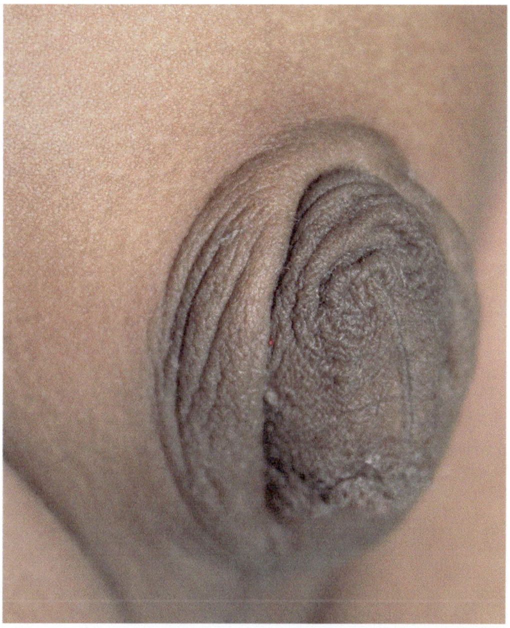

Fig. 11.4 A rare case of macroposthia with a highly wrinkled dark prepuce

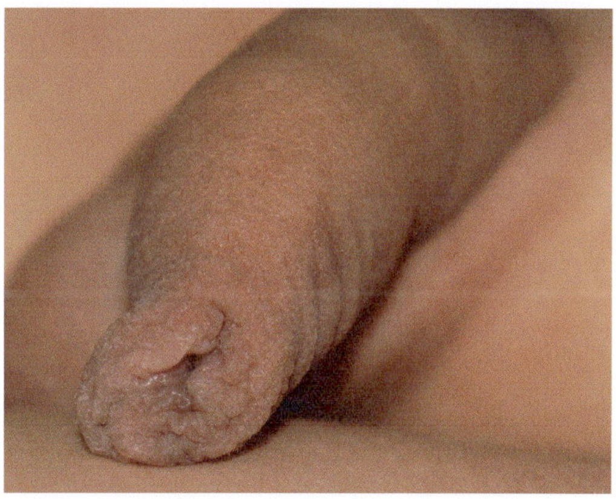

Fig. 11.5 Macroposthia with a wide preputial ring

trauma, contact dermatitis (Fig. 11.6), different sorts of infections; posthitis and balanoposthitis (Fig. 11.7). Repeated attacks of infection and healing by fibrosis, may end with losing the electricity of the preputial ring with a subsequent phimosis. This could explain the coincidence of phimosis and redundant long prepuce along mankind history, and this could justify the recommendation raised by some authors for committing circumcision for such cases.

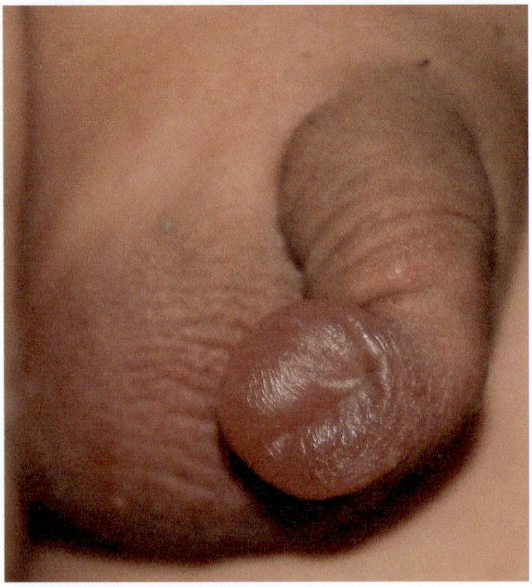

Fig. 11.6 Oedematous preputial tip, as a manifestation of contact dermatitis in macroposthia

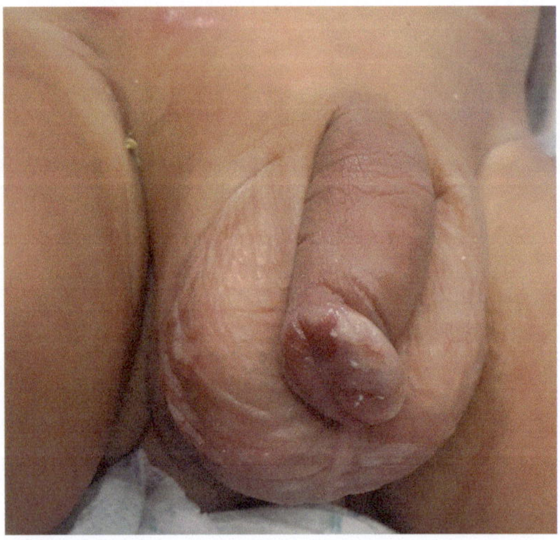

Fig. 11.7 Severe fungal infection at the tip of macroposthia

Velazquez et al. [6] found a 77% of non cancer population cases had long foreskin and that only 7% of those cases were phimotic. Cancer patients showed long foreskin in 78% of the cases, and phimosis was significantly frequent in this group (52%) as compared with the other ($p < 0.001$).

Elderly males with redundant prepuce, usually have a hyperplasia and hypertrophy of the prepuce. Men with an excessive prepuce could be at risk of premature ejaculation (PE), which may be due to higher penile sensitivity of the long preputial surface.

In his study, Gallo L. [7] founded that an excessive prepuce is very common in patients with lifelong PE: overall 59.1% of patients complaining of PE had an excessive prepuce. This high prevalence may reflect a scientific explanation in that men with an excessive prepuce have higher penis sensitivity, as the foreskin, as extensively discussed before, is the most sensitive part of the human penis.

Macroposthia if persist at adulthood it may presents with symptoms of dyspareunia, infection of urinary system, with a subsequent invasion of other genital system (epididymis, testis, seminal vesicle and prostate). A study results showed an association between foreskin length and the odds of chronic prostatitis/chronic pelvic pain syndrome (CP/CPPS). When the foreskin length covered up more than half of the glans penis, there were greater odds for CP/CPPS. This possible mechanism might result from interaction between pathogens and dendritic cells in the inner foreskin, consequently activating T-cells to mediate allergic inflammation in the prostate and producing the autoimmunizations causing CP/CPPS [8].

When the foreskin length reached an advanced level, the turbulent flow of urine will increase the pressure of lower urinary tract, causing the onset of voiding problems associated with the symptoms index.

Other important significance of macroposthia is the rate and varieties of complications following circumcision of an infant with long redundant prepuce; such cases may be subjected to redo after sometimes in response to the family wish, who are usually not seeing an exposed glans after incomplete removal of prepuce.

Also cases of macroposthia usually will end with a jeopardised frenulum after circumcision. Macroposthic child may be in need for excision of the excess preputial skin during the further penile growth along adulthood, when the penis grows up, so subsequantly such cases may had a scared or tethered penile skin.

Associated Anomalies

We don't believe that the degree of preputial meatus widening or retractability were dependent on the length of the foreskin. Some authors stated that "Circumcision is indicated in the presence of an unusually long foreskin." Others may be confounded between long prepuce and phimosis; and considering circumcision for both conditions [9].

Usually cases of macroposthia detected in anatomically normal penis, but few cases of MIP may be manifested with a large redundant foreskin, the abnormally wide urinary meatus may be hypospadiac or epispadic, so macroposthia may be an obvious manfestation of MIP [10] (Figs. 11.8 and 11.9).

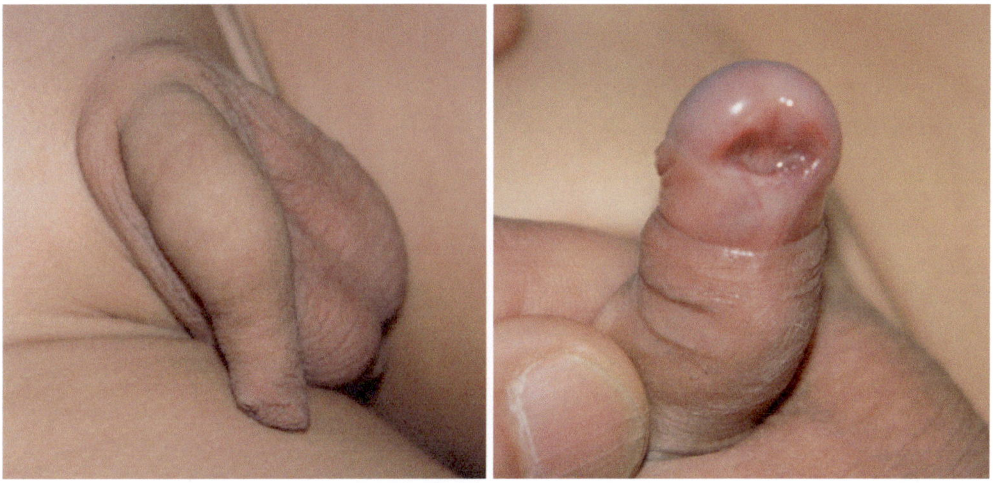

Fig. 11.8 A case of macroposthia with an intact prepuce hiding a megameatus

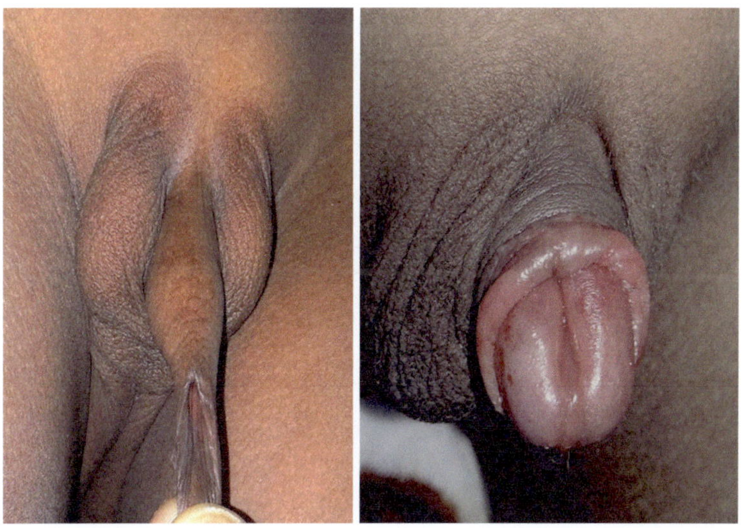

Fig. 11.9 A rare case of long macroposthic prepuce, when retracted revealed an isolated epispadias

Differential Diagnosis

The crucial point which is not yet settled; is how long prepuce at a specific age could be diagnosed as a normal variant? and how long is the prepuce which could be diagnosed as a pathological macroposthia?.

Cases of macroposthia have to be differentiated from cases of macrophallus and preputial lymphedema. Other cases which may leads to preputial enlargement as neoplasm and cysts are usually distinguishable. Also cases of macroposthia have to be differentiated from another misleading similar congenital entity of congenital megaprepuce.

Congenital Megaprepuce (CMP): "Preputial Bladder"

Megaprepuce is a congenital anomaly of the prepuce, which characterized by congenitally extensive redundancy of the inner preputial skin over a normal penile shaft and glans, which presented as an enormously capacious preputial sac, engulfing the whole penis or even the upper scrotum, with urine accumulation in this sac, prompting the term of "preputial bladder" (Fig. 11.10).

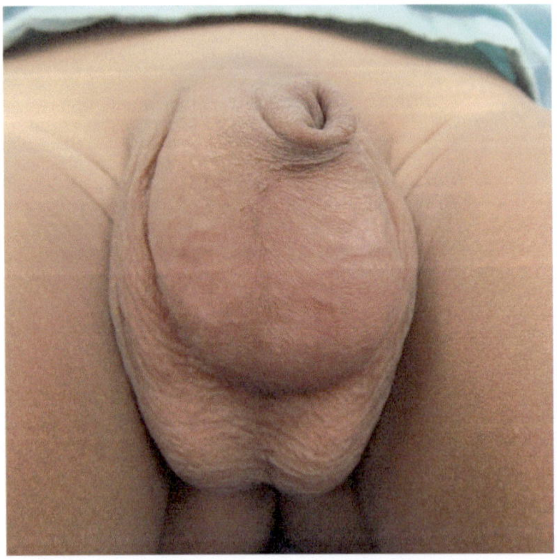

Fig. 11.10 A 12 months boy with a CMP and urine accumulates in the preputial sac giving a picture of a preputial bladder

Cardinal signs for diagnosis of CMP:

- Down ward ballooning of the preputial sac during micturition (Fig. 11.11).
- Squeezing of the accumulated urine reveals a redundant capacious prepuce (Fig. 11.12).
- Phimosis, and unretractable prepuce (Fig. 11.13).
- Extensive expansion of the inner prepuce (Figs. 11.14 and 11.15).

Other less frequent signs:

- Evidence of superimposed infection, usually from the retained urine in the preputial sac (Fig. 11.13).

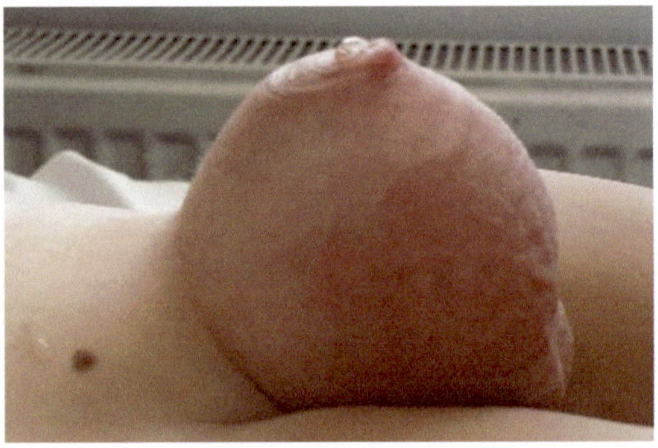

Fig. 11.11 Another case of CMP with a huge balloting of the preputial sac

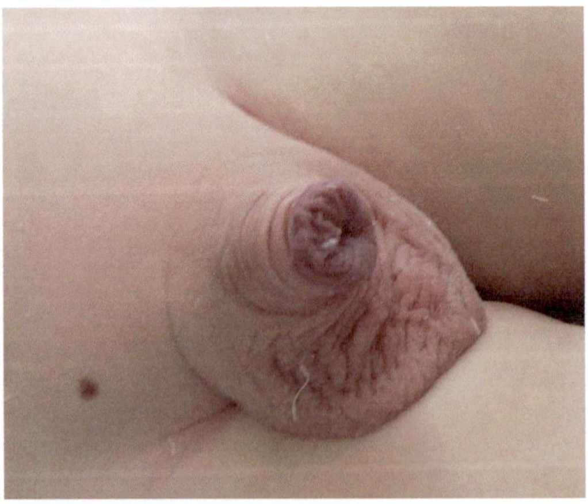

Fig. 11.12 The same case in Fig. 11.11 after evacuation of the preputial sac, redundant and congested inner prepuce is well seen from the preputial meatus

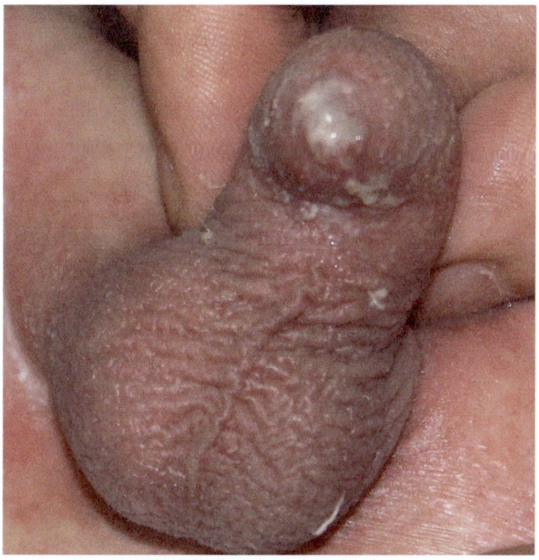

Fig. 11.13 A purulent discharge coming from a preputial meatus after evacuation of urine from the preputial bladder

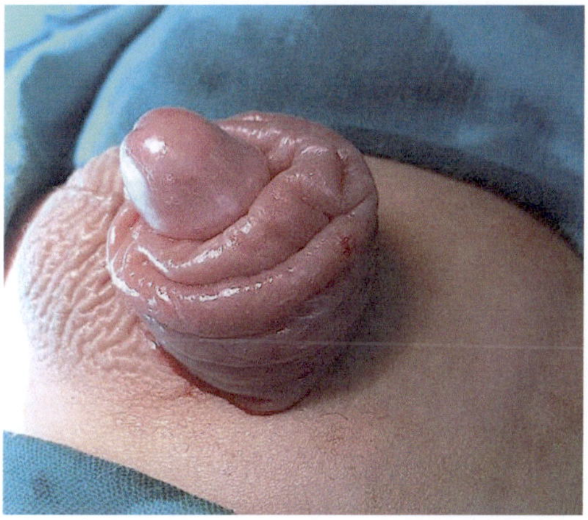

Fig. 11.14 Capacious redundant inner prepuce before surgical reconstruction

- Buried or concealed penis.
- Webbed penis.

Megaprepuce is not an old disease, as the first case was described only at 1994, and since then increasing numbers of patients with CM have been reported [11].

CMP can be especially confusing with cases of macroposthia, as this rare pathology are given an ill-defined nomenclature, various terms such as buried penis, trapped penis, webbed, concealed, or entrapped penis were all seemingly used interchangeably in the past. Till now; most cases of CMP are discussed under the titles of buried or concealed penis, and most of researches consider it as a subtype of buried penis, and most the discussion directed mainly to the different surgical procedures, without discussing the etiology, incidence or pathogenesis [12].

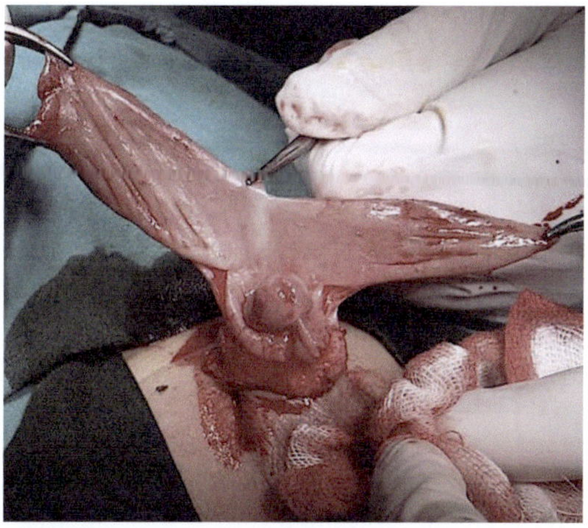

Fig. 11.15 Excision of the hugely extended inner prepuce encircling the coronal sulcus

Mike O'Brien [13] defined the condition as follow: A buried penis, sometimes referred to as a Congenital Megaprepuce, tends to present between 6 and 12 months of age with a history of significant, spherical ballooning on micturition.

Cases of CMP have to be differentiated from rare cases of megalopenis and megalourethra, our policy is to do a micturating cystourethrography not to confirm the diagnosis, but to rule out any possible associated anomalies.

Timing of Intervention

One of the most important aspects of CMP is early recognition and the proper age of surgical correction. It is reported that a common misbelief among parents that the child would eventually grow out of the appearance of their penis. Liu et al. recommended waiting until completion of toilet training to initiate surgical treatment [14].

As most cases may have a superimposed UTI and usually there is a difficulty in proper bladder evacuation; so our trend is an early surgical intervention. (Fig. 11.15).

The understanding of the aetiopathogenesis and the long-term outcomes of correctional repair of congenital megaprepuce (CMP) remains unestablished. Different techniques have been described, however optimum results have been difficult to achieve [15].

Proper excision of the excess inner prepuce, preservation of dartos fascia and either refashioning of the prepuce (preputioplasty) or circumcision according to families wishes is our trend (Fig. 11.15).

References

1. Cuckow PM, Rix G, Mouriquand PDE. Preputial plasty: a good alternative to circumcision. J Pediatr. 1994;29:561–3.
2. Hodges FM. The history of phimosis from antiquity to the present. In: Denniston GC, Hodges FM, Milos MF, editors. Male and female circumcision: medical, legal, and ethical considerations in pediatric practice. New York: Kluwer/Plenum; 1999. p. 37–62.
3. McGrath K. Variations in penile anatomy and their contribution to medical mischief. In: Denniston GC, Hodges FM, Milos MF, editors. Circumcision and human rights. Dordrecht: Springer; 2009. https://doi.org/10.1007/978-1-4020-9167-4_8.
4. Dickinson RL. Human sex anatomy: a topographical hand atlas. 2nd ed. Baltimore: Williams & Wilkins; 1949.
5. Kühn DCG, editor. Galenis de usu partium corporis humani, 11.13. Medicorum græcorum, vol. 3. Leipzig: Cnobloch; 1822, p. 898.
6. Velazquez EF, Bock A, Soskin A, et al. Preputial variability and preferential association of long phimotic foreskins with penile cancer. Am J Surg Pathol. 2003;27(7):994–8.
7. Gallo L. The prevalence of an excessive prepuce and the effects of distal circumcision on premature ejaculation. Arab J Urol. 2017;15:140–7. https://doi.org/10.1016/j.aju.2017.02.002.
8. Zhao YY, Xu DL, Zhao FJ, et al. Redundant prepuce increases the odds of chronic prostatitis/chronic pelvic pain syndrome (CP/CPPS). Asian J Androl. 2014;16(5):774–7. https://doi.org/10.4103/1008-682X.131706.
9. Huang C, Song P, Xu C, Wang R, Wei L, Zhao X. Comparative efficacy and safety of different circumcisions for patients with redundant prepuce or phimosis: a network meta-analysis. Int J Surg. 2017;43:17–25. https://doi.org/10.1016/j.ijsu.2017.04.060. Epub 2017 May 15.
10. Fahmy MAB. The spectrum of genital median raphe anomalies among infants undergoing ritual circumcision. J Pediatr Urol. 2013. http://www.sciencedirect.com/science/article/pii/S147751311200294X#FCANote.
11. O'Brien A, AMJ S, Frank JD. Phimosis or congenital megaprepuce. Br J Urol. 1994;73:719–20.
12. Werner Z, Hajiran A, Al-Omar O. Congenital megaprepuce: literature review and surgical correction. Case Rep Urol. 2019;2019:1–6. https://doi.org/10.1155/2019/4584609.
13. O'Brien M. In: Losty PD, et al., editors. Rickham's neonatal surgery. London: Springer; 2018. p. 1227. https://doi.org/10.1007/978-1-4471-4721-3_69.
14. Liu X, He D-W, Hua Y, Zhang D-Y, Wei G-H. Congenital completely buried penis in boys: anatomical basis and surgical technique. BJU Int. 2013;112(2):271–5.
15. Summerton DJ, McNally J, Denny AJ, Malone PS. Congenital megaprepuce: an emerging condition–how to recognize and treat it. BJU Int. 2000;86(4):519–22. https://doi.org/10.1046/j.1464-410X.2000.00509.x.

Prepucioplasty for Hooded Foreskin

12

Introduction

Prepuce is defined as the fold of skin that covers the head of the penis and it is also known as foreskin. Only about one in every 20 boys is born with a retractable foreskin. First known use of the term prepuce was in fifteenth century, in the meaning defined. The prepuce is attached to the glans by the inner prepucial skin fold called fraenulum. The prepuce covers the glans penis in the adult male either partially or completely and protects the glans penis from friction and dryness. Removal of the prepuce exposes the glans to foreign stimuli which changes the colour of skin, the texture and moisture of the glans and dulls the special sensitive receptors. The colour tends to change from a red-purple to a light pink in Caucasians and the texture changes from a glossy finish to a matte finish and becomes dull rather than shiny.

Development of Prepuce

The glans penis is at first naked, not covered by a developing prepuce and is demarcated from the shaft of the organ by a shallow groove. Development of the prepuce is initiated by ~12 weeks with the appearance of the preputial placode, a novel structure, a dorsal thickening of the epidermis on the dorsal aspect of the developing glans [1]. During differentiation of the cavernous tissue of the penis, growth of this tissue does not occur at as rapid a rate as that of the ectodermal tissues, and the latter becomes thrown into folds on the dorsum of the penis. Bilateral preputial laminae from the lateral aspect of the preputial placode expand ventrally and joins the preputial folds fusing in the ventral midline (foreskin) covering all of the glans at ~16 weeks gestation. The line of fusion between the prepucial laminae ventrally in midline forms the frenulum. Preputial development is in some way linked to urethral development within the glans since in hypospadias, preputial tissue is absent ventrally, and excessive dorsally (classic dorsal hooded foreskin) [1]. The most common location of hypospadias is at the junction of the glans and coronal margin defined as the junction of glans with the penile shaft [1]. This position corresponds to interface between the two disparate mechanisms of urethral development (urethral fold fusion events in the shaft and direct urethral plate canalization in the glans). Clearly, the tubular elements generated by these two disparate morphogenetic mechanisms must join at or near the glans/shaft interface, which presumably accounts for the high incidence of hypospadias at this location. In contrast, the less prevalent but more severe forms of hypospadias occur in the penile shaft where disruption of urethral fold fusion occurs. The human male urethra forms within the glans penis between 12 and 18 weeks of

M. A. B. Fahmy, *Normal and Abnormal Prepuce*, https://doi.org/10.1007/978-3-030-37621-5_12

gestation by a unique mechanism distinctly different from urethral development within the penile shaft. The process involves a sequential canalization of the urethral plate followed by mesenchymal confluence and epithelial remodelling to form a "stand alone" tubular urethra. The presence of androgen receptors in the morphogenetic processes in both the shaft and the glans is an important mechanistic theme requiring further investigation during normal penile development and in the aetiology of hypospadias. Hence developmental anomaly may be seen in any of the part of the prepuce namely the median raphe, fraenulum, and body of the prepuce itself.

Types of Prepuce

Aposthia (absent Prepuce) with normal development of urethra is very rare and the foreskin of the penis is missing in a normally developed penis and urethra. Microposthia is a condition of having a very small foreskin and diagnosis of it is clinched on the basis of partially seen glans in a flaccid penis. On the basis of the extent of retraction and exposure of glans the prepuce may be classified into five [2]:

- *Type 0*: Full retraction, not tight behind glans, or easy retraction, limited only by congenital adhesions to the glans
- *Type 1*: Full retraction of the foreskin, tight behind the glans
- *Type 2*: Partial exposure of glans, prepuce (not congenital adhesions) limiting factor
- *Type 3*: Partial retraction, the meatus just visible
- *Type 4*: Slight retraction, but some distance remains between the tip and glans, that is neither meatus nor glans can be exposed
- *Type 5*: Absolutely no retraction is possible.

Variation in Fraenulum and Median Raphe

The prepuce consists of body of the prepuce, median raphe and the fraenulum. The midline line of fusion between the prepucial laminae ventrally forms the fraenulum and outer skin fusion creates the median raphe. The prepuce is attached to glans by this fraenulum in the midline ventrally. Usually the fraenulum is single and attaches the prepuce to glans ventrally ~~only~~ but very rarely fraenulum is noted dorsally. This may cause partial (Fig. 12.1a, b) or even complete dorsal attachment

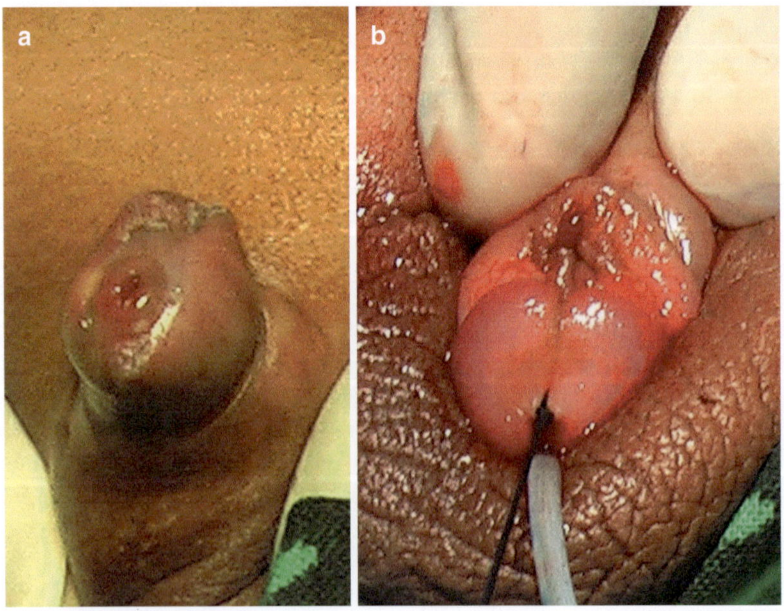

Fig. 12.1 Figure showing both dorsal and ventral fraenulum. (**a**) Dorsal hood with bifid at the top, (**b**) Retraction of prepuce showing dorsal Fraenulum

(Fig. 12.2). In cases with well formed prepuce dorsally the patient may have two frenulae. Dorsally formed prepuce with tight fraenulum may pose problem during sexual intercourse and may need division/resection. The deviation of median raphe towards right or left ending on the prepuce is an important sign of penile torsion (Fig. 12.3a). The deviance of median raphe at end prepuce is a guide to assess the degree of torsion specially where prepuce is not retractable (Fig. 12.3b). The deviation of median raphe may start from penoscrotal junction to corona. Site of deviation of median raphe is an important sign of origin of the embryological abnormal event. Even in intact prepuce the site of deviance of median raphe shows the site of bifurcation of spongiosum and length of hypoplastic urethra (Fig. 12.4a, b).

Hooded Foreskin

The terminology of hooded Foreskin is used where the foreskin of a boy is wide open. It is the mildest form of hypospadias, and is mainly a cosmetic defect. This is also called hooded prepuce without hypospadias (Fig. 12.5) but in real sense it the hooded prepuce with glanular hypospadias. Usually the disfigurement of penis in the baby is noted at birth but sometimes it may diagnosed in elder boys or even routine medical examination

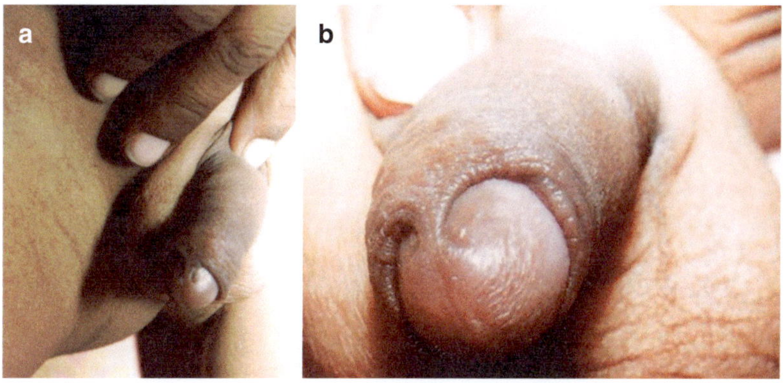

Fig. 12.2 Showing double fraenulum: (**a**, **b**) showing well formed tight fraenulum attached to mid-glans

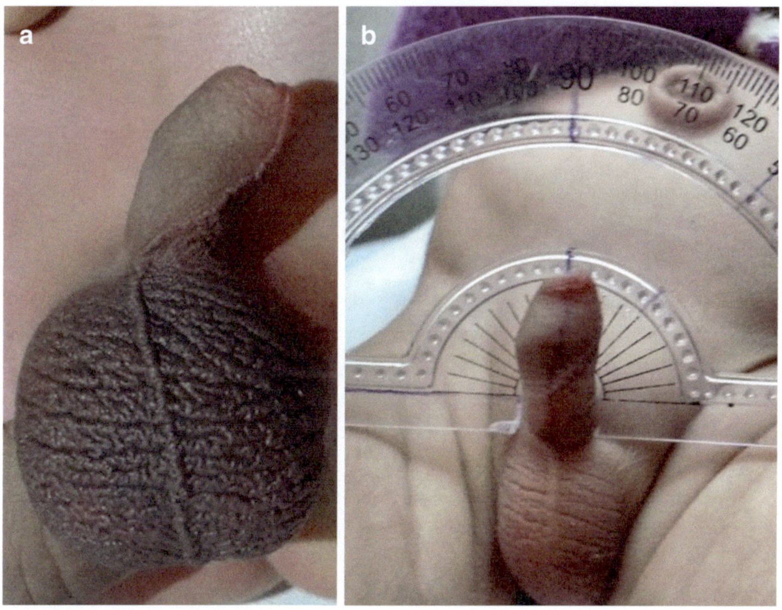

Fig. 12.3 Showing median raphe. (**a**) Deviance of median raphe towards left. (**b**) Measuring the degree of torsion by at the point of ending median raphe on prepuce

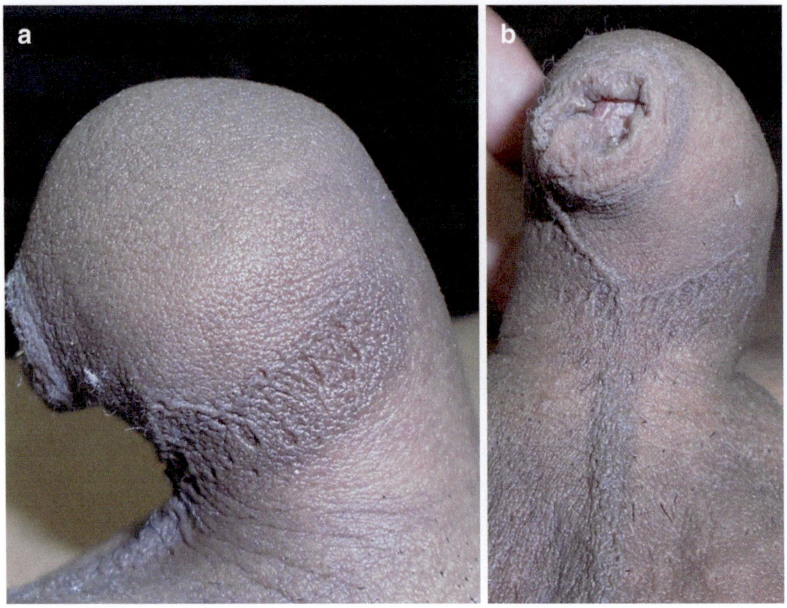

Fig. 12.4 (**a**, **b**) Intact prepuce with deviance of median raphe starting point embryological abnormality

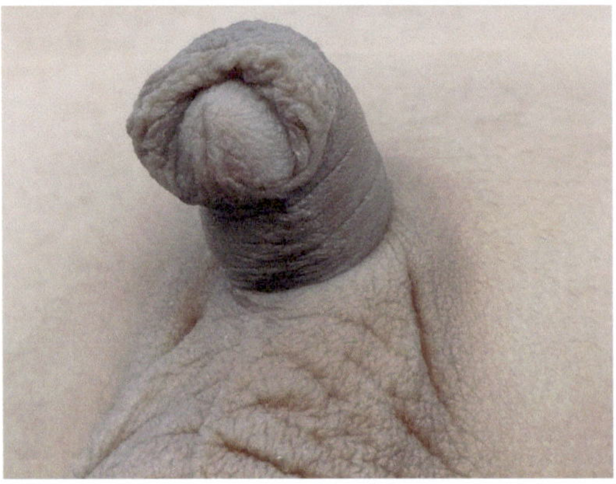

Fig. 12.5 Showing typical appearance of a hooded foreskin

at the time of service entry or during examination for another reasons.

Treatment options for hooded foreskin are:

1. No intervention: As the condition is of cosmetic concern only, may be left as such in childhood. This will allow the child to make a decision regarding if he wants treatment for the hooded foreskin at adulthood. The downside is that if he decides that he wants surgery when he is older, the operation will take more out of him.
2. Prepucioplasty: Penile disfigurement is not acceptable in modern day hypospadiology. Fore skin reconstruction creates aesthetically normal looking penis and give the chance to decide himself for circumcision later in life. The technique of prepucioplasty is same as in cases hypospadias.
3. Complete circumcision: If chosen by the parents the circumcision is a simple day care surgery. The technique of choice for circumcision in infants with preputial defect remains uncertain and usually is performed by conventional dissection technique but it can be done with the plastibell technique based on the usual manner or with minor modification. The disadvantage with plastibell technique is the incomplete coverage of bell by foreskin but does not alter the results. However, there is a theoretical risk of urethral injury if the ventral shaft skin is manipulated, as the corpus spongiosum is not well developed, and the urethra may be close to the skin. There are more chances of injury with this technique is patient has chordee. So the plastibell is only safe in child with hooded prepuce without hypospadias or mild hypospadias if chordee has been ruled out and this technique is choice of circumcision in such infants and children, if parents would prefer their son to be circumcised without glanuloplasty.

Classification of Prepuce in Hypospadias

Morphology of prepuce can have an impact on hypospadias repair. There are different types of prepuce with a difference in pattern of blood supply of the prepuce [3]. On the basis of length, prepuce is divided in to (Fig. 12.6):

1. Very Small
2. Small
3. Adequate
4. Normal Length
5. Normal prepuce

Morphology of prepuce in hypospadias: The prepuce is usually used for the neourethra and penile body skin reconstruction for severe hypospadias but where prepuce can be spared it is used for prepucioplasty. There is a definite correlation between the morphological and vascularization types of prepuces, so the morphological types may be guide to see the adequacy of the preputial skin for the longitudinal island flap and preputioplasty. Morphology of the prepuce and correlated vascular pattern help us to predict complications and, thus, to select the best operative technique of 1 or 2-stage surgery.

Based on the morphology and abnormalities of the prepuce in hypospadias are classified as

(a) Monk's hood" or "1 humped": There is an area raised on the dorsal called hump and this may range from being flat to big hump. A typical hypospadiac prepuce is shaped like a hood or hump. This deformity is the result of ventro-dorsal disproportion. Depending on the connection between the prepuce ridges during embryogenesis, one (Fig. 12.7) or two humps (Fig. 12.8) appear on the prepuce.

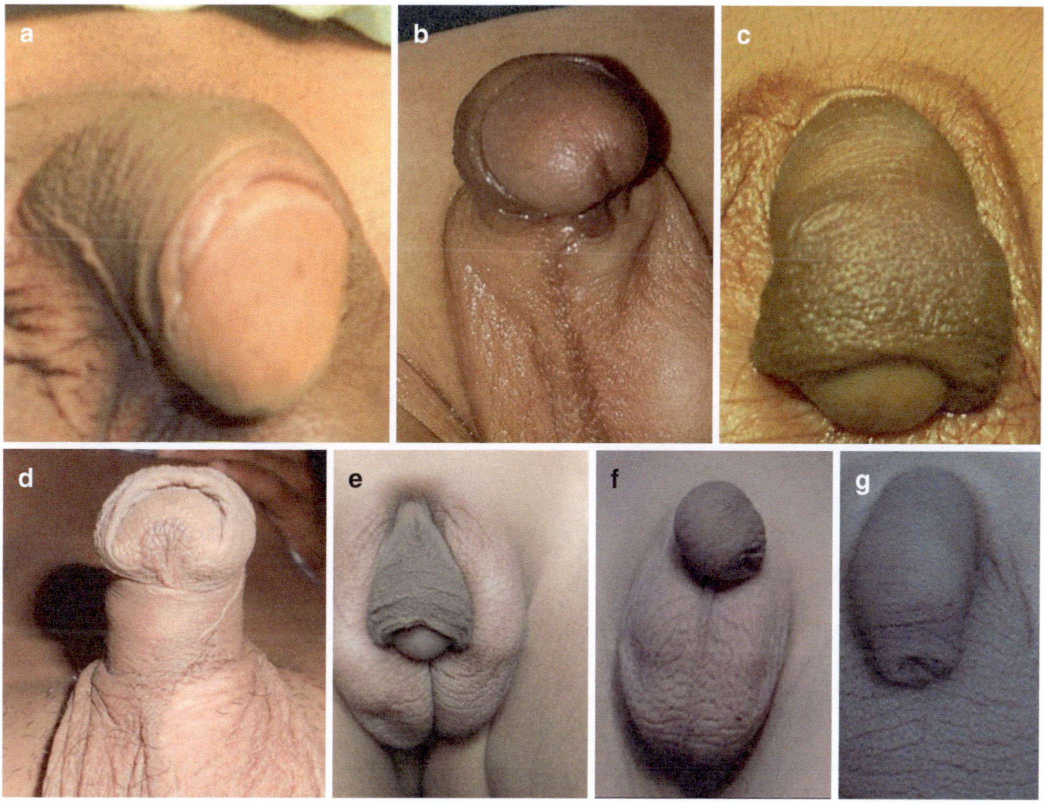

Fig. 12.6 Showing various sizes of the prepuce. (**a**, **b**) Small prepuce, (**c**) Adequate, (**d**) Collar Scarf, (**e**) Normal length, (**f**, **g**) Normal prepuce

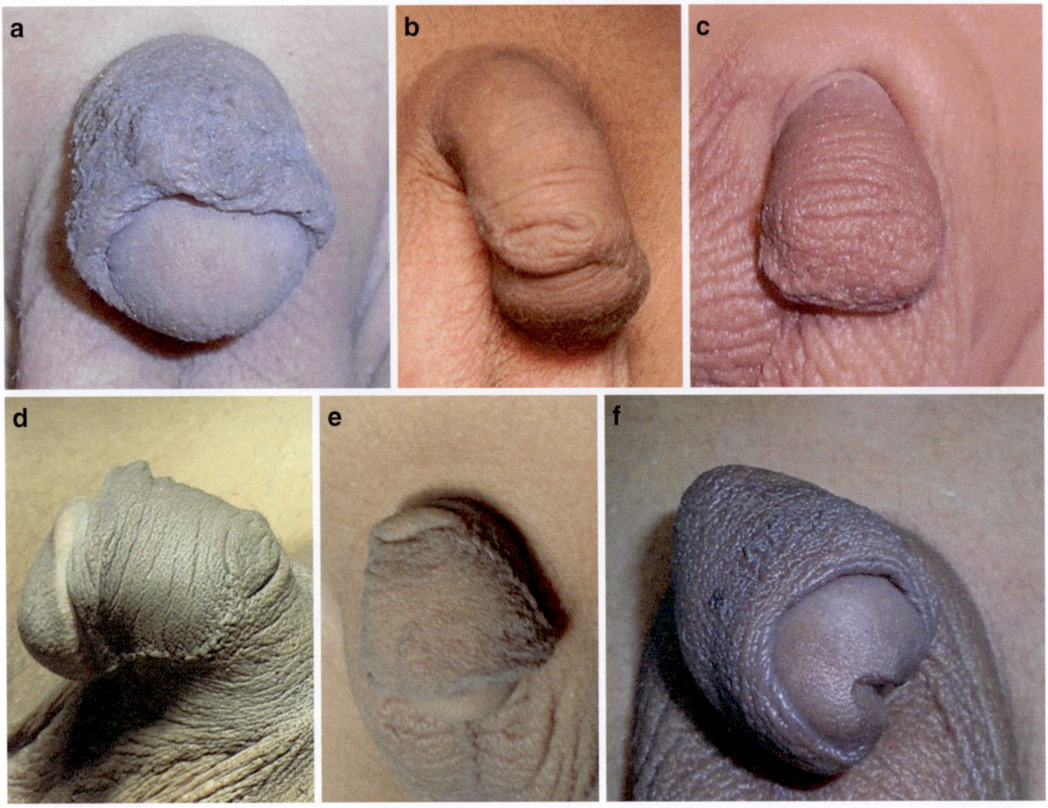

Fig. 12.7 Figure showing Monks Hood/Single Hood. (**a**–**c**) Distal one distal hypospadias, (**d**–**f**) Proximal one with severe hypospadias

This may be seen distal one at the site over the glans (Fig. 12.7a–c) and proximal to corona (Fig. 12.7d–f). The site of hump gives a clue of the severity of hypospadias as this is the site of staring of the embryological abnormality and large hump as shown in Fig. 12.7f may give problem in skin closure if we resect the hump and disfigurement if we keep the hump. The hump may be small or large and patients with large hump (Fig. 12.7e, f) may not be suitable for preputioplasty.

(b) "Cobra eyes" or Two hump: This is more common in distal hypospadias. These again can be divided in to distal as distal hypospadias (Fig. 12.8a–c) and proximal showing severe hypospadias (Fig. 12.8d–f). Site of hump is directly co-related with severity of hypospadias (Fig. 12.9a, b). Double bull prepuce may also be present in chordee without hypospadias with intact prepuce (Fig. 12.6f). Patients with big may not be suitable for preputioplasty as Bull's eye may be seen on prepuce postoperatively leading to disfigurement (Fig. 12.10a, b).

(c) Triple Hump: This anomaly is very rare, not reported in the literature. The embryology of this not known. There are three humps two and third one is seen at the margin of the prepuce. (Fig. 12.11). Preputioplasty in such cases is not feasible but since the hump has a good blood supply of inner prepuce these cases are suitable for inner prepucial flap urethroplasty, otherwise need circumcision for cosmesis.

(d) "Flat" and "V"-shaped: The flat and v-shaped (Fig. 12.6e) prepuces occur often in severe hypospadias. This results from a higher degree of ventral hypoplasia and arrests the development of the prepuce.

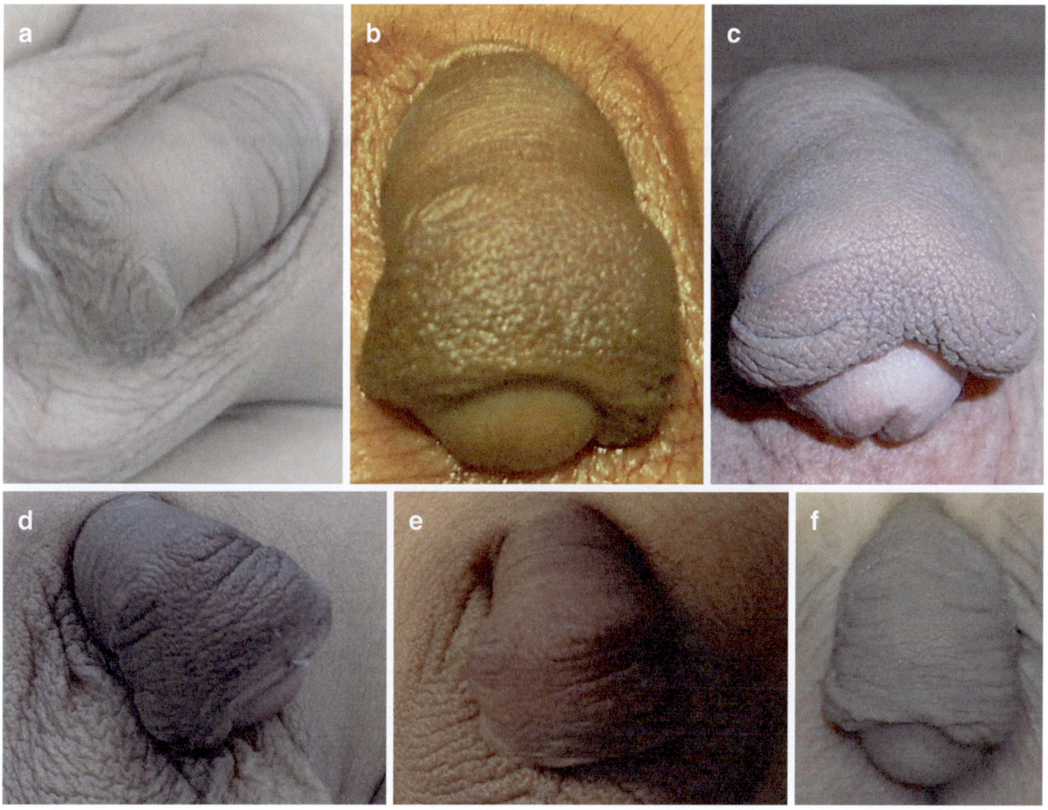

Fig. 12.8 (**a–c**) Showing cobra eyes or double hump with distal hypospadias, (**d–f**) Showing hump with proximal hypospadias

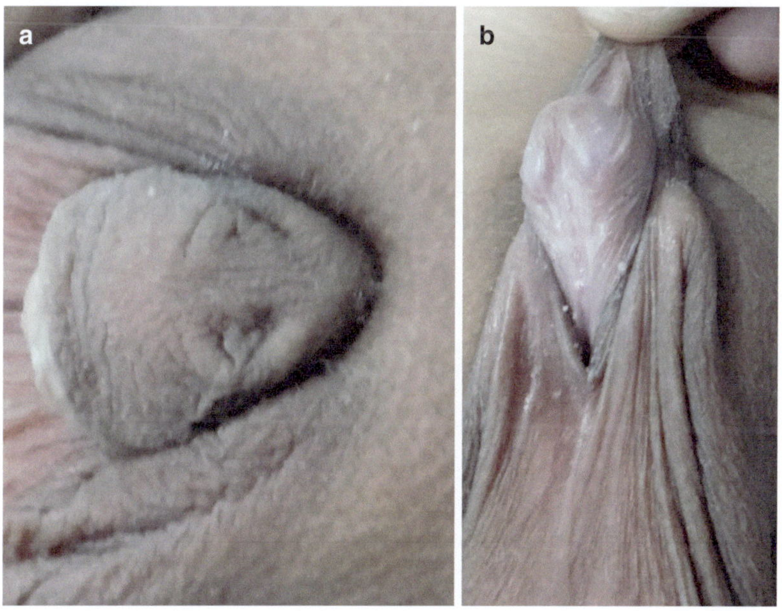

Fig. 12.9 Showing co-relation of site of hump and severity of hypospadias. (**a**) Hump at proximal penile region. (**b**) Penoscrotal hypospadias

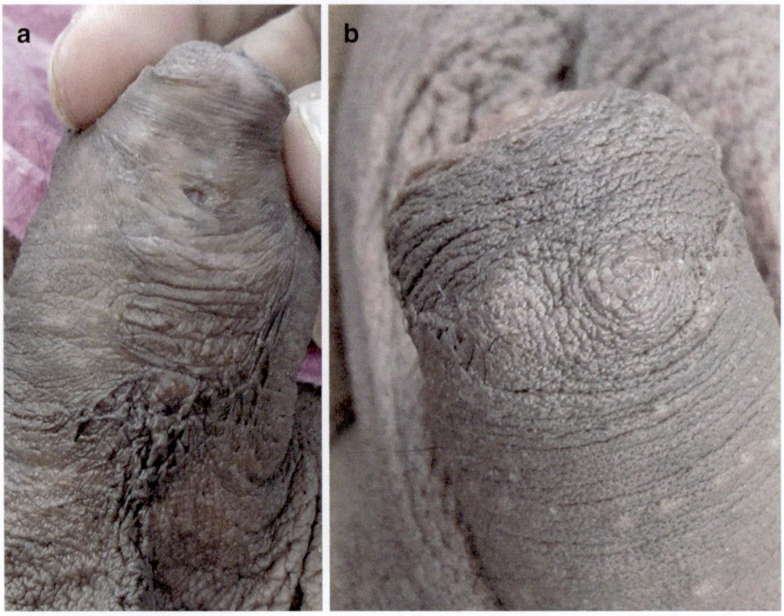

Fig. 12.10 Showing Post operative disfigurement in patients with prepucioplasty in double bull prepuce. (**a**) Preputial fistula, (**b**) Double bulls eye deformity

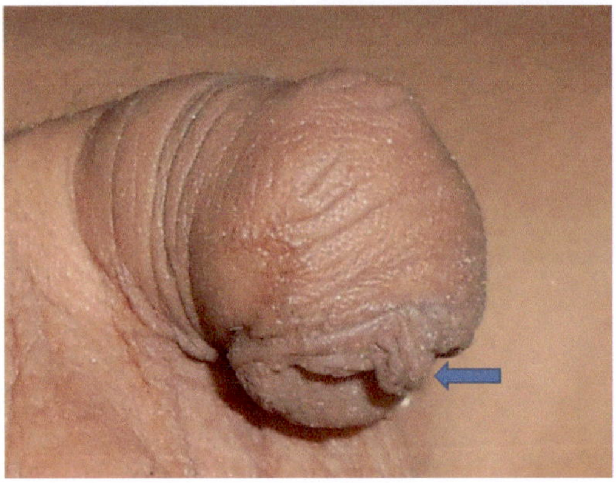

Fig. 12.11 Showing Triple hump Two humps on the dorsal surface, arrows marking the third hump at the margin of the prepuce

The v-shaped prepuce is usually present with penoscrotal transposition. Preputioplasty is not feasible in these cases and hypospadias surgery is even more complicated because the underdeveloped preputium is not appropriate to correct the ventral deficiency. There may be difficulty in covering the ventral surface skin. Therefore, in such patients two stage hypospadias repair is a better choice.

(e) "Collar-scarf": Such a prepuce resembles a collar with an adequate size (Fig. 12.6d) and is commonly seen in distal hypospadias. The collar-scarf prepuce has a close connection on the ventral side with pillars of the hypoplastic corpus spongiosum at the base of the open glans. These prepuce are best suited for preputioplasty. Prepucial hood is adequate and margins can easily approximated to create fraenulum as well as large prepucial orifice. Care is taken while raising the glanular and prepucial flap not to injure the inner prepucial skin. Operative preparation of this structure is difficult and may result in injury and defect of the ventral part of the internal preputial skin, which makes reconstruction of the sub-glanular part of the penile skin difficult, ie formation of the mucosal collar. This type of prepuce is suitable for inner prepucial flap urethroplasty also.

(f) "Normal" (intact): The normal prepuce may be found cases of variants of hypospadias like megameatus intact prepuce and chordee without hypospadias. Single or double hump be seen on the dorsal surface of shaft and the site of hump is indicative of severity of chordee without hypospadias (Fig. 12.6f).

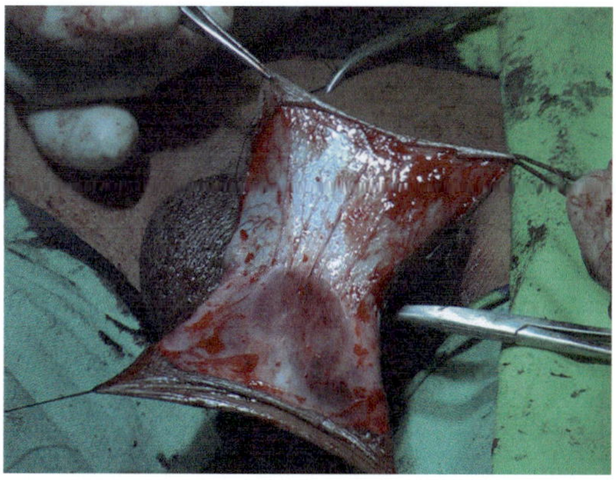

Fig. 12.12 Showing numerous vessels on the outer preputial skin

Prepuce may be classified based on vascular pattern of the prepuce

1. One blood vessel was predominant
2. Two blood vessels were predominant
3. Numerous blood vessels (≥3) were presented (Fig. 12.12)
4. No predominant blood vessel was presented (e.g., no definite axial vessel displayed a network distribution).

All types of predominant vessels were axially distributed, and then showed a transverse distribution and formed numerous reticular lateral branches at the junction of the inner and outer prepuce. The predominant vessels in the same pedicle displayed no obvious difference in their development, and a majority was symmetrically distributed along the middle line of the pedicle. Prepuce of type one with prominent single vessel and type IV without prominent vessel blood supply of margins of the dorsal hood may be compromised, hence these patients may not be suitable for preputioplasty.

Preputioplasty in Hooded Prepuce With/Without Hypospadias

Hypospadias is one of the most common congenital anomalies, having incidence of one in 300 male newborns [4]. With a common goal to achieve normal or near normal penile anatomy and good functional outcome, numerous techniques have been described in literature for hypospadias repair. Presently the most common procedure to be performed is TIP (Tubularized Incised Plate) urethroplasty wherein the prepuce is used over the dorsal dartos to form a water proof covering over the neourethra. This results in a circumcised penis [5, 6]. But in recent times, circumcision has become less acceptable to both the parents/patients as well as the treating physician. Hence, the rates of preputioplasty have increased significantly along with hypospadias repair. The prepuce can be preserved in cases where spongioplasty is done adequately and scrotal dartos or tunica vaginalis is left to cover the anastomosis.

Initially the only cases where preputioplasty was done were distal, coronal or glandular hypospadias cases without penile curvature and no requirement of penile degloving [7]. Since the advent of TIP repair the number of cases undergoing preputioplasty has increased significantly. It is now being done for both mid and proximal hypospadias with acceptable success. We had a well formed retractable prepuce with 88.9% satisfaction rate regarding outcome of surgery and cosmesis in the patients. The incidence of complications was also similar to complication rate in cases of proximal hypospadias repair without preputial reconstruction i.e., 11.10%.

Why Preputioplasty? The primary objective of hypospadias repair is reconstruction of a straight penis with the meatus at the tip along with normalization of erection. The urethral calibre should be adequate and uniform and the glans and shaft should appear symmetrical. The goal is to be as anatomically normal as possible. The human foreskin is highly innervated, and vascularised sensitive erogenous tissue. It plays an important role in normal human sexual response and is necessary for normal copulatory behaviour [8]. An understanding of this role is now emerging in the scientific literature. Removal of the foreskin (circumcision) may interfere with normal sexual function. Objectives in management of hypospadias are creating a straight penis, positioning of the meatus on the tip, normalization of erection and projectile stream in voiding, creating the urethra of adequate and uniform caliber, symmetry in appearance of glans and shaft and deceasing the complications. Basic Principle in management of any congenital anomaly is to restore the normal or near normal anatomy with the existing tissue or with supplementation of tissue. Many of the patients/parents want to preserve the prepuce in view of their religious sentiments. Prepucial reconstruction gives the child psychologically benefit of feeling equal to his colleagues for shape of his penis. Thirdly, as the foreskin is highly innervated and vascularised and plays an important role in normal sexual intercourse [8]. Dorsal dartos can be preserved by utilizing spongioplasty as a healthy tissue cover and then covering the neourethra with ventral dartos. In addition, a preserved prepuce can serve as a reserve of tissue in case the hypospadias repair is unsuccessful.

Preputioplasty in Hooded Prepuce With/Without Hypospadias Repair

Measuring Adequacy of Prepuce

Preputial reconstruction should be attempted in only those patients whose prepuce can be approximated in the midline without any tension at the level of coronal groove. If the ventral defect is large, reconstruction should not be attempted. There are different techniques to measure the adequacy of the prepuce for preputioplasty. The ideal one is to measure the glans breadth at corona and midglans (Fig. 12.13) and length and width of the prepuce (Fig. 12.14a, b) with the Vernier calipers, then decide the prepucioplasty. These dimensions also help in estimation of distal limit of preputial reconstruction. Though we can measure the exact length but it is cumbersome to measure with the callipers in a child. Other methods are the measuring by approximation of edges of preputial hood with finger and thumb or forceps (Fig. 12.15a, b) and three stay sutures. These are easy and can be done on table before proceeding for prepucioplasty.

Stay Suture Technique

The technique to assess prepucial width is by applying three stay sutures, one each at the level of the corona, the distal end of prepucial hood at the junction of inner and outer prepucial skin and the penile shaft skin at the level of corona after urethroplasty (Fig. 12.16a). The preputial skin is pulled over the glans by the second stay suture after fixing the inner prepucial skin at the corona

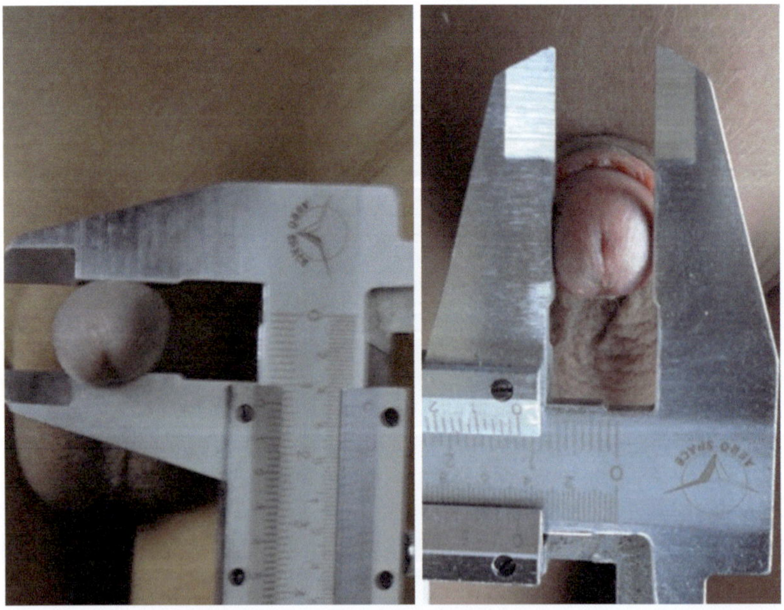

Fig. 12.13 Measuring the width of the glans using Vernier calipers

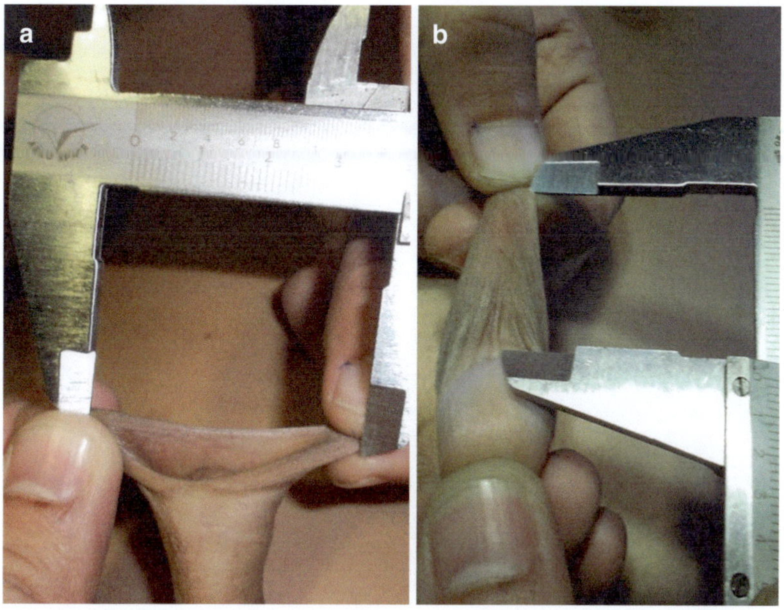

Fig. 12.14 Measuring the dimensions of the prepuce using Vernier calipers, (**a**) Measuring the width of prepuce, (**b**) Measuring the length of prepuce

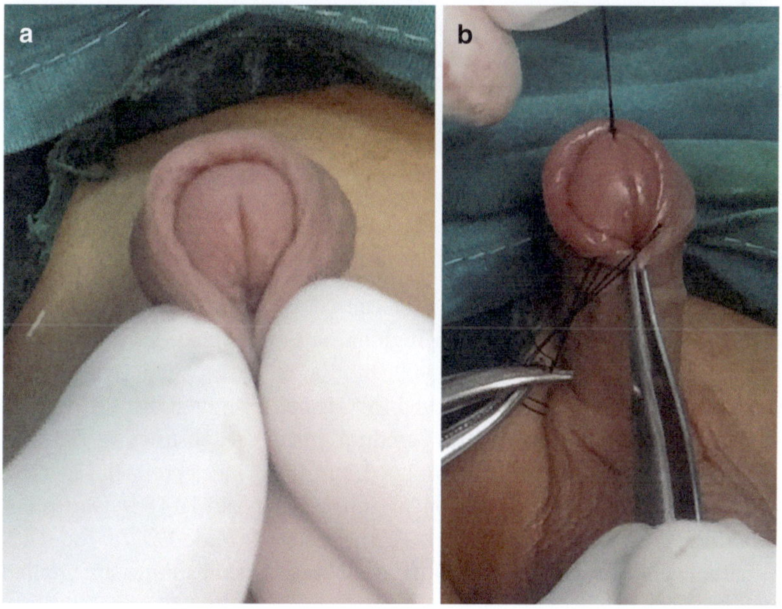

Fig. 12.15 Showing measurement of skin adequacy for prepucial reconstruction, (**a**) approximation with thumb and finger; (**b**) with forceps

by the first stay suture (Fig. 12.16b, c). Then the prepuce is retracted by the third stay suture. When the skin can easily be pulled over the glans and retracted, the prepucial hood is considered to be adequate, when the skin easily pulls up to cover glans and also retracts easily. After that suturing the inner preputial skin between first and second stay suture will reconstruct the fraenulum and inner layer of the prepuce; suturing of outer prepucial skin between stay suture second and third will reconstruct outer skin layer of the prepuce.

Surgical Techniques Three layer closure after three stay suture technique for tissue estimation is the most common technique used for preputial reconstruction. It can be performed in either general or regional anesthesia. General anesthesia is

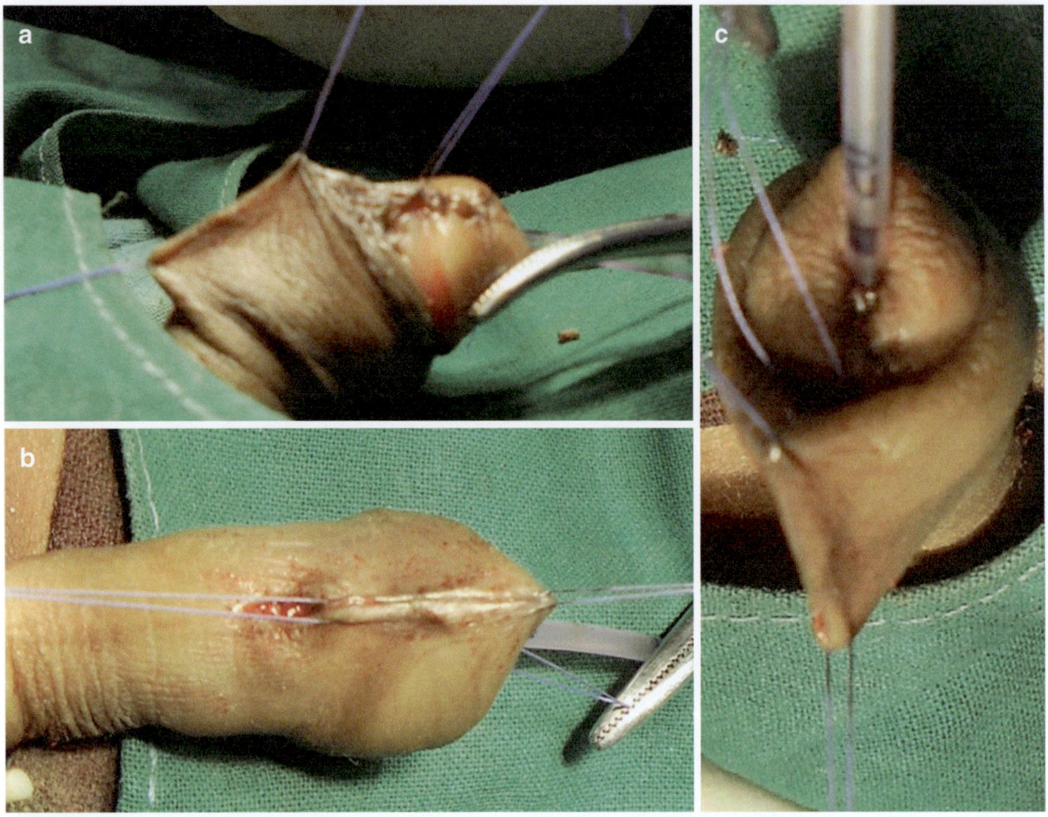

Fig. 12.16 Showing adequacy of prepuce for preputioplasty. (**a**) Photograph showing three sites of stay sutures. (**b**, **c**) Middle suture pulled up to see the adequacy of prepuce

preferable as it avoids the difficulty caused by penile engorgement occurring in regional anesthesia. After injecting one in 100,000 solution of adrenaline at the site of incision, and 'Y' shaped incision is given encircling the urethral plate (Fig. 12.17a). The incision is continued into the prepuce hood up to the junction of inner and outer prepucial skin (Fig. 12.17c). The next step is partial penile de-gloving (Fig. 12.17c). In those patients who also have chordee/torque incision is extended circumferentially in circumcoronal region along with Complete penile de-gloving is done (Fig. 12.18a, b).

Prepuce is reconstructed after neourethra is created by tubularization of urethral plate and spongioplasty (Figs. 12.17d and 12.18c, d). Waterproofing of neourethra with tunica vaginalis or scrotal dartos may or may not be done. The preputial edges are freshened and then the repair is performed in three layers. To begin, the first suture is placed at the corona (where the first stay suture is applied at the inner prepucial skin) and then sutured distally up to the second stay suture, thus reconstructing the fraenulum (Fig. 12.17d) and inner prepucial layer of prepuce (Figs. 12.17d, e and 12.18d). Dartos is sutured as the second layer (Figs. 12.17e, f and 12.18e, f) and then the outer skin sutures are applied from second to third stay suture to complete the preputioplasty (Figs. 12.17g and 12.18g). This procedure can be performed even in proximal hypospadias. First inner prepucial skin closure is done and then circumcoronal sutures are applied when complete penile degloving is done. This is followed by closure of dartos layer and skin closure (Figs. 12.17h, i and 12.18g, h). Suture material used is 5–7/0 polydioxanone according to the age of the child with interrupted sutures. Satisfactory results have been achieved.

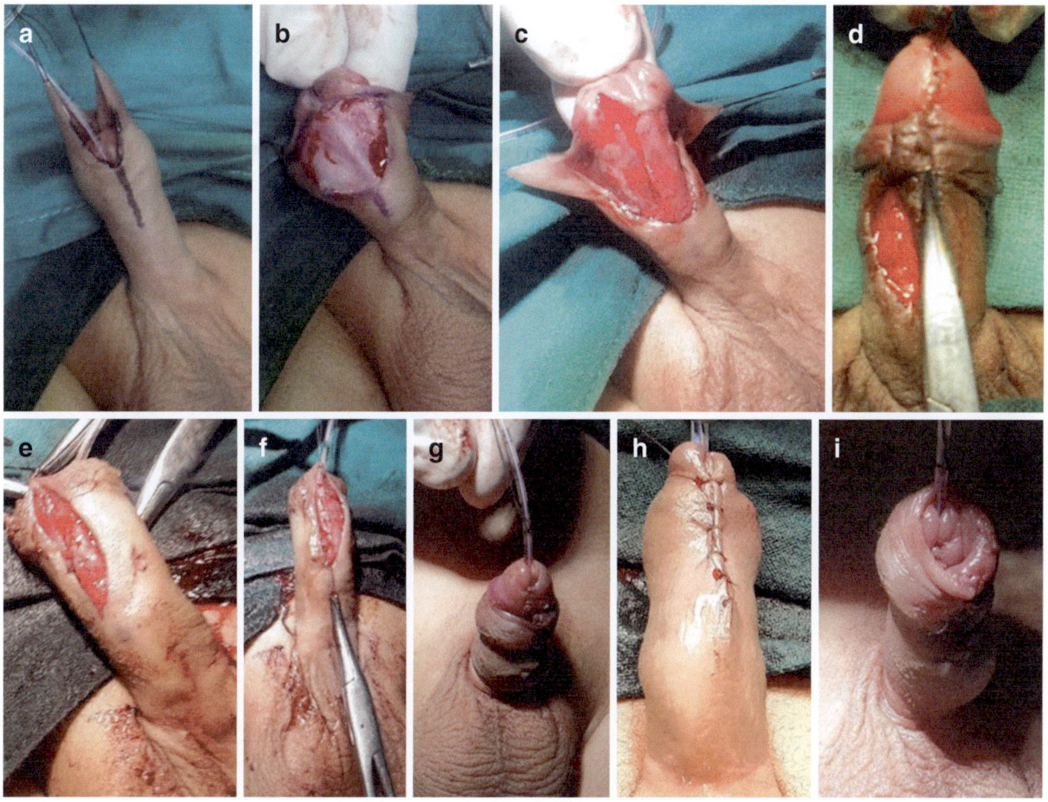

Fig. 12.17 Showing technique of preputioplasty in a case of Distal hypospadias. (**a**) Inverted U shaped incision, (**b**, **c**) Partial penile de-gloving, (**d**) Glansplasty and frenuloplasty, (**e**–**g**) Prepucioplasty, (**h**, **i**) Final postoperative appearance

Gilpin et al. described an alternative technique to close the outer skin layer of prepuce by utilizing Z-plasty to decrease the tension on the suture line and so the complications [9].

Follow Up

A thorough follow up after preputioplasty is essential to assess the cosmetic and functional outcome and diagnose complication. Our protocol involved follow up at 2 weeks, 1 month, 3 months, 6 months, 12 months postoperatively and then annually. Prepucial oedema may last 2–3 weeks postoperatively (Fig. 12.19a). It is important to counsel patients/parents strictly not to try retraction of prepuce by themselves. Retraction is best done for the first time by the operating surgeon himself when he considers it appropriate after examination after 6–8 weeks. After that the patient/parents are advised for daily gentle retraction during bathing. Glans may remain partially or completely covered according to the size of prepucial hood. Klijn et al. reported higher complication rate when they advised the parents/patients to start retraction from postoperative day ten [10].

Complications

Preputioplasty is a technically simple procedure which requires only 15–20 min of extra time during surgery. Postoperative edema (Fig. 12.19a, b) is commonly seen in most of the cases but can easily be managed with conservative treatment. Phimosis/tight prepuce is a common complication and is directly related to the procedure. It may get resolved with local application of corticosteroids

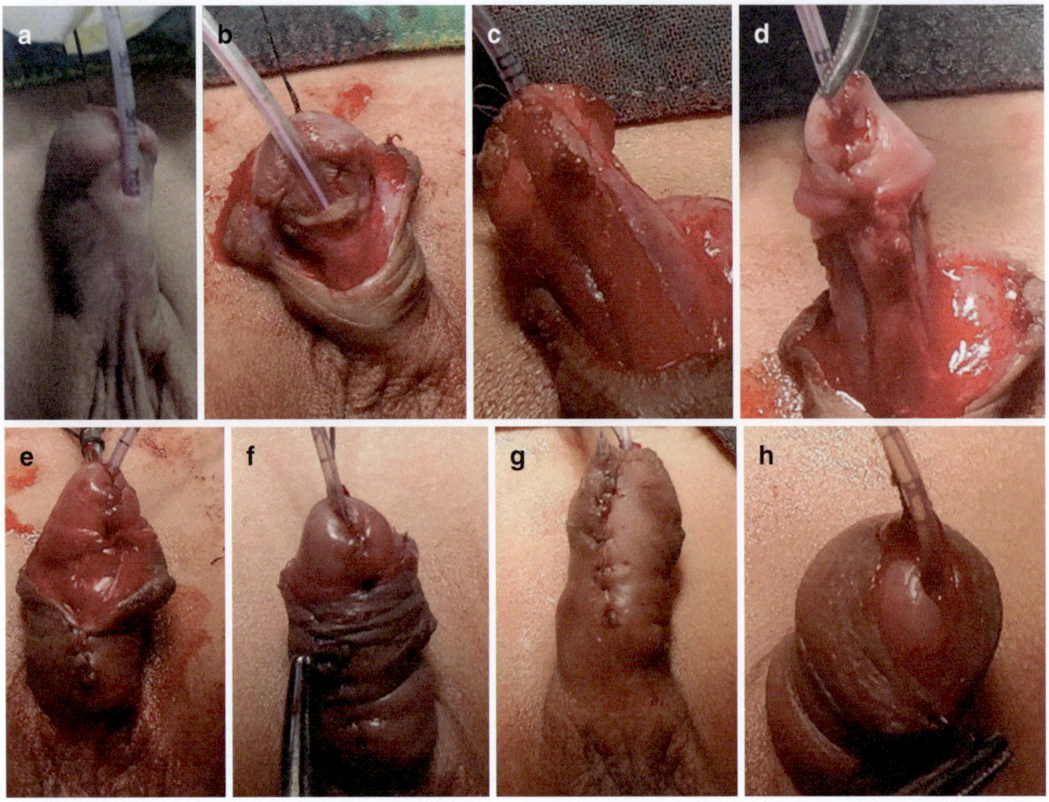

Fig. 12.18 Showing technique of preputioplasty in a case of distal penile hypospadias. (**a**) Pre-operative appearance showing distal penile hypospadias, (**b**) Complete penile Degloving, (**c**) TIP with spongioplasty, (**d**) Glansplasty, (**e**) Repair of penile shaft skin, (**f**) Reconstruction of prepuce, (**g**, **h**) final post-operative appearance after preputioplasty

Fig. 12.19 Complications of preputioplasty. (**a**) showing prepucial oedema from ventral side penis (**b**) Prepucial oedema showing at prepucial opening

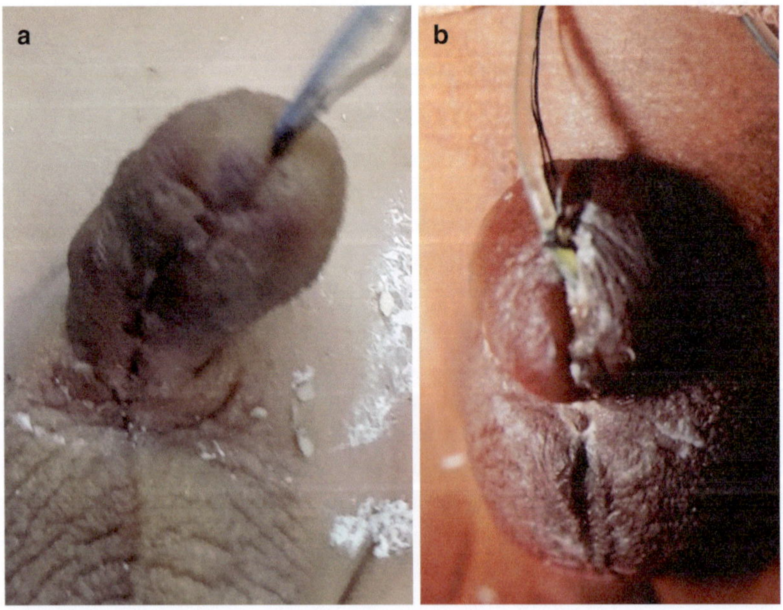

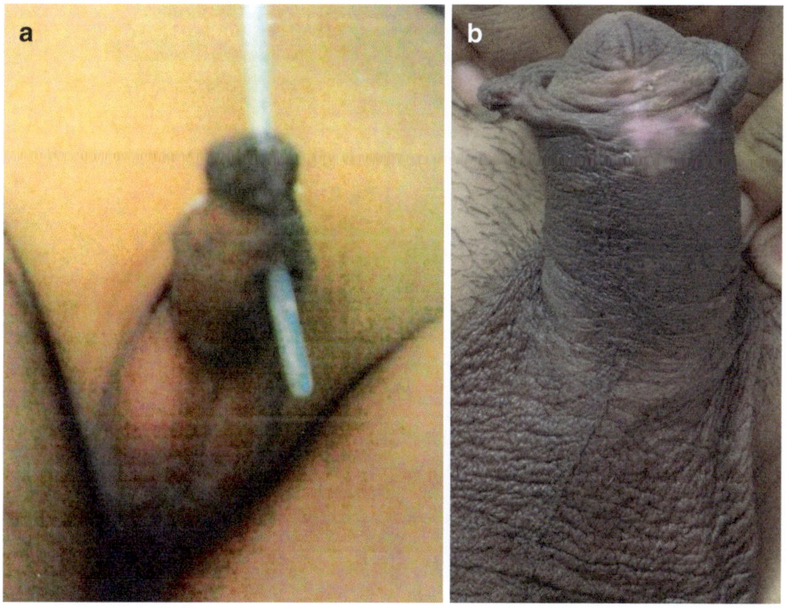

Fig. 12.20 Complications of prepucioplasty. (**a**) Preputial fistula/partial dehiscence, (**b**) complete preputial dehiscence

or eventually require circumcision if conservative management fails. Incidence of phimosis requiring circumcision ranged from 0.2 to 3.9% across various studies [11–13]. Other complications include partial dehiscence or preputial fistula (Fig. 12.20a), complete preputial dehiscence (Fig. 12.20b) and urethrocutaneous fistula. The incidence of prepucial dehiscence ranges from 4.5 to 7.4% [11–13]. Proximal hypospadias with penile degloving has a higher incidence of complications. The authors found acceptable complication rates even in proximal hypospadias cases. We had about 11% complication in proximal hypospadias with preputioplasty which was similar to that of without preputioplasty [14].

Conclusions

Prepuce is the mirror of urethral and penile shaft anomaly. Anomaly is to be seen in all three parts of prepuce median raphe, fraenulum and body of the prepuce. Ending of median raphe on the prepuce gives an information of degree of torque. Bifurcation of median raphe and site dorsal hump offer clues regarding the severity of hypospadias. Preputial reconstruction along with TIP is possible in all types of hypospadias and even cases with penile curvature and torsion. Preputioplasty is feasible even in cases of Mathieu repair and in proximal hypospadias with penile degloving. It does not increase complications associated with urethroplasty. Preputioplasty with urethroplasty and spongioplasty reconstructs an aesthetically normal looking penis and hence, is more acceptable to the patient and/or parents of the patient with hypospadias. Type of prepuce in hypospadias is an important variable to predict postoperative results in preputioplasty. The complications of preputioplasty are postoperative oedema, phimosis and dehiscence which may be partial or complete. Oedema can be managed conservatively with anti-inflammatory drugs and phimosis with application of steroid cream. Phimosis can be prevented measuring the adequacy of the prepuce and marking the margins of the prepucial flaps. Circumcision is rarely required for phimosis and partial or complete prepucial dehiscence.

References

1. Liu X, Liu G, Shen J, Yue A, Isaacson D, Sinclair A, et al. Human glans and preputial development. Differentiation. 2018;103:86–99.
2. Radojicic ZI, Perovic SV. Classification of prepuce in hypospadias according to morphological abnormalities and their impact on hypospadias repair. J Urol. 2004;172(1):301–4.

3. Zhao Z, Sun N, Mao X. Vascularization of vessel pedicle in hypospadias and its relationship to near-period complications. Exp Ther Med. 2018;16(3):2408–12.
4. Murphy JP. Hypospadias. In: Ashcraft KW, Holder TM, editors. Pediatric Surgery. 2nd ed. Philadelphia: WB Saunders; 1993. p. 694.
5. Mustafa M. The concept of tubularized incised plate hypospadias repair for different types of hypospadias. Int Urol Nephrol. 2005;37(1):89–91.
6. Snodgrass WT, Koyle MA, Baskin LS, Caldamone AA. Foreskin preservation in penile surgery. J Urol. 2006;176(2):711–4.
7. Erdenetsetseg G, Dewan P. Reconstruction of the hypospadiac hooded prepuce. J Urol. 2003;169(5):1822–4.
8. Taylor JR, Lockwood AP, Taylor A. The prepuce: specialized mucosa of the penis and its loss to circumcision. Br J Urol. 1996;77(2):291–5.
9. Gilpin D, Clements W, Boston V. GRAP repair: single-stage reconstruction of Hypospadias as an outpatient procedure. Br J Urol. 1993;71(2):226–9.
10. Klijn AJ, Dik P, De Jong TP. Results of preputial reconstruction in 77 boys with distal hypospadias. J Urol. 2001;165(4):1255–7.
11. Barber N, Chappell B, Carter P, Britton J. Is preputioplasty effective and acceptable? J R Soc Med. 2003;96(9):452–3.
12. Esposito C, Savanelli A, Escolino M, Giurin I, Iaquinto M, Alicchio F, et al. Preputioplasty associated with urethroplasty for correction of distal hypospadias: a prospective study and proposition of a new objective scoring system for evaluation of esthetic and functional outcome. J Pediatr Urol. 2014;10(2):294–9.
13. van den Dungen I, Rynja S, Bosch J, de Jong T, de Kort L. Comparison of preputioplasty and circumcision in distal hypospadias correction: long-term follow-up. J Pediatr Urol. 2019;15(1):47.e1–9.
14. Bhat A, Gandhi A, Saxena G, Choudhary GR. Preputial reconstruction and tubularized incised plate urethroplasty in proximal hypospadias with ventral penile curvature. Indian J Urol. 2010;26(4):507–10.

Preputial Lymphedema 13

Abbreviations

LGV Lymphogranuloma venereum
PL Preputial lymphedema

Classification of Preputial Lymphedema

PL could be classified to an acute or chronic condition, and according to the etiology to either primary or secondary.

Acute cases are usually transient, self-limiting and reactive to surgical and non surgical trauma, venous thrombosis and angioneurotic oedema.

Transient penile oedema was described in relation to relation to repeated vigorous sexual intercourse, secondary to chronic masturbation and has also been also described in relation to human papillomavirus infection [1].

Chronic PL is a persistent, long standing devastating condition either primary congenital or secondary to parasites or other pathogens, and usually deserve a surgical intervention.

Primary Penile lymphedema: (usually in western countries) it is congenitally inherited in 15% of the cases, in either an autosomal dominant form (Milroy's disease), or a sporadic form (in 85% of the cases) that occurs at puberty (Meigs' disease) [2] (Fig. 13.1).

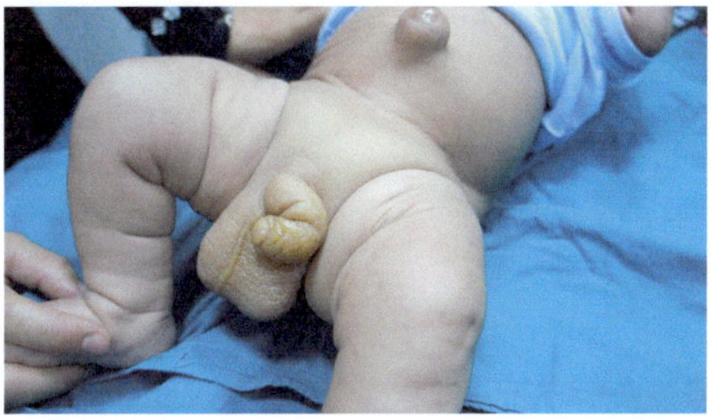

Fig. 13.1 An infant with a primary congenital lymphedema affecting genitalia and lower limbs

Secondary: which develops more frequently than primary lymphedema, and usually caused by acquired infection in Africa and Asia e.g., lymphogranuloma venereum, chlamydia trachomatis or filarial infestation with Wuchereria bancrofti, and other causes will be discussed.

Chronic Penile Lymphedema

The chronic lymphedema–elephantiasis-of penis commonly occurs in association with lymphedema of scrotum but it can occur alone indicating that the penile lymphatic drainage may be distinct from scrotal lymphatic drainage.

Singh et al. [3] reported 48 patients of filarial male genital lymphedema which included 14 patients of isolated penile and 34 patients of penoscrotal lymphedema.

M. A. B. Fahmy, *Normal and Abnormal Prepuce*, https://doi.org/10.1007/978-3-030-37621-5_13

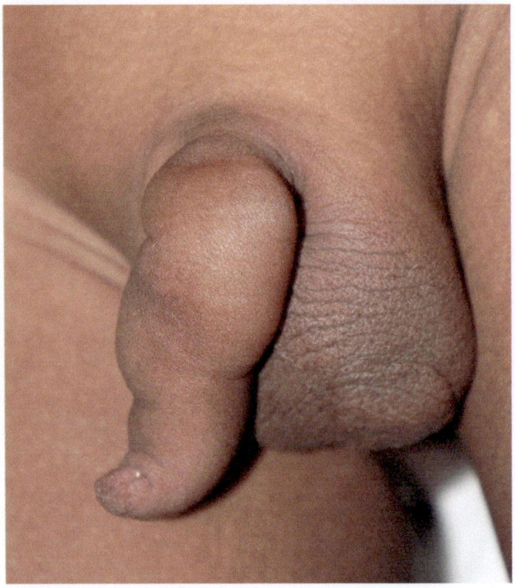

Fig. 13.2 Penile chronic lymphedema confined mainly to the prepuce and penile sheath, without scrotal affection

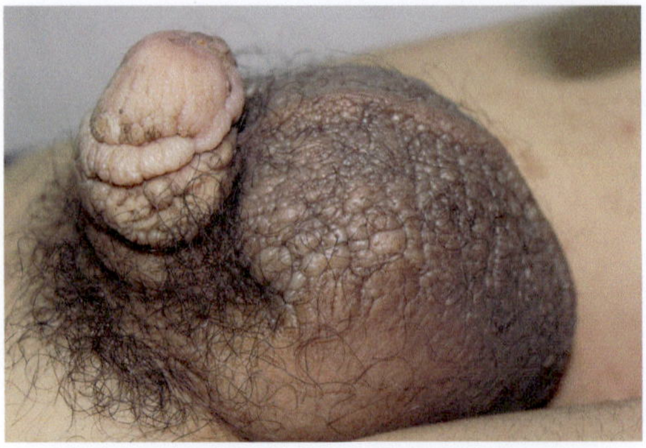

Fig. 13.3 A case of lymphedema affecting the circumcised mucosal remnants, penile and scrotal skin, caused by lymphogranuloma venereum

PL is a disease of integuments of penis as the erectile tissue of the glans and shaft cannot be affected as there are no lymphatics in these parts of penis. Lymphatic obstruction is limited to penis and scrotum and is not seen in adjacent organs such as lower extremities, abdomen and buttock.

The length of prepuce is increased, and due to lymphedema and after a subsequent fibrosis, the prepuce may lose its retractile property to expose the glans ("filarial phimosis"). Dirty blackish smegma may accumulate in the prepucial sac mainly in post-coronal sulcus. Rarely the prepuce may become nodular (Fig. 13.2).

Regardless of the cause of scrotal and penile lymphedema, this disease can lead to physical and spiritual weakness and its treatment is difficult particularly in the aged.

Etiology

The aetiopathogenesis of penile lymphedema must be carefully considered in each individual case, as several factors may be involved [4].

1. *Infection*: In this group the lymphatic filariasis is the commonest cause in tropical and subtropical countries. It causes lymphedema due to adenolymphatic obstruction of inguinal lymphatics. Other infections which can cause inguinal lymphatic obstruction include tuberculosis and lymphogranuloma venereum (LGV), which caused by Chlamydia trachomatis infection (Fig. 13.3).
2. *Malignancy*: The metastatic disease of inguinal lymph nodes and its treatment with node dissection or radiotherapy may also cause penile lymphedema–elephantiasis. The infections involving the inguinal lymph nodes are the commonest cause in tropical and underdeveloped countries while malignancy involving these lymph nodes is the commonest cause in western nations.
3. *Primary lymphedema*: This type of lymphedema of penis is attributed to developmental defect of lymphatics, i.e., hypoplasia [5].
4. *General anasarca*: PL may be manifested as a part of general anasarca that occurs in congestive heart failure, cirrhosis of liver, chronic renal disease, and hypoproteinemia. This swelling disappears following successful treatment of the cause.
5. *Other causes*: de Godoy et al. [6] described a case of lymphedema of penis and scrotum following surgery of pancreas. Penoscrotal oedema has also been attributed to continuous ambulatory peritoneal dialysis, amputation of septic limbs in diabetes, acute necrotizing pancreatitis, streptococcal infections, and Crohn's disease, which may be occult and asymptomatic [7].

6. *Idiopathic*: Edema of penis and scrotum can occur without a known cause.

   A persistent lymphatic insult from whatever cause could result in an inflammatory process affecting genital and pelvic lymphatic vessels and nodes. Imaging of lymphatic channels is not particularly helpful [8].

Clinical Presentation

The clinical picture of PL is widely heterogeneous. It is frequently chronic and there are often exacerbations and remissions associated with cellulitis. All the patients will reveal a gross oedema affecting the foreskin, penile shaft, and scrotum; in a different grades and combinations [9].

Patients with chronic penile oedema present with chronic swelling of the genitalia, pubic mound, buttocks and thighs, which may be warm and red. There may be intercurrent attacks of cellulitis and/or erysipelas with systemic upset [10].

Ahmed [11] has described three types of penile involvement in chronic filarial lymphedema:

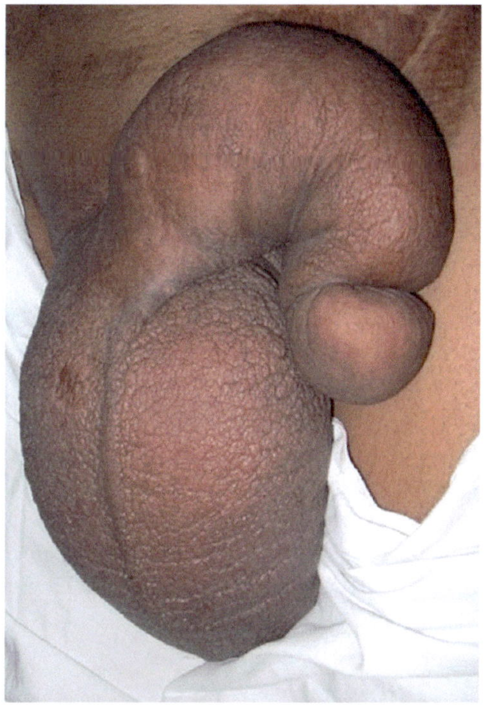

Fig. 13.4 Genital lymphedema leading to saxophone penis with scars of previous surgeries seen in groins

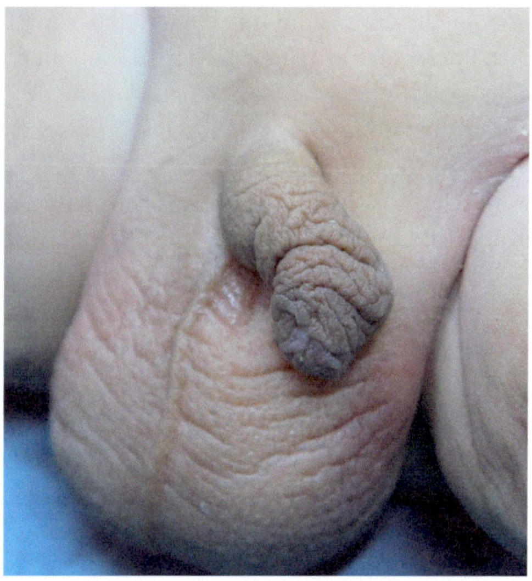

Fig. 13.5 Lymphedema with a straight hypertrophied penis and prepuce with a phimotic preputial meatus

1. *Ram-horn penis*: It is also named as a saxophone penis (Fig. 13.4). The lymph accumulates more in the distal part of penis than in its proximal part. With passage of time fibrosis sets in this fluid due to increasing protein levels. Due to unequal fibrosis and contraction of the scar tissue the swollen prepuce becomes distorted and angulated giving it a ram-horn shape or like that of a snail. It is the commonest type of elephantiasis of penis.
2. *Straight hypertrophied penis*: This type is chronic lymphedema of penis is characterized by lymphedema and elephantiasis of distal penile skin without distortion (Fig. 13.5). It is relatively uncommon type and may be a stage earlier than ram-horn penis, usually this type results in stenosis of the preputial ring and lymphedema phimosis.
3. *Buried penis*: The penis is gradually buried in the anterior wall of progressively enlarging scrotum due to chronic filarial lymphedema–elephantiasis. It is usually possible to deliver the penis on the surface by manipulation and pressure, but it returns to its buried position as soon as the manipulating hand is lifted up. It is the commonest clinical presentation of chronic filarial penoscrotal lymphedema–elephantiasis.

In the first two types of elephantiasis the penis cannot be buried into the scrotum as the penile skin has lost its elasticity and stretchability and cannot be pulled into it by the enlarging scrotum. Hai et al. [12] described 195 cases of filarial lymphedema of male external genitals; with 15 patients had penile lymphedema and 45 cases of buried penis in elephantoid scrotum.

Complications

There may be intercurrent attacks of cellulitis and/or erysipelas with systemic upset. Acute attacks require admission to hospital and treatment with systemic broad-spectrum antibiotics; a short course of prednisolone may also be helpful. Investigations should be directed at elucidating possible underlying causes.

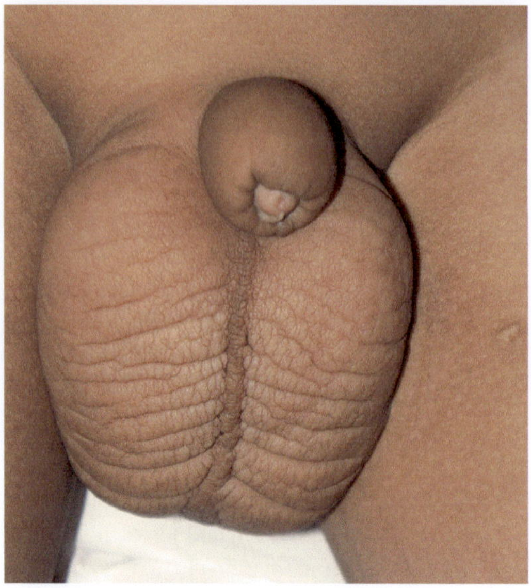

Fig. 13.6 Penoscrotal congenital lymphedema not improved after circumcision

Treatment

All cases of chronic penoscrotal oedema should be treated aggressively at first presentation, because the more chronic the genital lymphedema the more difficult it is to treat, both medically and surgically. Aims of management of chronic penile oedema must be prophylaxis against further infective episodes and aggressive treatment of relapses. Long-term treatment with antibiotics appears to ameliorate and stabilize the process, and improves the appearance and function of the penis. The patient with filariasis should given a course of diethylcarbamazine 100 mg three times daily for 3–4 weeks and further attacks of filariasis should be prevented.

Minimal genital swelling may be reduced by doing self-massage of swollen penis and with continuous use of a cotton–polyester compression garment [6].

Medical control with antibiotics then allows surgical intervention in the form of circumcision, if the patient or the parents accepting this, but it should be clear that although circumcision may give a chance for glans exposure and cleaning, but the penile shaft lymphedema may be aggravated after circumcision or it least it may not improve (Fig. 13.6).

Plastic repair may be necessary after excision of affected tissue [13].

Nodo-Venous Shunt

It is a drainage operation which may help in mild to moderate lymphedema without fibrous proliferation, in this procedure bilateral inguinal nodo-venous shunt is combined with circumcision.

Excision of Elephantoid Tissue

The operation is done under general or spinal anesthesia. The buried type of penis is brought out of the swollen scrotum during surgical treatment.

The other two types of penile elephantiasis are treated by excision of all elephantoid tissue including the outer layer of prepuce by a racket incision at the root of penis and a circumferential incision around the prepucial orifice with both the incision joined together by a longitudinal dorsal midline incision. Usually there is a good plane of cleavage between the normal and elephantoid tissue which is quite avascular. Hence, the excision is not difficult. The distal limit of the excision is the distal junction of external and inner layers of prepuce. The whole elephantoid tissue is excised to give proper shape to the penis, preventing injury to its vessels and nerves [14].

Resurfacing of the penis is required after excision of elephantoid tissue of penis, and there are many methods of doing it:

- Use of excised skin of the penis (after debulking) as a full thickness graft, but this skin should not be used as it is not healthy.
- Use of inner layer of prepuce, the raw area of the penis is commonly covered by inner layer of prepuce which is turned back on the penis to cover it like a pillow cover and its edge is stitched to the cut edge of the skin around the root of penis. Also to prevent a circumferential scar at the root of penis; a Z-plasty is usually required.
- Use of skin flaps from suprapubic, inguinal, or femoral region and even the scrotum, but they make the penis bulky. Also it requires staging of the procedure.
- Use of partial thickness skin grafts 0.7–0.8 mm thick. The graft is stitched at the root of penis in a zigzag manner to avoid a circular scar and on the ventral surface also in a zigzag manner to prevent scar contracture. However the contracture of any scar can occur, but the scar contracture on the dorsal surface usually is not troublesome [15].

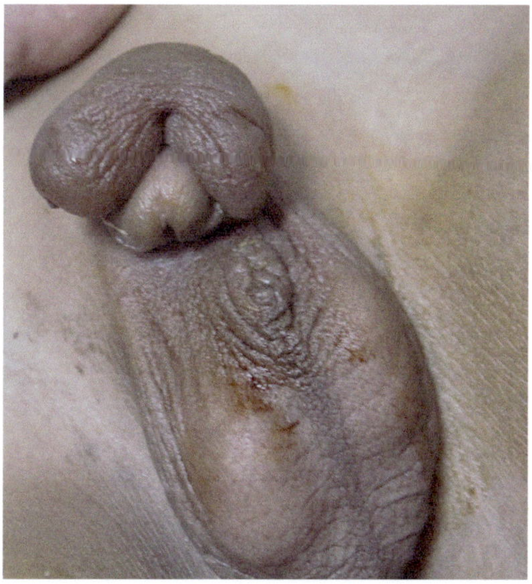

Fig. 13.7 Postoperative preputial oedema, the unreconstructed prepuce (hooded) developed severe oedema, which persist for one week after surgery

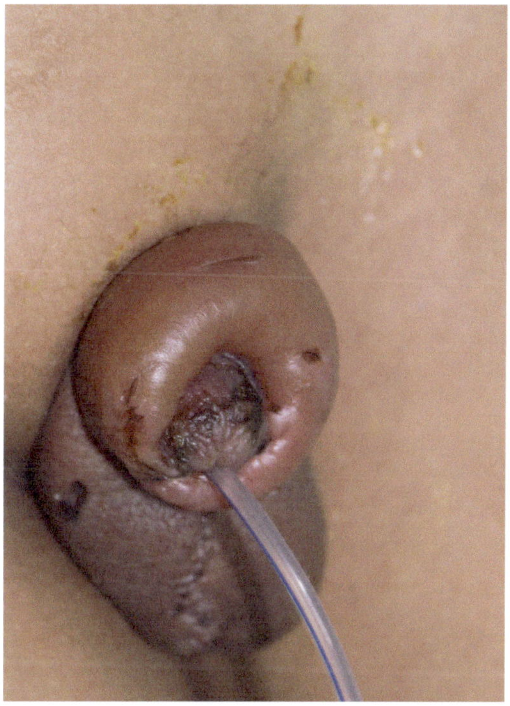

Fig. 13.8 Reconstructed prepuce after hypospadias repair developed a marked lymphedema

Postoperative Preputial Edema

Preputial edema is a common complication after penile, preputial and urethral surgery, specially after hypospadias repair surgery; whether the prepuce left without repair (Fig. 13.7), or after preputial reconstruction (Fig. 13.8), with a higher incidence rate in children than in adults. Although preputial edema is just moderate symptom and does not affect urination, it worries or even distresses the patient and the family both physically and psychologically. In recent years, rapid achievements have been made in prepuce surgery, as in circumcision, hypospadias surgery, preputial neoplasm excision, and penile degloving repair, which can now be accomplished with shorter time and higher efficiency (Fig. 13.9). Despite constant improvement in the methods and techniques for prepuce surgery, postoperative edema remains difficult to be totally prevented. Pathogenic factors for postop-

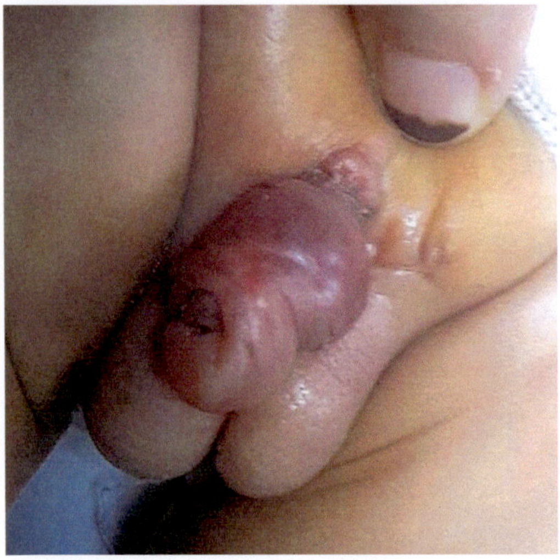

Fig. 13.9 Preputial oedema extended to the penile shaft after scrotal transposition surgery

erative preputial edema vary from disturbance of blood circulation to inflammatory factor-induced change in capillary permeability, lymphatic circulation disorders, and neurogenic edema [16]. Elimination of the pathogenic factors and precautionary measures after surgery count significantly to the prevention and management of postoperative preputial edema.

References

1. Noble H, Goh BT. Chronic penile oedema secondary to chronic masturbation. Int J STD AIDS. 2004;15:489–90.
2. McDougal WS. Lymphedema of the external genitalia. J Urol. 2003;170:711–6.
3. Singh V, Sinha RJ, Sankhwar SN, Kumar V. Reconstructive surgery for penoscrotal filarial lymphedema: a decade of experience and follow up. Urology. 2011;77:1228–31.
4. Shim TN, Doiron PR, Francis N, et al. Penile lymphoedema: approach to investigation and management. Clin Exp Dermatol. 2019;44:20–31. https://doi.org/10.1111/ced.13609.
5. Sandeepa S, Rao K, Hemalatha AN, Shenoy V. A rare case of isolated primary penile lymphedema. Indian J Appl Res. 2015;5(3):449–50.
6. de Godoy JMP, Facio FN Jr, Matias de Carvalho EC, de Godoy Mde FG. New compression mechanism in penilelymphedema and sexual rehabilitation. Urol Ann. 2014;6(1):88–90.
7. Saha M, Edmonds E, Martin J, Bunker CB. Penile lymphoedema in association with asymptomatic Crohn's disease. Clin Exp Dermatol. 2009;34:88–90.
8. Muehlberger T, Homann HH, Kuhnen C, et al. Aetiology, clinical aspects and therapy of penoscrotal lymphoedema. Chirurg. 2001;72:414–8. (in German).
9. Weinberger L, Zirwas M, English J. A diagnostic algorithm for male genital oedema. J Eur Acad Dermatol Venereol. 2007;21:156–62. https://doi.org/10.1111/j.1468-3083.2006.02025.x.
10. Porter WM, Dinneen M, Bunker C. Chronic penile lymphoedema. Arch Dermatol. 2001; 137:1108–10.
11. Ahmed N. Filarial penis – its variations and treatment. Indian J Surg. 1941;3:16–22.
12. Hai AA, et al. Filarial lymphoedema of male genitalia. In Second international conference on surgery in tropics, Bombay Hospital Institute of Medical Sciences; 1987. pp. 22–27.
13. Bunker CB, Neill SM. The genital, perianal and umbilical regions. In: Burns T, Breathnach S, Cox N, Griffiths C, editors. Rook's textbook of dermatology, vol. 1. 8th ed. Oxford: Blackwell Publishing; 2010. ISBN: 978-1-405-16169-5.
14. Goel TC, Goel A. Chronic lymphedema–elephantiasis of penis. In: Lymphatic filariasis. Singapore: Springer; 2016. https://doi.org/10.1007/978-981-10-2257-9_23.
15. Khanna NN. Surgical treatment of elephantiasis of male genitalia. Plast Reconstr Surg. 1970;46(5):481–7.
16. Kong F-Y, Liu X-L. Pathogenesis, prevention and management of edema after prepuce surgery. Natl J Androl. 2018;24(8):740–3.

14 Preputial Haemangioma and Vascular Malformations

Abbreviations

MALT	Minimal access laser therapy
Nd:YAG	Neodymium:yttrium-aluminum-garnet
VMs	Vascular malformations

Classifications

Genital hemangiomas, like other haemangiomas, are classified to either "capillary", "cavernous" or "mixed" lesions based on the following definitions [1]:

- A "capillary" hemangioma is represented by a bright red, raised lesion, ranging from few millimetres to several centimetres in diameter. It is always well circumscribed, and only partially compressible.
- A "cavernous" hemangioma instead, is a more nodular one, that could be larger in diameter, width and depth as well. It is often bluish or purple and easy compressible.
- The "mixed" lesions, indeed, have components of both.

The penis and prepuce may be affected by different forms of Vascular Malformations (VMs). These lesions are congenital but are usually not diagnosed until the teenage years or young adulthood. These lesions are presented as a faint blue patch or a soft blue mass. VMs can be also subdivided into either slow-flow (capillary, lymphatic, venous) or fast-flow (arterial, arteriovenous) type.

Strawberry hemangiomas are the most common type and result from proliferation of immature capillary vessels. These are also categorized as cutaneous hemangiomas because they occur on the skin. Although the lesions may undergo a period of rapid growth lasting for 3–6 months, but gradual involution is common (Fig. 14.1).

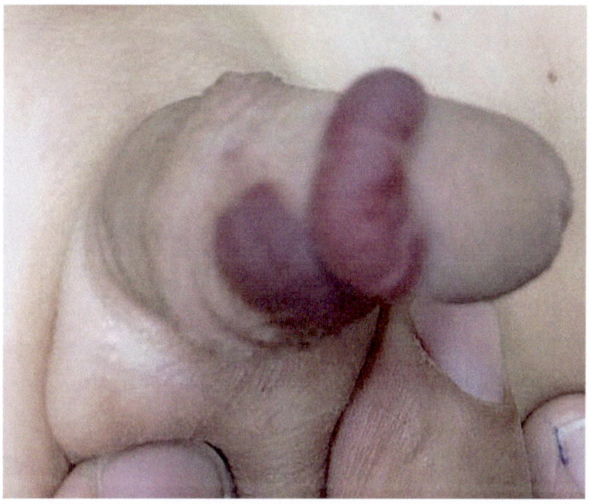

Fig. 14.1 Strawberry hemangioma of the post circumcision preputial remnants and penile shaft [2]

M. A. B. Fahmy, *Normal and Abnormal Prepuce*, https://doi.org/10.1007/978-3-030-37621-5_14

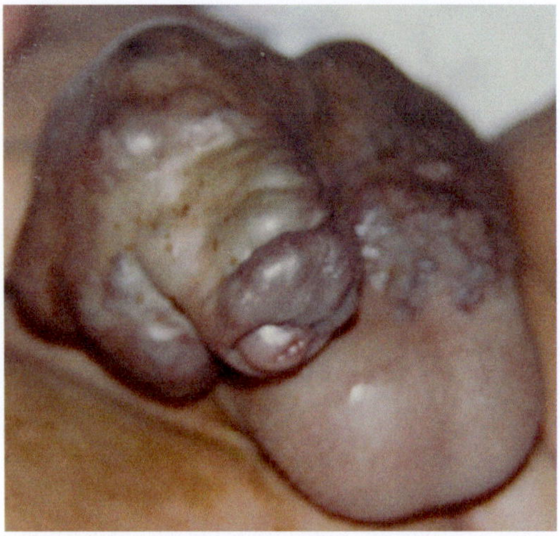

Fig. 14.2 Extensive arteriovenous malformation of the penile skin, prepuce and scrotum

Cavernous hemangiomas, are much less common in genital area, and are probably more appropriately classified as a vascular malformation. They may be detected at birth or later in life. Cavernous hemangiomas tend to enlarge gradually and should be treated with care. Physical examination reveals a "bag of worms" sensation similar to that of a varicocele, although the lesions tend to be firm and do not decompress when the patient is recumbent [3] (Fig. 14.2).

Genital Haemangioma in Association with Other Syndromes

Klippel-Trénaunay-Weber Syndrome

Klippel-Trénaunay-Weber syndrome is a triad of cutaneous vascular malformation, most commonly in the form of nevus flammeus, in combination with soft tissue and bone hypertrophy. The anomaly manifests at birth, usually involving a lower extremity, but it may also involve the trunk, upper limb or face. Abdominal wall and genitalia are affected in 3% of the cases. These vascular lesions have a propensity to bleed. In a review of 214 patients from a single institution, Husmann et al. found that 30% of the confirmed cases had genitourinary cutaneous or visceral involvement. Of the 48 (22%) who had cutaneous genital involvement, 29% developed intractable bleeding [4]. Genital VMs associated with this syndrome could be managed conservatively with sclerotherapy injection or laser to alleviate its annoying manifestations on the genitalia, as excision of such hemangiomas was associated with significant blood loss.

Kasabach-Merritt Syndrome

Penoscrotal area may be affected along the VMs of Kasabach-Merritt syndrome which is a rare type of vascular lesion with peculiar characteristics based upon three basic findings; enlarging haemangioma, thrombocytopenia and consumption coagulopathy [5] (Fig. 14.3).

Segmental Haemangioma

Hemangiomas found in developmental segments are referred to as "segmental lesions". These segmented hemangiomas are commonly associated with other extracutaneous abnormalities. The PELVIS/SACRAL syndrome denotes the association of segmented hemangiomas of the loins (sacrolumbar region, buttocks or perineum and napkin hemangioma) with spinal dysraphia affecting the sacrolumbar spine, the terminal medullary cone, the genitourinary organs and the anal region to a varying degree. The acronym "LUMBAR", indeed, is proposed by several authors to describe the association between **L**ower body hemangioma and other cutaneous defects, **U**rogenital anomalies, ulceration, **M**yelopathy, **B**ony deformities, **A**norectal malformations, or Arterial and **R**enal anomalies [6].

Also cavernous haemangioma of the prepuce is reported in a patient with enchondromatosis and D-2-hydroxyglutaric aciduria [7].

Clinical Presentation

Symptoms of preputial haemangioma can be various and include skin discolouration, local swelling and disfigurement, bleeding, thrombophlebitis, lymphorrhea and pain, depending on the affected vascular components, location,

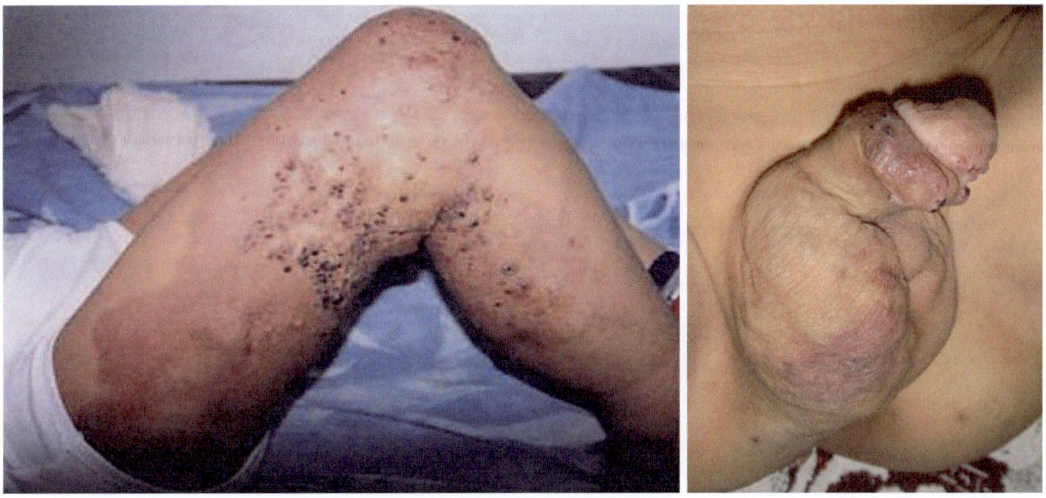

Fig. 14.3 Kasabach-Merritt syndrome affecting the right lower limb, with involvement of the scrotum, penis and preputial remnants [2]

and size. Close to 80% of penile cutaneous hemangiomas are located, at least in part, in the glans [8].

Even a small haemangioma if located at the tip of the prepuce of a neonate, it is more liable to trauma and bleeding, and necessitates intervention (Fig. 14.4).

Investigations

Ultrasonography with color Doppler imaging, computed tomography (CT), or MRI is recommended, specially in cases suspected to be a cavernous haemangioma, to delineate the size of the hemangioma because clinical examination does not disclose the extent of the lesion [9].

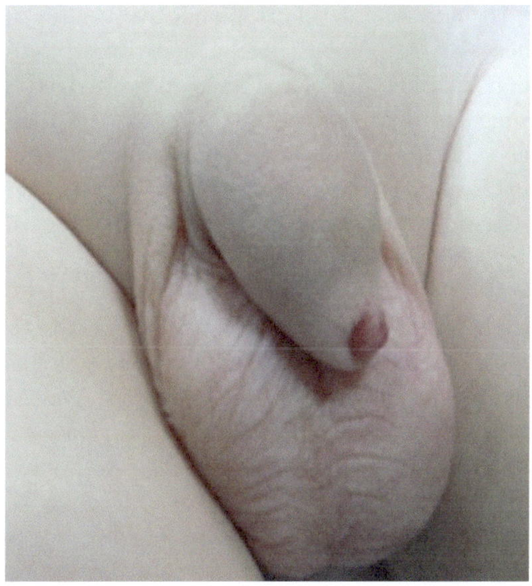

Fig. 14.4 A small haemangioma at the tip of the prepuce, which is liable for bleeding

Complications

Penile haemangioma in general, and preputial one in particular, are usually superficial in nature, histologically, they are composed of aggregates of closely packed, thin-walled vessels, lined by flattened endothelial cells and usually blood-filled with a high nucleocytoplasmic ratio (Fig. 14.5). Bleeding, ulcerations, disfigurement, poor healing, and scar formation are a frequent complications of genital haemangiomas.

Treatment

Ordinarily active treatment is usually postponed when patients are infants. Nevertheless, for the preputial hemangiomas total excision of the tumor by circumcision was preferred by some authors. Treatment options include conservative approaches, interventional treatment, open surgical repair, or any combination thereof [10].

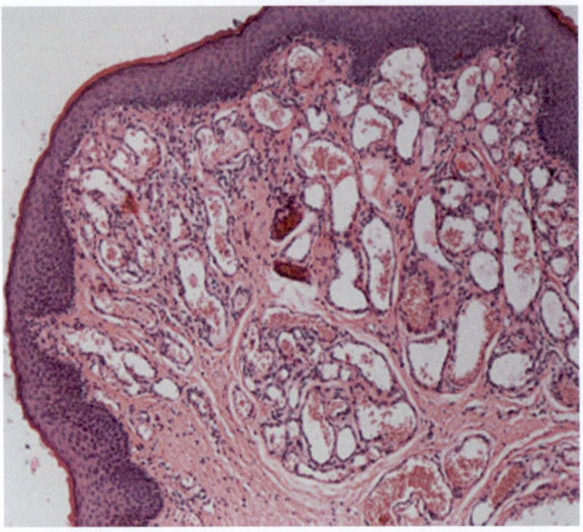

Fig. 14.5 Preputial hemangioma, higher magnification (40×), newly formed blood vessels with an abnormal cuboidal shape of endothelial cells and a high nucleocytoplasmic ratio are noticeable [15]

If ulceration develops, urgent intervention is necessary to prevent complications from bleeding. The most popular form of therapy, in this situation, is short-term oral corticosteroid therapy. Treatment with laser therapy allows selective photothermolysis and destruction of superficial blood vessels. In some cases, surgical excision is necessary [9].

Wait and see trend, which was generally applicable for haemangioma detected early in life, is not applicable for genital haemangioma. Psychologically; external genitalia VMs can lead to a negative self-image; and the physiological function can be profoundly affected. Restriction of the health-related quality of life may be another indication for treatment.

Surgery has been the classical therapeutic approach. Because of their high vascularity, surgical excision of these tumors carries the risk of bleeding not only during the excision, but also in the postoperative period with nocturnal erection. In addition to poor healing, scar formation is a frequent complication of surgery to the glans penis. Despite these disadvantages, surgical excision still is an option for preputial haemangioma, especially in peripheral hospitals, where it can be performed with minimal available infrastructure with acceptable results. Other possible therapies besides surgical excision, are laser therapy, and sclerotherapy include electrofulgration and cryotherapy.

Complete excision is often not possible due to technical or anatomical problems, in this setting, sclerotherapy has technical superiority. In case of recurrence, surgery gets more complication each time performed, and the rate of complications raises.

Minimal access laser therapy (MALT) with a commercial Nd:YAG laser device seems to be a promising alternative in the treatment of this specific condition. Sclerotherapy may have a higher rate of punctures in repetitional interventions but seems to have no higher rate of procedural complications.

Neodymium:yttrium-aluminum-garnet (Nd: YAG) laser treatment in a case of glans penis hemangioma was first described by Jimenez-Cruz and Osca [9]. The Nd:YAG laser emits light with a wavelength of 1060 nm, which is poorly absorbed by body pigments. Despite its excellent tissue coagulation without fibrosis, the tissue penetration rate is deeper. The potassium thiophosphate (KTP) laser may be preferable for large lesions or for children because it is absorbed in the hemoglobin and produces less scar formation. However, even after 4 weeks of Nd:YAG laser application, tissue healing is excellent, and no scar is evident. Reports of laser treatment for these lesions with the patient under local anesthesia have described good functional and cosmetic results. Laser treatment has been performed on an outpatient basis with almost no blood loss or complications [11].

Because both cryotherapy and laser therapy cause non-selective tissue damage, accurate control of the depth of treatment is essential to prevent bleeding during and after the procedure. A degree of scarring is inevitable with these therapies.

Sclerotherapy

Compression results in direct apposition of the treated vein walls to produce more effective fibrosis. Compressing the treated vessel decreases the extent of thrombus formation that inevitably occurs with the use of all sclerosing agents, and thereby decreases the risk of recanalizaion of the treated vessels. Sclerosing agents recommended for VMs are mainly ethanol, polidocanol, or sodium tetradecyl sulfate (STS); treatment of VMs are possible with OK-432, doxycycline or bleomycin [12].

Compared with lasers, sclerotherapy is less expensive and easily available, it has proved to be an effective, low-cost, and easy-to-perform procedure. Moreover, it is repeatable in case of failure. However, intralesional sclerotherapy can be associated with complications such as cutaneous necrosis, ulceration, and hyperpigmentation, anaphylaxis, and superficial thrombophlebitis [13].

In extensive cutaneous hemangiomas, sclerotherapy may cause major skin necrosis which could lead to infection or bleeding and prevent primary wound healing.

Definitive treatment for cavernous haemangioma is by en bloc resection is advised, and preoperative angioembolization may reduce the size of the mass and the risk of bleeding. Careful excision of venous malformation is effective but if the lesion affects the glans penis, the neodymium:yttrium-aluminum-garnet laser may yield a better result [14].

References

1. Hassanein AH, Mulliken JB, Fishman SJ, Greene AK. Evaluation of terminology for vascular anomalies in current literature. Plast Reconstr Surg. 2011;127:347–51. https://doi.org/10.1097/PRS.0b013e3181f95b83.
2. Fahmy M, *Congenital Anomalies of the Penis*, Springer International Publishing Switzerland, 2017. https://doi.org/10.1007/978-3-319-43310-3_17
3. Ferrer FA, McKenna PH. Cavernous hemangioma of the scrotum: a rare benign genital tumor of childhood. J Urol. 1995;153:1262–4. https://doi.org/10.1016/S0022-5347(01)67582-7.
4. Husmann D, Rathbun S, Driscol D. Klippel-Trénaunay syndrome: treatment of genitourinary sequelae [abstract]. J Pediatr Urol. 2005;1:161.
5. Hall GW. Kasabach-Merritt syndrome: pathogenesis and management. Br J Haematol. 2001;112:851–62. https://doi.org/10.1046/j.1365-2141.2001.02453.x.
6. Bourrat E, Lemarchand-Venencie F, Jacquemont ML, El Ghoneimi A, Wassef M, et al. [PELVIS/SACRAL syndrome with livedoid haemangioma and amniotic band]. Ann Dermatol Venereol. 2008;135:855–9.
7. Yeetong P, Phewplung T, Kamolvisit W, et al. Widespread and debilitating hemangiomas in a patient with enchondromatosis and D-2-hydroxyglutaric aciduria. Skelet Radiol. 2018;47:1577–82. https://doi.org/10.1007/s00256-018-2963-z.
8. Tsujii T, Iwai T, Inoue Y, Kubota T, Kihara K, Oshima H. Cutaneous hemangioma of the penis successfully treated with sclerotherapy and ligation. Int J Urol. 1998;5:396–7. https://doi.org/10.1111/j.1442-2042.1998.tb00377.x.
9. Ramos LM, Pavon EM, Barrilero AE. Venous malformation of the glans penis: efficacy of treatment with neodymium:yttrium-aluminum-garnet laser. Urology. 1999;53:779–83. https://doi.org/10.1016/S0090-4295(98)00578-0.
10. Kulungowski AM, Schook CC, Alomari AI, Vogel AM, Mulliken JB, Fishman SJ, et al. Vascular anomalies of the male genitalia. J Pediatr Surg. 2011;46:1214–21. https://doi.org/10.1016/j.jpedsurg.2011.03.056.
11. Ulker V, Esen T. Haemangioma of the glans penis treated with Nd:YAG laser. Int Urol Nephrol. 2005;37:95–6. https://doi.org/10.1007/s11255-004-4695-3.
12. Brill R, Guntau M, Stangl F, Teusch V, Schramm D, et al. Image-guided percutaneous sclerotherapy of vascular malformations of the male genitalia - a retrospective study. Am J Intervent Radiol. 2019; 3(3):1.
13. Savoca G, De Stefani S, Buttazzi L, Gattuccio I, Trambetta C, Belgrano E. Sclerotherapy of hemangioma of the glans penis. Urology. 2000;56:153. https://doi.org/10.1016/S0090-4295(00)00481-7.
14. Kaufman D, Feber KM, Palmer LS, et al. Venous malformations of the genitals: a therapeutic dilemma. Aesthet Surg J. 2010;30(1):71–3. https://doi.org/10.1177/1090820X09358079.
15. Ozcan CU, Ozcan T, Yaman B, Yazici S. An unusual localization: preputial hemangioma. Ped Urol Case Rep. 2015;2(5):1–4. https://doi.org/10.14534/PUCR.2015512748.

15 Igloo Prepuce

Nomenclature

Igloo like prepuce (ILP).

Definition

A rare preputial anomaly; it may be congenital or acquired, in which the dorsal preputial surface overgrowth the ventral surface, directing the preputial ring and orifice to the undersurface of the penis, giving the prepuce a look resembling an igloo (Fig. 15.1). The prepuce is usually enlarged and curved like an umbrella handle.

Historical Background

This anomaly is not well known in the old textbooks, the term 'igloo-like prepuce' (ILP) was coined by Lopez in 1998 to describe a congenital malformation in non-twin brothers, consisting of overdevelopment of the prepuce on the dorsal side and underdevelopment on the ventral side of the penis, resulting in anomalous ventral displacement of the preputial ring [1].

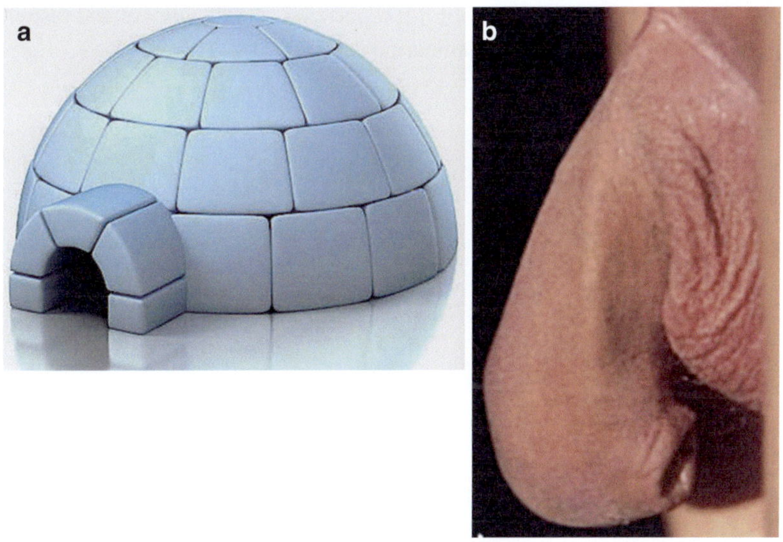

Fig. 15.1 (**a**) An igloo, also known as a snow house (A public Domain Photo). (**b**) Typical case of igloo prepuce

M. A. B. Fahmy, *Normal and Abnormal Prepuce*, https://doi.org/10.1007/978-3-030-37621-5_15

Presentation

In communities discarding the prepuces along circumcision, there is no concern about the abnormalities and disfigurements of the prepuce, but with an increasing interest about the health, beauty and the semblance of the prepuce in western countries; we could suspect detection and reporting of many abnormalities such as ILP. We had a collection of such cases with a spectrum ranging from only a minimal downward direction of the preputial ring, to a full picture with long phimotic prepuce (Figs. 15.2, and 15.3). Igloo prepuce may be presented as:

- Enlarged disfigured prepuce
- Extremely downward urinary stream
- Post-void dribbling
- Painful intercourse
- Balanoposthitis
- Phimosis, which may be complicated with paraphimosis

Aetiology

This case is a developmental anomaly of the prepuce, due to incommensurate distribution of the preputial constituents; mainly muscles and elastic fibers, with a ventral deficiency of one or more layers of the prepuce. Sbano et al. [2] reported in their case an ultrastructural examination confirming that prepucial ventral lesion formed of hypertrophic large amount of smooth-muscle fibers, without subjacent structural alterations. On the contrary, elastic tissue was practically absent in the area involved by smooth-muscle fibers proliferation. These findings suggested that the cause of ILP is a smooth-muscle hamartoma of the dartos involving a small localized area of the ventral side of the prepuce, and this hamartoma with a virtual absence of elastic fibers results in asymmetric dorsal growth of the prepuce, as well as ventral displacement of the preputial ring. Isolated smooth muscle hamartoma is not rare, but few cases are reported in the genitalia; either as a congenital anomaly or as an acquired disease [3].

Some authors consider these cases are an acquired deformity secondary to distension of the foreskin during repeated erections in a phimotic and ventrally webbed penis [4].

Associated Anomalies

- Akroposthia is a common association with ILP (Fig. 15.3)
- Webbed Penis
- Penile chordee (Fig. 15.2)
- Scrotal transposition
- Undescended testicle
- Hypospadias

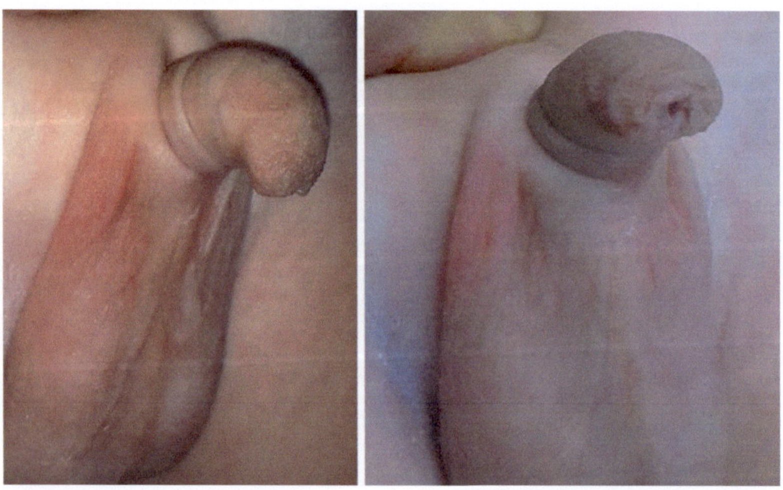

Fig. 15.2 Minimal degree of igloo like prepuce, with penile curvature distal to the coronal sulcus

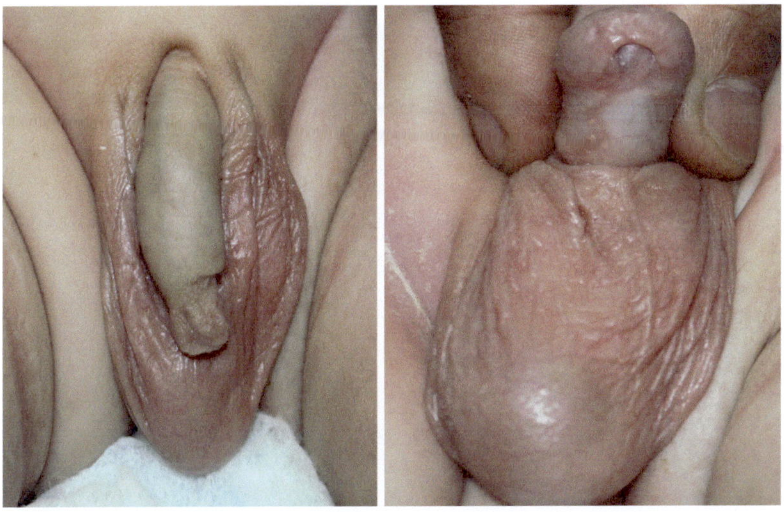

Fig. 15.3 ILP with a marked akroposthia, a minimal degree of scrotal transposition is noticeable

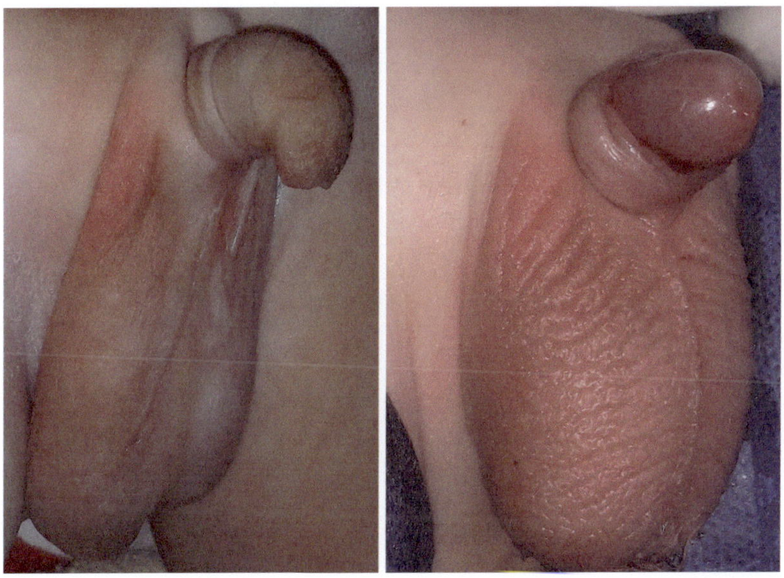

Fig. 15.4 Asymmetrical circumcision with minimal ventral skin resection could restore the normal penile look

Management

If the family agree to accept circumcision; young aged cases can be managed with asymmetrical dorsoventral postectomy, with a meticulus fine suturing (Fig. 15.4). Another technique for correction of disproportionate preputial growth with phimosis is described with multiple z plasty to overcome the associated webbed penis and tethered ventral penile skin [5].

References

1. Lopez Aramburu MA, Rosa Arias J, Arroyo Munoz JL. Prepucio semejante a un "iglu". Actas Urol Esp. 1998;22:175.
2. Sbano P, Sbano E, Alessandrini C, Criscuolo M, Fimiani M. Igloo-like prepuce: a peculiar aspect of smooth muscle hamartoma of the genitalia? J Cutan Pathol. 2005;32:184–7.
3. Hsiao GH, Chen JS. Acquired genital smooth-muscle hamar-toma. Am J Dermatopathol. 1995;17: 67–70.
4. Ferro F. Unusual phimosis: a simple surgical solution. Br J Urol. 1999;84:869–70.
5. Singh RB, Pavithran NM, Bakshi N. A new technique for correction of disproportionate preputial growth with phimosis. Pediatr Surg Int. 2004;20:799–800. https://doi.org/10.1007/s00383-004-1160-4.

16 Rare Preputial Anomalies

Abbreviations

PCD Penile extra-gastrointestinal Crohn's disease
PG Pyoderma gangrenosum

Rare Anomalies of the Prepuce

The normal preputial configuration and its anatomical variants was described in Chap. 6. During our survey for the congenital anomalies of the penis and prepuce we encountered some other very rare conditions, which give the prepuce an abnormal semblance:

- *Notched Prepuce*: It is a midline notch or cleft at the dorsum of the prepuce; which start at a wide preputial ring and extend proximally to a different distances, it may be hyperpigmented and associated with incomplete frenar band or a hooded prepuce with a normally positioned urethra and meatus (Fig. 16.1). This notch may results in an incomplete preputial cleft (Fig. 16.2), or it may appear just like a line of depression at the midline (Fig. 16.3).

  There no obvious other associated anomalies detected along these cases and it may be explained as failure of the normal development of the prepuce. Such cases will deserve a formal anatomical preputial reconstruction,

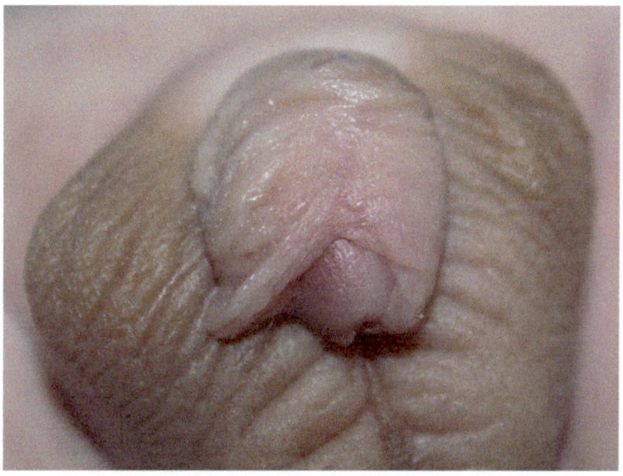

Fig. 16.1 Notched incompletely formed prepuce

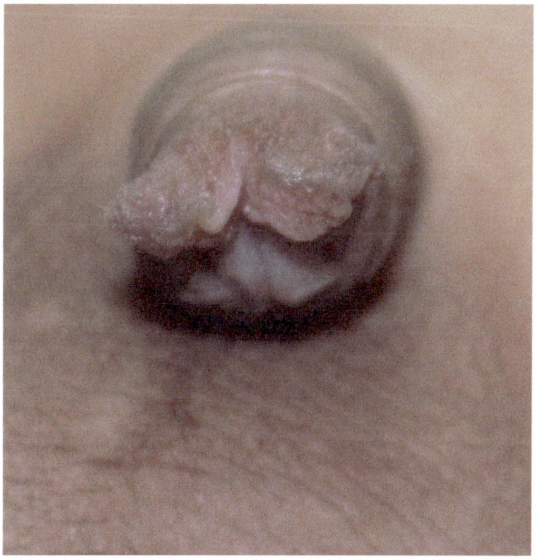

Fig. 16.2 Dorsally splitted hooded prepuce with a normal urethra and meatus

M. A. B. Fahmy, *Normal and Abnormal Prepuce*, https://doi.org/10.1007/978-3-030-37621-5_16

specially if the child is not from a communities supporting circumcision.

- *Angulation of the prepuce*: Penile rotation is not a rare anomaly, the incidence of isolated penile torsion is variable from 1.7 to 27%, and torsion of more than 90° is reported in only 0.7% of the cases, penile rotation commonly started at the root of the penis secondary to improper penile attachment or disproportional growth of the two corpora [1].

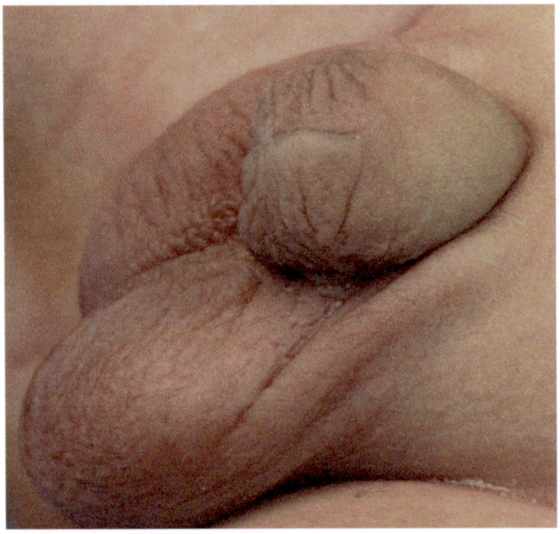

Fig. 16.3 A deep groove at midline at dorsal surface of the prepuce

Congenital torsion and chordee have to be distinguished from Peyronie's disease in adults, where *curvature* is acquired progressively, and it is due to fibrous plaques in the corporal bodies. Penile rotation can range from mild to severe. The penis is almost always rotated to the left (counter-clockwise). Penile torsion can be a stand-alone medical issue, or associated with other congenital conditions of the penis.

Isolated preputial rotation or distortion in relation to the penis is not reported before, in such cases the penile shaft and skin is normal with a normal urethra, but the prepuce lies at a different planes from the rest of the penis, preputial deviation is to the left side in the presented two diagnosed cases (Fig. 16.4).

Isolated downward angulation of glans penis and the prepuce is not also reported before, what was mentioned in literature are different forms of penile chordee, the case in Fig. 16.5 shows a downward direction of the prepuce and preputial meatus, with an abnormal urinary stream, again this is an isolated anomaly; where the prepuce is not in the same line with the penile shaft (Fig. 16.5).

Congenital curvature becomes usually symptomatic at puberty, when erections makes it obvious. The need for treatment has

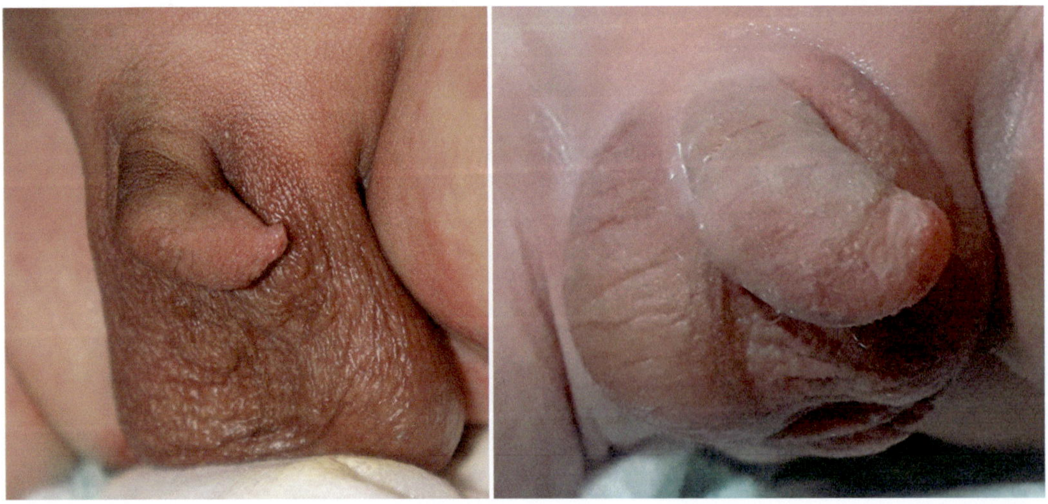

Fig. 16.4 Left sided isolated preputial deviation, with a normal penile alignment

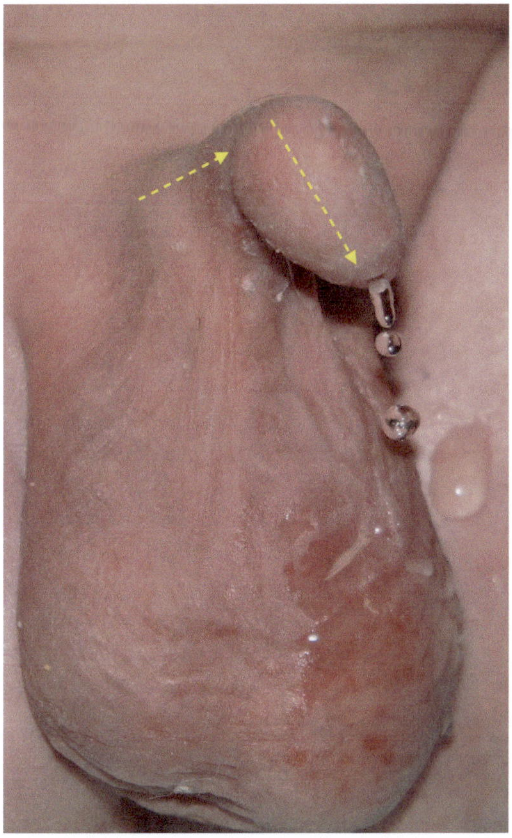

Fig. 16.5 Downward angulation of the prepuce, with an associated bending of the glans penis, prepuce and glans penis are at a right angle with penile axis

to be assessed according to the symptomatology. Curvatures making intercourse impossible require indeed surgical correction. Usual clinical practice recommends correction of curvature if the bending is superior to 30 degrees [2].

- *Abnormal preputial corrugations*: Normally the prepuce acquire the same corrugations of the scrotum secondary to the attachment of the dartos muscle fibers to the skin, but the cases in Fig. 16.6 showing a one side (left) preputial corrugation with a smooth skin in the right half of the prepuce, this unilateral preputial corrugation is associated with an ectopic testicle in the same side (Fig. 16.6).
- *Median raphe anomalies* are so wide and it may affect the preputial raphe as well, [3] but the case seen in Fig. 16.7 is an extremely rare raphe anomaly; where the scrotal median raphe is abnormally prominent and anchored the preputial meatus to the scrotal skin (Fig. 16.7).

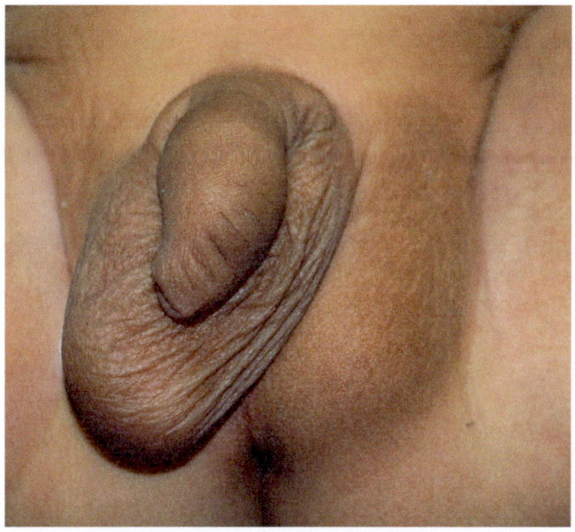

Fig. 16.6 One side (left sided) preputial corrugation associated with an ipsilateral ectopic testicle

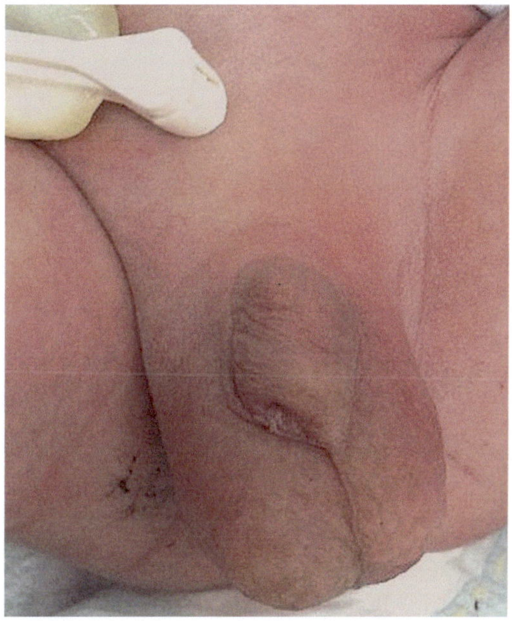

Fig. 16.7 Very rare case of preputial adhesion with a prominent median raphe, result in severe penoscrotal adhesion

- *Congenital Preputial perforation* or double preputial meatuses: Perforation of prepuce has been previously reported as a sequel of both

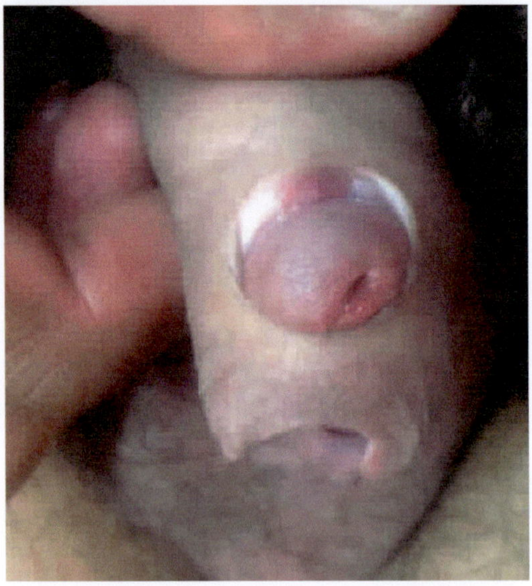

Fig. 16.8 Glans protruding through a large defect on the dorsal aspect of prepuce and narrowed primary opening of prepuce positioned on the ventral aspect of penis

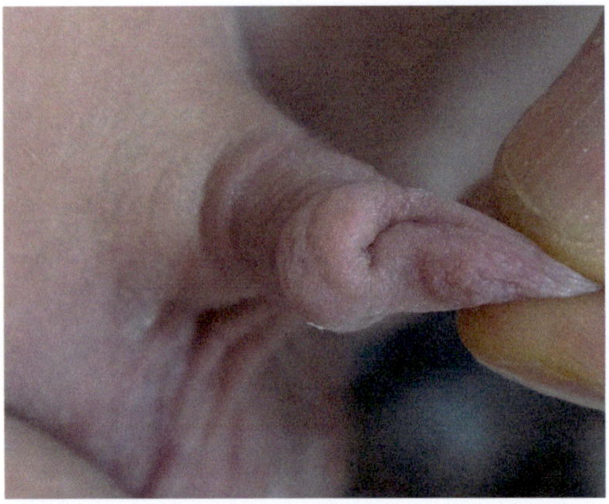

Fig. 16.9 A neonate with two preputial openings, one to the right patent with urinary meatus and another one as a dimple at the tip of the prepuce

infectious and noninfectious diseases, and herpetic perforation of prepuce recently reported [4] (Fig. 16.8).

But there is no previous report about a congenitally double preputial meatuses, in Fig. 16.9; the prepuce had a normal opening at the tip, but it is an obliterated one, where another opening detected at the right side communicated to the urinary meatus (Fig. 16.9).

Preputial Cutaneous Horn (Angiokeratoma)

Generally the cutaneous horn (Latin: cornu cutaneum) is a rare clinical entity that appears as a conical protuberance over the human skin surface and resembles a minuscule animal horn. The scientific name of this lesion, based on its histological characters is angiokeratoma.

Historically

The first description of cutaneous horn accredit to a German pathologist called Baron Carl von Rokitansky, The Danish anatomist Thomas Bartholin was the first to have a correct theory of the etiology of these horny growths, and the English surgeons John Hunter and Everard Home confirmed his findings in the late eighteenth century. Preputial horn is a very rare acquired lesion reported infrequently [5].

Definition

It is a circumscribed conical markedly hyperkeratotic lesion in which the height of the keratotic mass amounts to at least half of its largest diameter. On the other hand, angiokeratoma has a pleomorphic appearance varying from papules, nodules, or plaques which may be single or multiple. They are of different shapes and sizes and in some cases the main lesion may have another smaller satellite horns (Fig. 16.10).

Clinically

Many clinical variants had been described, solitary angiokeratoma represents an acquired disorder presenting as single warty papule, which is scarcely described in the literature, but they still remain novel to many clinicians especially when located in unusual areas like the prepuce. Cutaneous horn occurs mainly in males above 50 years of age and preputial horns are no exception to this rule [6].

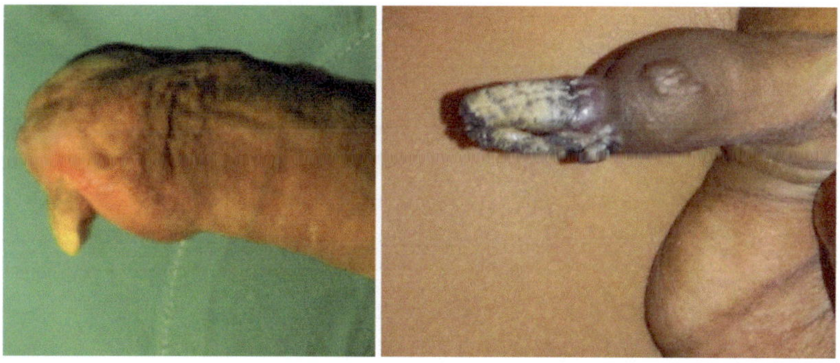

Fig. 16.10 Different sizes of preputial horns

Horns are usually appear in uncovered areas from constant irritation over the exposed skin, possible underlying factors which may lead to appearance of genital horns include phimosis, post surgical trauma, and radiotherapy.

Differential Diagnosis

Penile horns are a common misleading pathology, despite the typical appearance, there are a wide range of pathologies, from benign, premalignant to malignant which may mimc it; at older age malignant verruca, and condylomata acuminata at middle age should be differentiated from the preputial and penile horns, benign verruca or seborrheic keratosis should be also considered. It is a great cause for apprehension to many patients. In younger age group, only one case of a 20 years old male with a penile horn over the ventral surface of penis has been reported, cutaneous penile horn in pediatric age group is extremely rare [7].

Histology

The horn is composed of compacted keratin. The base of the horn may be flat, nodular, or crateriform. On histology, various lesions have been documented at the base of the keratin mound, and histologic confirmation is often necessary to rule out malignant changes. Histological appearance characterised by hyperkeratosis, papillomatosis and marked acanthosis with inwardly bending broad rete pegs enclosing cavernous blood vessels with fibrin thrombi.

A study analyzing 643 cases of horns affected many body areas; had reported that the most common cutaneous horns are benign (61.1%), followed by premalignant (23.2%) and malignant (15.7%) in that order [8].

To date, a little more than 150 cases of penile horns have been reported in the literature. It is reported that penile horn may be benign in 42–56% of cases, premalignant in 22–37%, or frankly malignant in 20–22%. There is no precise clinical information to make a distinction between benign and malignant cutaneous horns, but malignancy could be suspected if the horn had a large base or long height to base ratio, tenderness, present at unusual sites such as genitalia, and if discovered at advanced age. The presence of a malignancy elsewhere in the body supports the probability of cutaneous horn to be malignant [9].

Pilonidal Sinus and Cyst

A pilonidal cyst or sinus is an abscess or a chronic draining sinus usually containing hairs. To date there have been fewer than 20 cases of pilonidal sinus of the penis reported worldwide. The first was reported at 1833. Diagnosis of a pilonidal sinus of the penis or foreskin is generally made from postoperative histopathological findings rather than from preoperative findings [10].

Clinically they may present as a classic case of inflammation with pain, local infection, and redness, but may also show chronic ulceration or a draining sinus. Rarely, squamous cell carcinoma may develop. It is therefore important to consider pilonidal sinus as a differential diagnosis for a penile lesion and distinguish it from balanoposthitis, epidermal cyst, and carcinoma [11].

The theory on pathogenesis of pilonidal sinuses is that it is an acquired pathology, mechanical forces lead to hair being pushed beneath the skin into tiny abrasions or scars in the skin, forming a one-ended tunnel where bacteria and necrotic debris may collect. This leads to inflammation and infection resulting in cyst formation, which subsequently becomes oedematous and ruptures. A sinus will then form to drain the suppuration. In the penis, although rare, the theory of formation is that the coronal sulcus acts as a cleft where the hair accumulates and is pushed into the shaft of the penis by mechanical forces and the rolling movement at the junction of the glans penis and the uncircumcised prepuce.

Pilonidal sinuses of the penis affect men aged between 21and 59 years, and who are usually uncircumcised. The lesion is usually located between the coronal sulcus and prepuce. It is related to phimosis and most commonly occurs dorsally (60%), however, it does occur ventrally in 33% of reported cases. Risk factors for pilonidal sinus occurrence include young age, a hirsute body structure, sedentary occupations, poor personal hygiene, family history of pilonidal sinus and a high body mass index [12].

On ultrasound as a mode of radiological imaging; the diagnostic imaging features include sinus anatomy with presence of both isoechoic and hypoechoic components and strands of hair present within.

Simple excision with primary closure or healing by granulation tissue and sinus tract excision is usually the treatment for pilonidal sinus elsewhere. However, this option would most likely be unsightly on the penis and therefore a circumcision is usually undertaken.

Preputial Phlebectasia

Phlebectasia is an abnormal dilatation of the veins of the penis, very rarely it may affect the prepuce.

Etiology

Local anatomic alterations are typically implicated as the primary causes of phlebectasia formation. These lesions can be considered as hamartomas, so it is an embryonic remnants, but usually revealed at older age by hormonal and physiologic stimuli at puberty.

The condition is rather unusual; its incidence increases after puberty.

Clinical Appearance

It appears as asymptomatic enlarged vessels on foreskin or on glans, either as a violaceous, raised, and serpiginous tract or as a bluish and soft nodule; single or multiple lesions approximately 0.5–1 cm in diameter. The nodules are usually tender and disappear under slight pressure but reappear when the pressure released.

Clinical Course

The presence of phlebectasia has no significant functional impact on intercourse, but psychically it may results in apprehensive state. Occasionally, vascular occlusion may occur causing the development of erythematous or dark painful swellings.

Diagnosis

Anamnesis and clinical appearance are enough for diagnosis, but Doppler ultrasonography may be used to better define the anatomical and physiological features. Rarely a direct phlebography may be indicated, which could confirm the clinical diagnosis [13].

Management

Recommended techniques are surgical resection and percutaneous radiographic embolization. Sclerosis of phlebectasia could be carried out by interventional radiology using ethanol made radiopaque with suitable agent and controlled with fluoroscopy. Such therapy permitted recovery of treated lesions, leaving light scars [14].

Preputial Crohn's Disease (PCD)

Anogenital lesions occur in approximately 30% of patients with intestinal Crohn's disease, either as a direct extension of active intestinal disease or as metastatic disease. Preputial Crohn's disease may presents many years before intestinal involvement, and in some cases there is a manifested preputial oedema only, with no evidence of granulomatous inflammation. The more usual presentation is ulceration, abscess, sinus and fistula formation, with a granulomatous histology. There may be deep linear fissures (knife cut sign) along the skin creases [15].

Four categories summarize the cutaneous manifestation of Crohn's disease; (a) granulomatous cutaneous disease, including perianal, peristomal and metastatic disease; (b) aphthous like and linear ulcerations, mucosal cobblestoning and nodules with granulomas; (c) nutritional changes, including acquired zinc deficiency, striae and changes associated with malabsorption; (d) a diverse group of disorders such as pyoderma gangrenosum, erythema nodosum, necrotizing vasculitis and finger clubbing. These manifestations sometimes are mistaken for contact dermatitis, candidiasis; and sexual abuse.

Treatment: If genital Crohn's disease is the presenting problem it is important to involve a gastroenterologist in management, as those patients need a full work-up to assess if there is intestinal disease as well. In ulcerative disease it is essential to exclude any fistulous tracts. In patients who have no systemic disease topical measures may be sufficient to control the cutaneous lesions, that is an ultrapotent topical steroid or topical tacrolimus. Severe disease may respond to oral steroids but recalcitrant ulcerative anogenital lesions and fistulous tracts may require infliximab [16].

Prophylaxis with phenoxymethyl penicillin/erythromycin was effective at preventing further episodes. Tumor necrosis factor-a inhibitors are recommended at an early stage [17].

Preputial Histoplasma

Cutaneous Histoplasma infection is very uncommon, though systemic Histoplasmosis is endemic in the southeastern and midwestern United States. A few reports have described penile Histoplasmosis, most commonly among immunocompromised patients and secondary to hematogenous spread in the context of systemic involvement. It presents as painless noduloulcerative lesions of the glans and shaft of the penis, if the prepuce affected; it is commonly presented with a picture of phimosis, and given the term "Histoplasmic Phimosis", a diseases which had no regional lymphadenopathy. The diagnosis can be made based on histomorphology and anti-Histoplasma immunostaining.

Treatment is with itraconazole 200 mg daily for a month [18].

Preputial Porokeratosis

Porokeratosis is a rare penile condition that present as spreading plaques with thin ridge-like borders and central atrophy. It is often misdiagnosed as condyloma, syphilis, granuloma annulare, lichen simplex chronicus, or eczema. Therefore, it has been suggested that this condition is underreported due to treatment as a sexually transmitted disease.

Biopsy shows comoid lamella with underlying dyskeratotic cells and management by cryosurgery, carbon dioxide laser, surgery, or local 5-fluorouracil.

Topical diclofenac has provided a resolution of some lesions but not all. Topical glucocorticoids or retinoids achieved only symptomatic relief. It is also important to follow up these patients as malignant transformation has been reported in nearly all types of porokeratosis but has not been reported in genital porokeratosis [19].

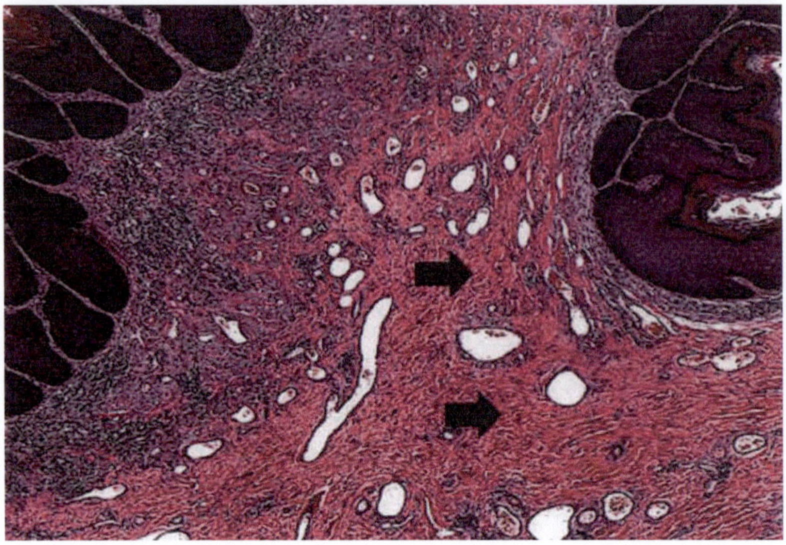

Fig. 16.11 Foreskin with localized amyloidosis showing sheets of eosinophilic, amorphous, fissured material in dermis and subcutaneous tissue (arrow)

Preputial Amyloidosis

The cutaneous form of amyloidosis is an uncommon lesion with asymptomatic, benign and indolent behaviour, that is easily differentiated from other genital lesions such as condyloma, verrucous carcinoma, and pearly penile papules. The characteristic microscopic features on H&E, and the positivity for Congo red and amyloid P component usually confirm the diagnosis. It is important to exclude systemic amyloidosis by investigating myelomatous (AL type), infectious (AA type), familial (ATTR type) or another systemic disease (b2 microglobulin). The management by local excision alone has been reported to be curative with no progression or systemic involvement [20] (Fig. 16.11).

Pyoderma Gangrenosum

Pyoderma gangrenosum (PG), is an extremely rare inflammatory ulcerative disease that usually occurs with systemic manifestations and rarely affects the penis. The diagnosis is by biopsy to exclude other causes of genital ulcers-infectious diseases (syphilis, chancroid, genital Herpes).

Rare neoplastic lesions like; apocrine hidrocystoma, preputial xanthoma and neuroma were discussed in Chap. 24.

References

1. Sarkis PE, Muthurajan S. Incidence and predictive factors of isolated neonatal penile glanular torsion. J Pediatr Urol. 2007;3:495–9.
2. Eroglu E, Gundogdu G. Isolated penile torsion in newborns. Can Urol Assoc J. 2015;9(11–12):E805–7. https://doi.org/10.5489/cuaj.2833.
3. Baky Fahmy M. The spectrum of genital median raphe anomalies among infants undergoing ritual circumcision. J Pediatr Urol. 2013;9(6):872–7. https://doi.org/10.1016/j.jpurol.2012.11.018.
4. Sumit Sethi S, et al. Herpetic perforation of prepuce. Indian J Dermatol Venereol Leprol. 2018;84:65. https://www.researchgate.net/publication/321954749.
5. Bondeson J. Everard home, john hunter, and cutaneous horns: a historical review. Am J Dermatopathol. 2001;23:362–9.
6. Agarwala MK, Mukhopadhyay S, Sekhar MR, Menon A, Dincy Peter CV. Solitary angiokeratoma presenting as cutaneous horn over the prepuce: a rare appearance. Indian J Dermatol. 2016;61:236.
7. Barolia DK, Sethi D, Sethi A, Ram J, Meena S, Rachhoya P. Penile cutaneous horn—a rare case. Int J Med Res Rev. 2015;3:1102–4.
8. Yu RC, Pryce DW, Macfarlane AW, Stewart TW. A histopathological study of 643 cutaneous horns. Br J Dermatol. 1991;124:449–52.

9. Mantese SA, Diogo PM, Rocha A, Berbert AL, Ferreira AK, Ferreira TC. Cutaneous horn: a retrospective histopathological study of 222 cases. An Bras Dermatol. 2010;85:157–63.
10. Randhawa K, Thomas S, Keanie J, Shukla CJ. Pilonidal sinus of the penis: merits of preoperative radiological diagnosis. J Clin Urol. 2019:205141581984015. https://doi.org/10.1177/2051415819840151.
11. Kulaylat MN, Gong M, Doerr RJ. Multimodality treatment of squamous cell carcinoma complicating pilonidal disease. Am Surg. 1996;62:922–9.
12. Ercil H, Alma E, Eflatun Deniz M, et al. Recurrent pilonidal sinus cyst on penis. Arch Iran Med. 2018;21:131–3.
13. Edington GH. Some malformations of the penis. Br Med J. 1907;2(2438):725–9. JSTOR, www.jstor.org/stable/20295897.
14. Balato N, Montesano N. Acquired phlebectasia of the glans penis. J Am Acad Dermatol. 1985;13:824–6.
15. Bhoyrul B, Hilmy M, Lyon C. Crohn's disease of the penis and scrotum: a prospective study. Eur J Gastroenterol Hepatol. 2018;30:1528–9.
16. Casson DH, Eltumi M, Tomlin S, et al. Topical tacrolimus may be effective in the treatment of oral and perineal Crohn's disease. Gut. 2000;47:436–40.
17. Tally MR, Orenstein SR, Cohen BA. Crohn's disease of the vulva in an 8-year-old girl. Pediatr Dermatol. 1988;5:103–6.
18. Paixao M, Miot HA, Avancini J, Belda Junior W. Primary cutaneous histoplasmosis developed in the penis of an immunocompetent patient. An Bras Dermatol. 2015;90:255–7.
19. Liang C, Batra P, Patel R, Kamino H. Genital porokeratosis. Dermatol Online J. 2009;15:23.
20. Ritter M, Nawab RA, Tannenbaum M, Hakky SI, Morgan MB. Localized amyloidosis of the glans penis: a case report and literature review. J Cutan Pathol. 2003;30:37–40.

Part III

Acquired Diseases of the Prepuce

17 Smegma

Nomenclature and Definitions

The word smegma is from Greek "smēgma" meaning soap or an ointment. It produced in both male and female mammalian genitalia; in males smegma accumulated commonly under the foreskin and in female it is collected around the clitoris and in the folds of the labia minora. Also smegma can be found in other genital intertrigo. It is just a genital form of body sebum. Its production increases in puberty and remains high in adults to decline in old age.

Historical Background

French physician, Claude-François Lallemand (1790–1853), pronounced that smegma could provoke erections that would lead to 'disastrous pleasures'.

American physician Roberts Bartholow (1831–1904) formulated the theory that smegma produced 'hyperæsthesia' of the glans.

American urologist Abraham Wolbarst (1872–1952), who updated the demonization of the foreskin and promulgated the idea that it harboured 'carcinogenic secretions'.

Smegma was originally thought to be produced by sebaceous glands near the frenulum called Tyson's glands. The English Anatomist Edward Tyson (1650–1708) described a modified sebaceous glands in the coronal sulcus, which he stated were responsible for smegma production. He never published his observations, but he noted them in a syllabus that was distributed to his students. Tyson inserted the words 'Glandula Mucilaginosa' under the heading 'Urethra Ejus' with a footnote stating that he had discovered such glands [1]. A modern interpretation indicated that his observations might have been in reference to primates rather than humans. Tyson might have described the condition that is at the present known as papillomatosis corona penis (Pearly penile papules), which is not related to sebaceous glands [2, 3].

Composition

Wright [4] states that smegma is produced from minute microscopic protrusions of the mucosal surface of the foreskin and that living cells constantly grow towards the surface, undergo fatty degeneration, separate off, and form smegma. According to Wright, little smegma is produced during childhood, although the foreskin may contain sebaceous glands. She also says that production of smegma increases from adolescence until sexual maturity when the function of smegma for lubrication assumes its full value, and from middle-age production starts to decline and in old age virtually no smegma is produced.

The smegma is cheese-like sebaceous matter is a combination of shed skin cells, skin oils, and moisture. A natural secretion of skin cells and oils that collects under the foreskin in both males

M. A. B. Fahmy, *Normal and Abnormal Prepuce*, https://doi.org/10.1007/978-3-030-37621-5_17

and females. If allowed to grow stale, it may have a pungent aroma (commonly compared to cheese in males or fish in females) [1].

Newly produced smegma has a smooth, moist texture. It is thought to be rich in squalene [5].

The presence of fructose and acid phosphatase in subpreputial material and the absence of urea, leads Prakash S and Jeyakumar [6] to indicates the presence of seminal vesical and prostatic secretions in smegma, they also reported that smegma is a subpreputial collection of desquamated epithelial debris, mixed with mucin, and secretions with a composition including fat (about 27%) and protein (about 13%), which consistent with necrotic epithelial debris.

Others claim that smegma contains prostatic and seminal secretions, desquamated epithelial cells, and the mucin content of the urethral glands of Littré [7].

Those who claim an immunological function of smegma reported finding of chymotrypsin, neutrophil elastase, cytokines cathepsin B, and lysozymes, which aid the immune system [8, 9].

Bacteriology

There are few studies investigating the colonisation and exact nature of smegma that had never been exposed to the outside in the subpreputial space between the inner prepuce skin and glans surface before prepuce excoriate. In one study smegma is found to be sterile [10].

In a study from Nigeria, they founded bacterial isolates in smegma swabs from 52 boys ranging in age from 7 days to 11 years. A single isolate was found in 34 boys (65.4%), eight had a mixed isolate (15.4%), while no bacteria was isolated in 10 boys (19.2%). The commonly isolated gram-positive bacteria were Staphylococcus epidermidis (44.8%) and S. aureus (41.4%) and the most commonly isolated gram-negative bacterium was E. coli (90.5%). Most of the bacterial isolates were multi-drug resistant. They suggested the differences in the organisms from other studies, means a local variation due to differences in climate and diet, but also the socio-economic differences in the various populations [11].

Some authors in order to prove the role of smegma in induction of UTI, they claimed that virgin smegma in the subpreputial space of children was colonized by many kinds of uropathogen of E. coli, which may predispose to UTI and leads to increased its high prevalence in uncircumcised boys [10].

Functions

Smegma beneficially serves to preserve subpreputial wetness. The main function of smegma is moisturising and lubricating the cavity between the foreskin and the glans that is the subpreputial space, facilitating erection, preputial eversion and penetration during sexual intercourse. This natural lubricant allows for prolonged intercourse and eliminates the need for artificial supplemental lubrication during normal coitus or masturbation [12].

Smegma had a pheromonal (sexual attractant), this is obvious in certain animals, but it is uncertain in human and perhaps it had bacteriostatic functions. The power of an accumulation of smegma to erogenously stimulate the nervous system was consistent with the accepted theory of reflex 'irritation', a term then understood to mean 'stimulation' rather than its modern connotation of discomfort [1].

It may contain anti-bacterial enzymes including lysozyme and hormones like androsterone, although this is equivocal [13].

It also may contain immunologically active chemical compounds such as cathepsin B, lysozyme, chymotrypsin, neutrophil elastase, cytokines, specially lysozyme, which probably originates from the prostate and seminal vesicles, to destroy bacterial cell walls and inhibit and destroy some candidal species [13].

Hazards

When the foreskin is not retractable smegma can accumulate between the inner surface of the foreskin and the glans and looks like a yellowish-white, clearly defined, soft mass

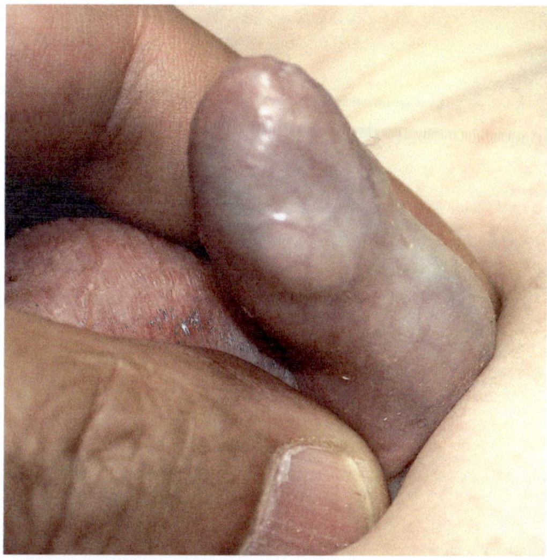

Fig. 17.1 Clumps of smegma aggregation under a nonretractable prepuce

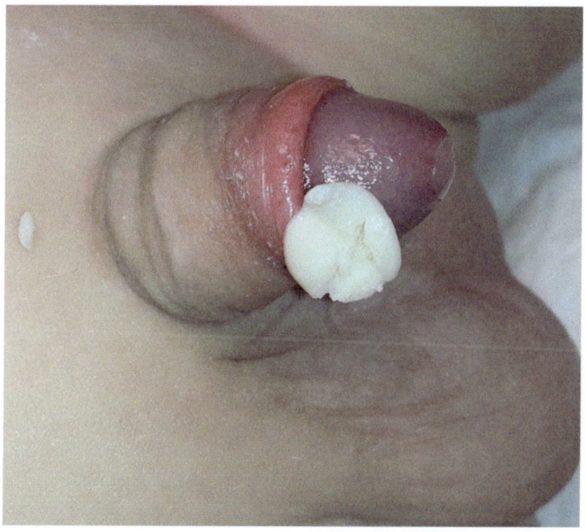

Fig. 17.2 Protruded smegma mass after managing the prepuce to retract

(Fig. 17.1). During retraction of the foreskin without forcing, this mass becomes evident and sometimes protrudes over the free edge of the foreskin (Fig. 17.2).

Smegma may aggregates to form a lump or it may become hard to form a smegma stone or smegmoliths, smegma may be entrapped between the edges of the circumcision wound to form a different shapes and sizes of smegma cysts (Fig. 17.3).

Smegma cysts of different sizes may be also formed in the circumcised penis distal to the

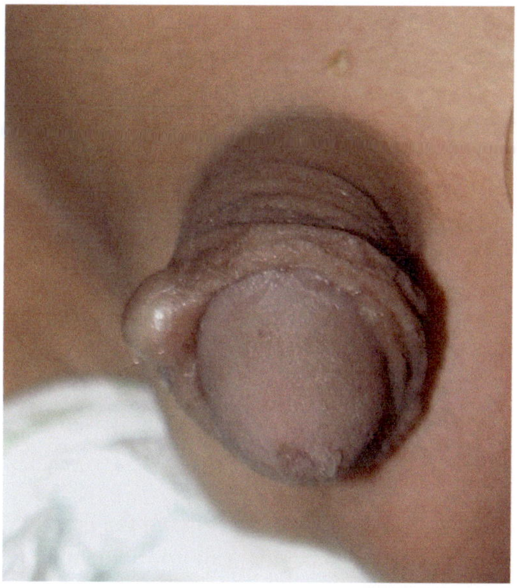

Fig. 17.3 Small smegma cyst formed between the edges of circumcision wound

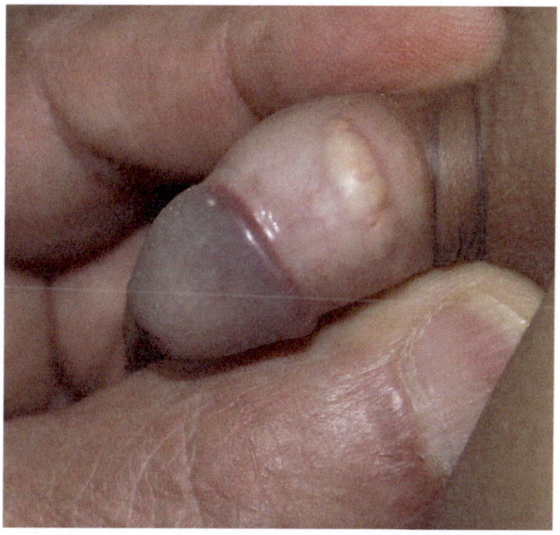

Fig. 17.4 Entrapped smegma cysts under the preputial remnants

edges of the wound, this may be due entrapment of smegma particles between penile or preputial skin layers (Fig. 17.4).

Smegma accumulations may induce irritation with a subsequent dermatitis (balanitis or balanoposthitis), also aggregated smegma may be colonised with different pathogenic bacteria and became a source of infection.

Circumcision will not abolish smegma secretion, but it will reduce the chance of its accumulations, circumcised boy may still accumulates smegma, if it is not cleaned and washed frequently.

Figure 17.5 showing a normally produced smegma in a circumcised boy, we can also notice the adjacent inflammation in the preputial remnant. Someone may argue that this because the circumcision is incomplete and the preputial remnant is predisposing for such complication, but in Fig. 17.6 an infant with excessive preputial removal, without any remnant, but he still had a liner smegma accumulated at the coronal sulcus. A smegma produced in circumcised boys in the same way as in uncircumcised one (Fig. 17.7).

Smegmoliths: (Fig. 17.8).

It is a concretions of smegma in the preputial sac, consisted of smegma with uric acid, and to a lesser extent calcium phosphate. It is seen with a different consistency and sizes, of greyish-yellow or tawny color, of roundish shape or oval, and consist of all or only some of those elements which make up the smegma and arranged in the form of concentric layers.

Majocchi [14], reported several cases of smegmoliths in male boys and he reffered that smegmoliths are also founded in the preputial sac of horses. He believed that B. coli acting upon urea makes ammonia which combines with the fat in the smegma and forms ammonia soaps. Urinary salts and epithelial debris are deposited around this nucleus which increases the size and the density of the smegma stones [15].

Smegma cysts discussed in Chap. 25.

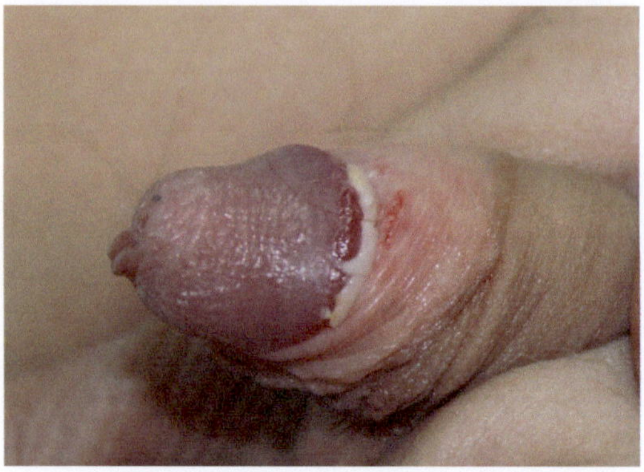

Fig. 17.5 A Circumcised boy with smegma at the coronal sulcus and minimal posthitis in the preputial remnant

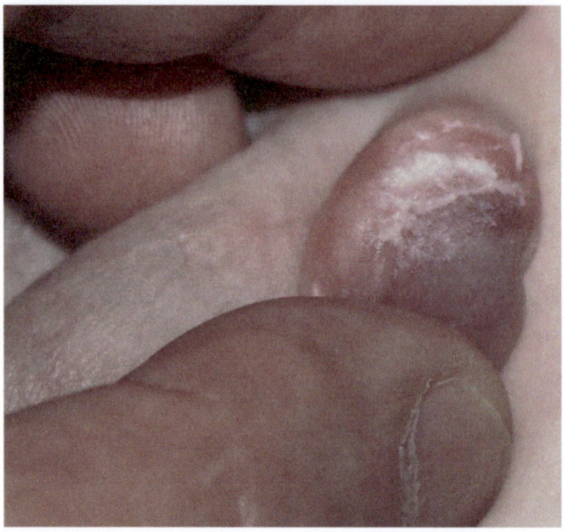

Fig. 17.6 Over circumcised infant with a smegma at the coronal sulcus

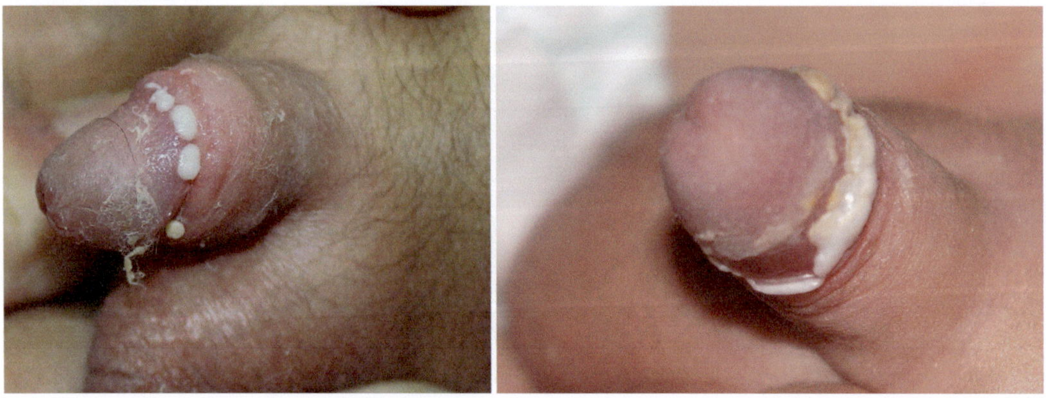

Fig. 17.7 Smegma produced by a circumcised boys in a same configuration as it is produced in uncircumcised one

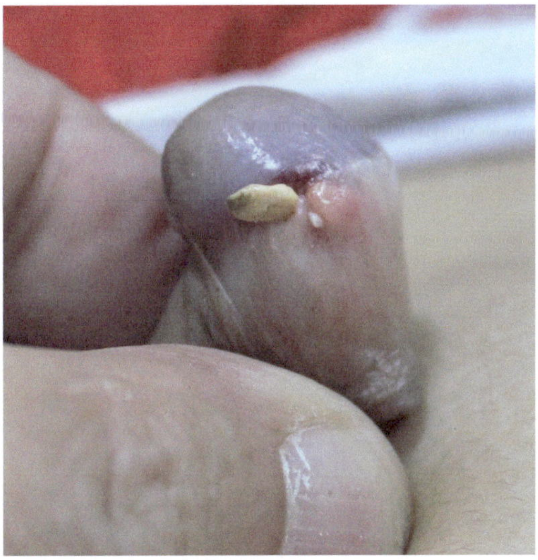

Fig. 17.8 A small smegmolith

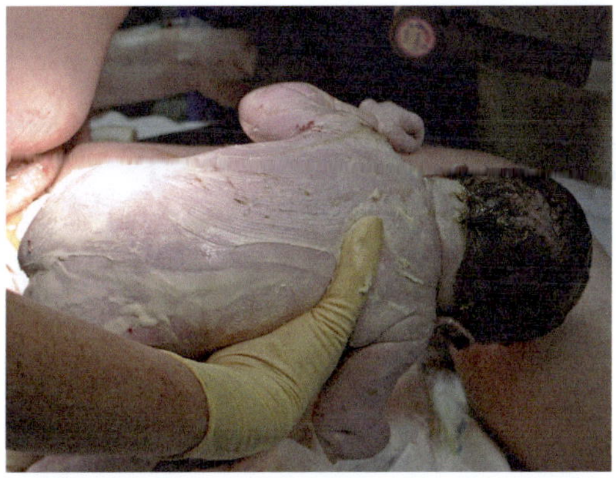

Fig. 17.9 Vernix caseosa at the back of a just born baby, it is physically similar to smegma. A public domain photo from Wikipedia, the file licensed under the Creative Commons Attribution-Share Alike 4.0 International license

When Smegma Starts to Form?

Smegma is a natural emollient secretion of skin cells and oils that collects under the foreskin in both males and females, it is firstly seen in the enlarged posterior extremity of the glandar lamella, (the future coronal sulcus in adult), approximately at sixth month of foetal life. Prepuce completely covering and fusing with the glans structure at around 24th week of gestation.

Smegma like the earwax and vernix caseosa, also known as vernix, which is the waxy or cheese-like white substance found coating the skin of newborn human babies. It is produced by dedicated cells and is thought to have some protective roles during fetal development and for a few hours after birth. There is a great similarity between smegma and vernix in texture and physical characters (Fig. 17.9).

Smegma had no relation to the glandopreputial membrane and it is not formed by the shaded or desquamated cells of this membrane, as smegma formed and become detectable as early as the prepuce formed, and before any separations of the glandopreputial membrane, what was reported in some studies about desquamated cell detected histologically with smegma are just cells in the scene from which the smegma samples collected [7].

Researchers at Botkin's Hospital in Moscow have asserted that smegma is produced from minute microscopic protrusions of the mucosal surface of the foreskin. According to those scientists, living cells constantly grow towards the surface, undergo fatty degeneration, separate off, and form smegma [1].

Smegma quantities and aggregations are so variable between individuals; Cowper stated that sebaceous glands producing smegma were more numerous and larger in the individuals who have a larger prepuce [16].

Many neonates delivered with an obvious smegma, or even a different forms of preputial aggregations (Fig. 17.10).

Smegma may be scanty, or bulky, very rarely to be absent or deficient, it is commonly arranged in row or streaks at the coronal sulcus (Fig. 17.11), rarely it may be visible at the preputial ring, or adherent to the glandular surface in a radial form (Figs. 17.12 and 17.13).

Øster [17] reported that the incidence of absent smegma increased from 1% among 6- to 7-year-olds and 8- to 9-year-olds to 9% among 14- to 15-year-olds and 16- to 17-year-olds (an overall incidence of 5%).

In one survey, out of 18 self-selected intact men never saw smegma; 1 saw it after a week unwashed, 6 after 2 days, 8 after 1 day, and 1 after less than a day [16].

Smegma is mainly confined to the preputial sac, but it is also produced at any genital intertrigo, this gives us a strong believe that smegma

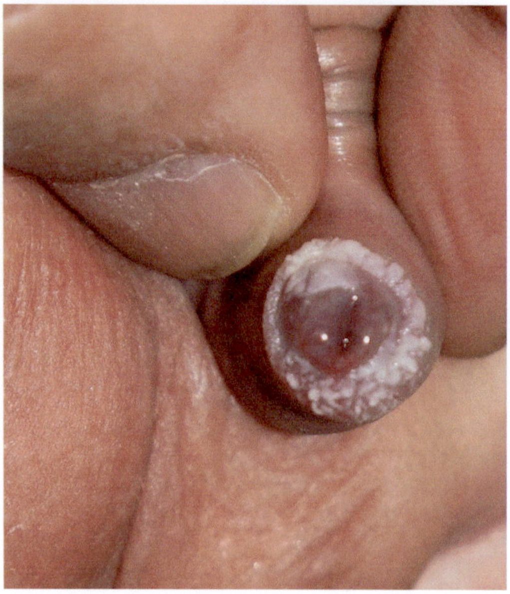

Fig. 17.10 A neonate with a small smegma particles emerging from the preputial ring

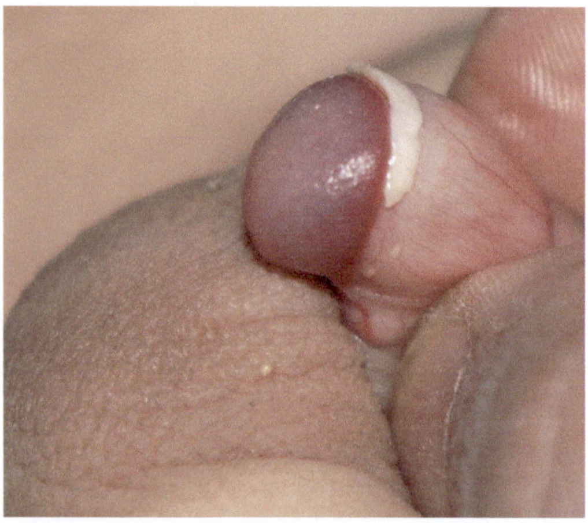

Fig. 17.11 Smegma commonly distributed as a streaks at the coronal sulcus

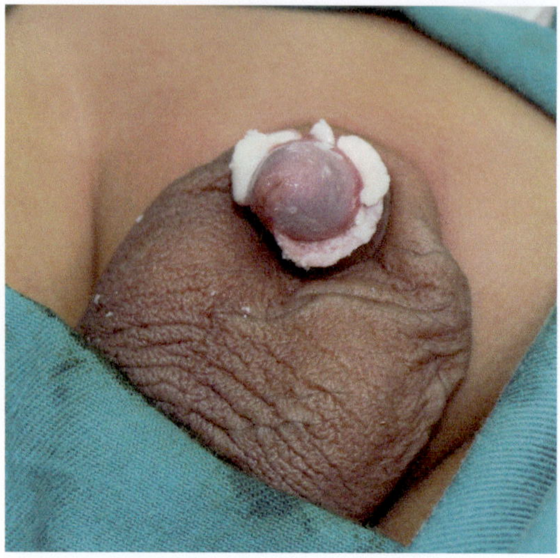

Fig. 17.12 Plenty of smegma at the base of inner prepuce

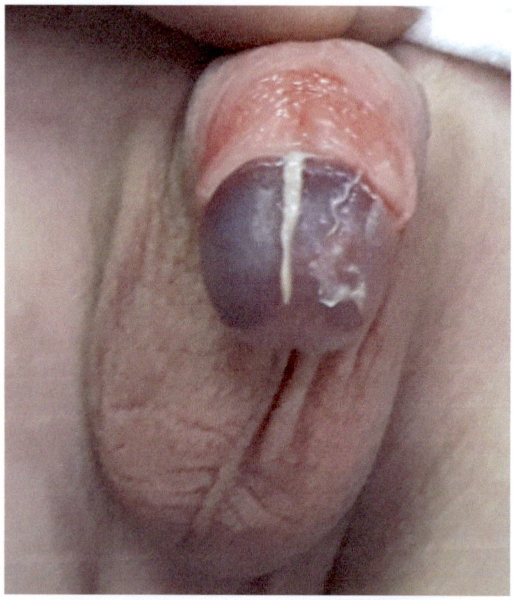

Fig. 17.13 Rare distribution of the smegma as a liner streaks arranged radially over the glans

is just a modified sebum secreted from the sebaceous glands of the genital area in both male and female, not only at the coronal sulcus or the preputial sac, but also from any skin crease in the genital area (intertrigo).

It is mentioned earlier by Cowper who stated that specialised sebaceous glands were located mainly at the coronal sulcus where the preputial mucosa reflected to form the inner prepuce [16].

So it is reasoning to have another similar glands producing the same smegma in other genital skin creases.

In Fig. 17.14 a neonate female with a prominent sebaceous gland and scattered area of

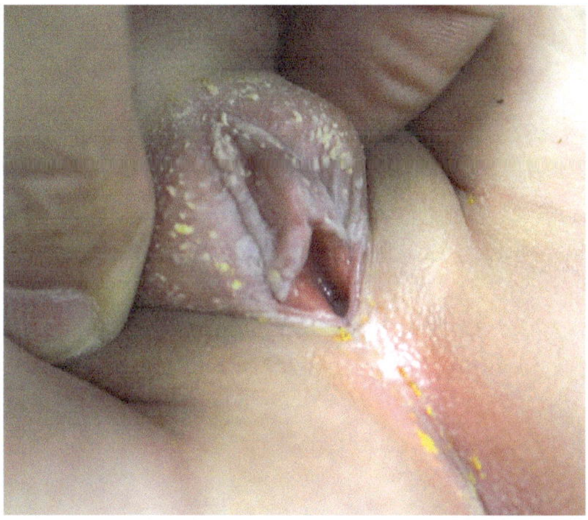

Fig. 17.14 A neonate girl with a prominent yellow papules and ectopic smegma scattered in the labia major

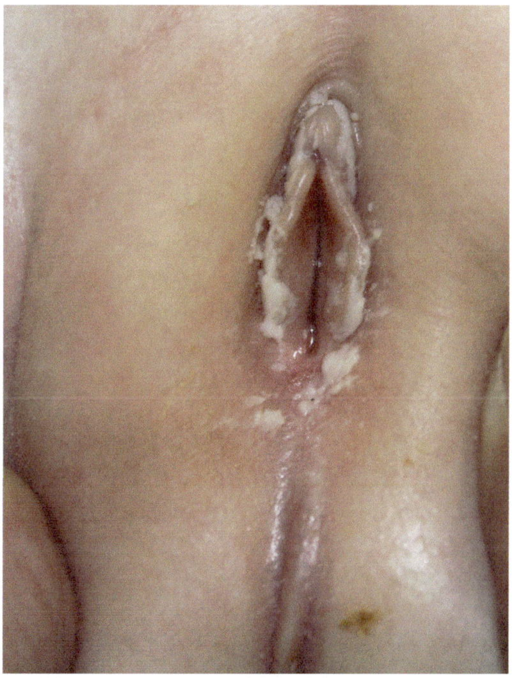

Fig. 17.15 An infant girl with smegma around the whole introits

smegma at the labia majora, this is also obvious in an older girl with a smegma not only confined to the clitoris and preputial area, but also all around the introits (Fig. 17.15).

In normal children, who had a skin crease at the root of the penis, a different aggregation of smegma can be appreciated at these creases (Figs. 17.16 and 17.17). Many cases of hypospadias also may have smegma at the penile root (Fig. 17.18).

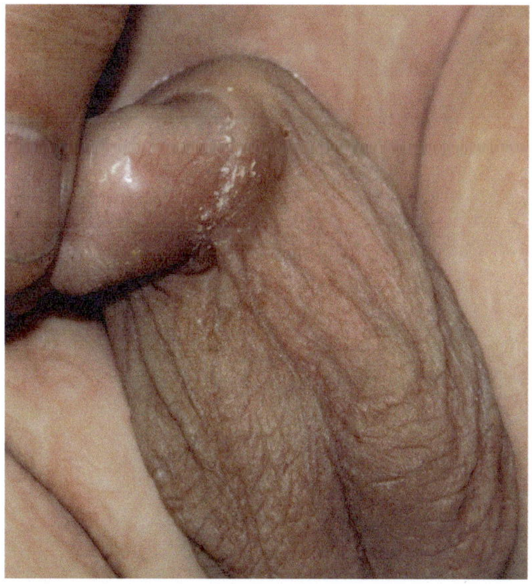

Fig. 17.16 Smegma in a skin crease at the root of the penis

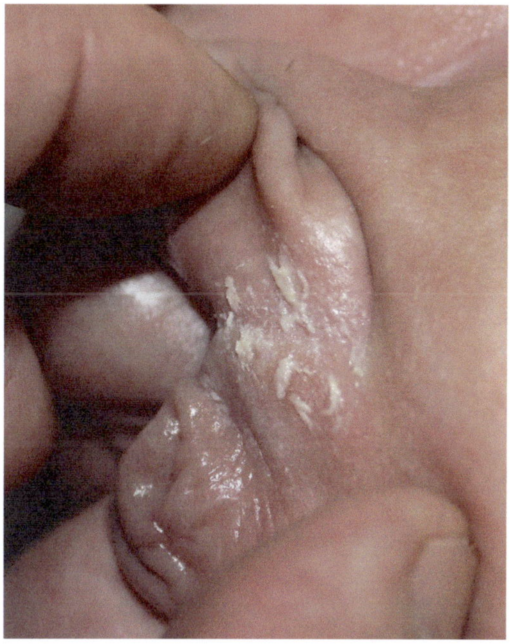

Fig. 17.17 Three months old boy with many smegma secreted at the root of the penis

An explicit example for the presence of smegma in an ectopic area is the case in

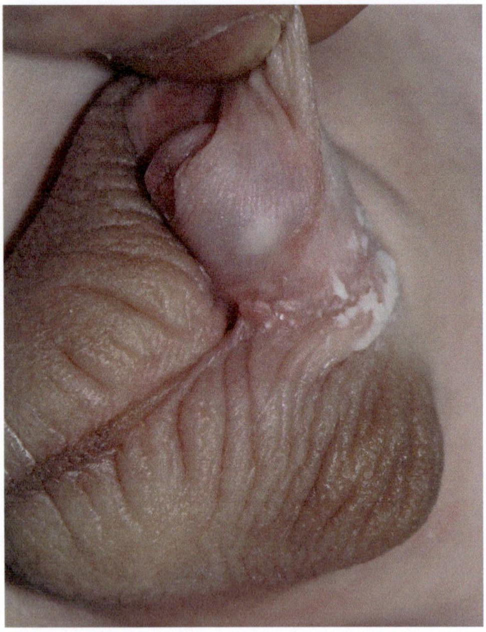

Fig. 17.18 A case of hypospadias with smegma at the root of the penis

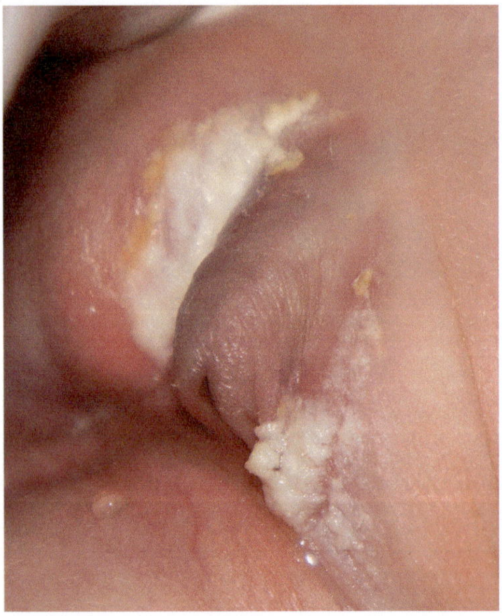

Fig. 17.19 An interesting case of a girl with adrenogenital hyperplasia, and extensive smegma at the furrows between the enlarged clitoris and labia

Fig. 17.19, a young girl with an adrenogenital hyperplasia with a prominent clitoris, and she had an extensive smegma at the furrows between the phallus and labia. This a clear prove that smegma is not a preputial secretion and of course it could not be eliminated with circumcision (Fig. 17.19).

Conclusion

Few years earlier I published my concept about smegma and its distribution in my illustrative textbook of the congenital anomalies of the penis [18], and herein I could refine this concept in few points:

- Smegma is secreted during the late intrauterine period, as many neonates, and even a preterm babies may had an accumulated smegma in their first day of life.
- Smegma is a secretion of a modified sebaceous gland, which are mainly located at the coronal sulcus, but any intertrigo in the genital area may also produce smegma in both male and female.
- Smegma is the natural secretion of the prepuce, like other body secretions, (like ear wax). So it is not harmful by itself, unless it is contaminated with other pathogens; either bacterial colonisation, virus overgrowth or combined organisms, or associated with phimosis.
- Circumcision will not stop smegma production or ameliorate its effect, if any, circumcision will just help in exposing smegma for regular wash. Smegma will continue to produce and even it may accumulates in circumcised boys if not cared.
- Smegma secretion and distribution had a great variations between individuals, without a clear explanation.
- Some boys may present with one or more yellowish lumps on the penis that are often diagnosed by the general practitioner as a sebaceous cysts or lipoma of the penile shaft, but on assessment, these prove to be collections of retained smegma trapped by the surrounding preputial adhesions.
- During circumcision and other penile surgery, smegma should be cleaned and removed meticulously with a saline wash, otherwise any retained small pieces will accumulate between the edges of perpetual remnants and results in different forms of smegma cyst, which may acquire a larger size and be troublesome.

References

1. Van Howe RS, Hodges FM. The carcinogenicity of smegma: debunking a myth. J Eur Acad Dermatol Venereol. 2006;20:1046–54.
2. Hyman AB, Brownstein MH. Tyson's "glands." Ectopic sebaceous glands and papillomatosis penis. Arch Dermatol. 1969;99:31–6.
3. Velazquez EF, Cold CJ, Barreto JE, Cubilla AL. Penis and distal urethra. In: Mills SE, editor. Histology for pathologists, vol. 965. Philadelphia: Lippincott Williams & Wilkins; 2007.
4. Wright J. How smegma serves the penis: Nature's assurance that the uncircumcised glans penis will function smoothly is provided by smegma. Sexology. 1970;37(2):50–3.
5. O'Neill HJ, Gershbein LL. Lipids of human and equine smegma. Oncology. 1976;33(4):161–6. https://doi.org/10.1159/000225134.
6. Parkash S, Jeyakumar S. Human subpreputial collection: its nature and formation. J Urol. 1973;110(2):211–2. https://doi.org/10.1016/s0022-5347(17)60164-2.
7. Fleiss PM, Hodges FM, Van Howe RS. Immunological functions of the human prepuce. Sex Transm Infect. 1998;74(5):364–7. https://doi.org/10.1136/sti.74.5.364.
8. Anyanwu LJ, Kashibu E. Microbiology of smegma in boys in Kano, Nigeria. J Surg Res. 2012;173(1):21–5. https://doi.org/10.1016/j.jss.2011.04.057.
9. Frohlich E, Schaumburg-Lever G, Klessen C. Immunelectron microscopic localization of cathepsin B in human exocrine glands. J Cutan Pathol. 1993;20:54–60.
10. Chung JM, et al. Microbiology of smegma: prospective comparative control study. Investig Clin Urol. 2019;60:127–32. https://doi.org/10.4111/icu.2019.60.2.127.
11. Anyanwu LJ, Kashibu E, Edwin CP, Mohammad AM. Microbiology of smegma in boys in Kano, Nigeria. J Surg Res. 2012;173:21–5.
12. O'Hara K, O'Hara J. The effect of male circumcision on the sexual enjoyment of the female partner. BJU Int. 1999;83:79–84.
13. Fröhlich E, Schaumburg-Lever G, Klessen C. Immunelectron microscopic localization of cathepsin B in human exocrine glands. J Cutan Pathol. 1993;20:54–60.
14. Majocchi D. Ueber die smegmogenen Concretionen des Präputialsackes "Smegmolithen" und über die Analogie zwischen diesen und anderen Epidermisconcretionen des Menschen und einiger Säugethiere. Arch F Dermat. 1902;59:9–26. https://doi.org/10.1007/BF01822886.
15. D'arcy McCrea E. Chapter XIII - Injuries of the penis. Phimosis and paraphimosis. Preputial calculi. In: Diseases of the urethra and penis. Amsterdam: Butterworth-Heinemann; 2013. p. 232–45. https://doi.org/10.1016/B978-1-4831-6791-6.50016-8.
16. Batistatou A, Panelos J, Zioga A, Charalabopoulos KA. Ectopic modified sebaceous glands in human penis. Int J Surg Pathol. 2006;14(4):355–6. https://doi.org/10.1177/1066896906291779.
17. Øster J. Further fate of the foreskin. Incidence of preputial adhesions, phimosis, and smegma among Danish schoolboys. Arch Dis Child. 1968;43(228):200–3. https://doi.org/10.1136/adc.43.228.200.
18. Fahmy M. Chapter 36: Smegmoma "smegma collection in health and disease". In: Congenital anomalies of the penis. Cham: Springer; 2017. https://doi.org/10.1007/978-3-319-43310-3.

18 Phimosis

Introduction

Many medical authorities, specially in the United States have claimed that every newborn male suffers from phimosis, a disease that many experts, along the medical history, presume that it is the cause of a wide range of other incurable diseases; from club foot to insanity.

Since its emergence in the nineteenth century, the modem concept of phimosis has been the focus of a carefully orchestrated campaign of legitimisation. Traditionally, doctors in the United States, who favour involuntary circumcision of the newborn, have claimed that phimosis is ubiquitous in that it apparently occurs as a congenital deformity in nearly all newborn males. In Britain, the ubiquity is reduced to some 30,000 cases a year, but this nonetheless represents an equal or higher rate of disease than the annual rate of breast cancer or lung cancer in Britain [1].

It has been demonstrated that the squamous mucosa of the glans, coronal sulcus, and prepuce are fused during the embryologic development of the penis, and they can be considered as one tissue compartment. The fused mucosa of the glans and inner lining of the foreskin separate gradually over years, as a spontaneous biologic process, this separation is variable between individuals and usually completed by the age of 17 years [2].

Definition

Along the recorded medical history ambiguity over the term phimosis continues, so that many children are thought to have a pathological condition when often there is none. Greater understanding among paediatric surgeons and general practitioners of the definition, diagnoses and proper management of phimosis should lead to a decreased rate of referral and reduce the anxiety of parents and patients.

The word phimosis is from the Greek *phimos* (φῖμός) which means a muzzle, and phimosis means muzzling (closure or stenosis of the mouth of a tube or a hose).

Phimosis by definition is the inability or difficulty to retract prepuce secondary to tight preputial hiatus; this tightness may be physiological or pathological, and it is completely different from the adhesion between inner prepuce and glans penis, which is called “Synechia”. Phimosis is not a synonyms of preputial non retractability or preputial synechiae [3].

Subsequently, preputial non retractability may be physiological either due to preputo-glandular adhesion or a stenotic preputial hiatus or a short frenulum (Frenulum brave) (Chap. 32).

The first recorded use of the word phimosis was in Roman times. Various medical writers used the term simply to indicate a condition of being muzzled, irrespective of the body part

M. A. B. Fahmy, *Normal and Abnormal Prepuce*, https://doi.org/10.1007/978-3-030-37621-5_18

affected, ancient Greek physicians, such as Galen, and others, used the term to refer to inflammatory strictures of the anus, vagina or the eyelid, but not the prepuce. The first known author to use the word *phimosis* in reference to the prepuce was the Roman author Aulus Celsus in the first century CE, he used the term to indicate an abnormal induration of the foreskin.

The second known use of the word is found in the extant writings of the second century CE Greek physician Antyllus, who defines phimosis as a condition where the foreskin cannot be retracted because of inelastic scar tissue on the foreskin or because of a "fleshy growth [4]."

Pierre E. Dionis (died in 1718) [5], a French surgeon, hypothesised that there were two types of phimosis: natural and accidental, Dionis defined phimosis as a condition in which "the extremity of the prepuce is so tight that it will not permit the glans to be uncovered.

John Hunter (1728–1793) [6] even refined the definition of phimosis to refer only to a symptom of the venereal disease chancre, which presented itself as an abnormal inflammation and thickening of the cellular membrane of the foreskin.

British medicine has been the driving force behind the narrowing European definition of phimosis. The European thinking on phimosis has taken a radical departure from its nineteenth-century roots and from current American ideology. Phimosis is no longer a disease in itself or a cause of disease. Instead, it is a symptom of a single dermatological conditions; mainly the balanitis xerotica obliterans (BXO).

In Britain, the argument that the definition of phimosis should be divested of any notions of retractability, balanopreputial attachment, or abnormal preputial length, has been most successfully made by Rickwood [7] of Alder Hey Children's Hospital in Liverpool, who refined the definition of "true phimosis" to designate a condition where the tip of the prepuce is scarred and indurated and has the histological features of balanitis xerotica obliterans.

But I think this another hyperbole of the phimosis terminology, if we limit the term for use only in cases of BXO.

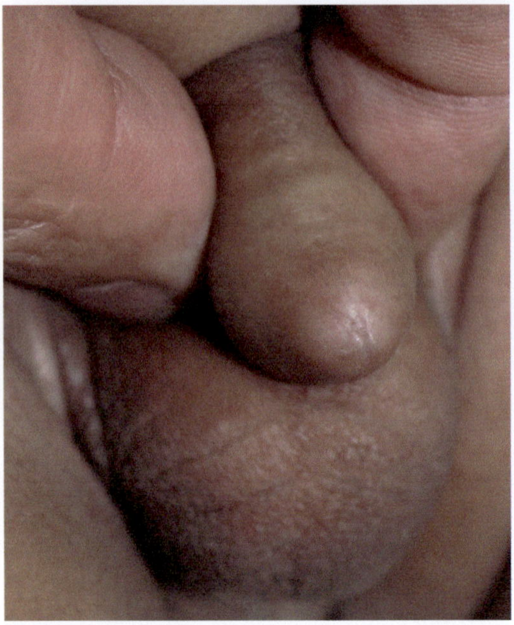

Fig. 18.1 Pathologically tight preputial hiatus hindering preputial gliding to expose the glans

My preferable defination for phimosis is: Phimosis is a pathologically tight preputial hiatus hindering preputial gliding to expose the glans penis, this tightness may be a congenital anomaly or an acquired disease (Fig. 18.1).

Synonyms

Preputial stenosis.

Historical Background

Phimosis prevented Louis XVI of France from impregnating his wife for the first 7 years of their marriage. She was 14 and he was 15 when they married in 1770. Some scholar claimed that he had phimosis, however, the presence and nature of his genital anomaly is not considered certain, and other scholars (such as Vincent Cronin and Simone Bertiere) assert that surgical repair would have been mentioned in the records of his medical treatments if this had indeed occurred.

US president James Garfield was assassinated by Charles Guiteau in 1881, Guiteau's autopsy report indicated that he had phimosis. At that time, this led to the speculation that Guiteau's murderous behaviour was due to a phimosis-induced insanity [8].

Phimosis in Animals

Phimosis is not only confined to humans, but also it is not rare in small domestic and wild animals, it is specially common in dogs, cats, guiana pigs, stallions and rhesus monkeys, and usually detected during breeding seasons and after weight loss, but paraphimosis is often related to breeding accidents [9].

Congenital cases of animal phimosis can result from a developmental anomaly of the penis or prepuce. Such anomalies include a short penis or retractor penile muscle, persistent adhesions connecting the prepuce to the penis, stenosis or absence of the preputial orifice. Acquired phimosis in dogs most commonly results from lacerations after trauma, preputial sucking by littermates, or licking by the dam. In addition, neoplasia such as mast cell tumors, transmissible venereal tumors, squamous cell carcinoma, and perianal gland adenomas accounts for many cases [10] (Fig. 18.2).

Phimosis in animals usually supervened by paraphimosis, preputial necrosis, and it is commonly results in secondary infection, and pooling of urine which causes cystitis.

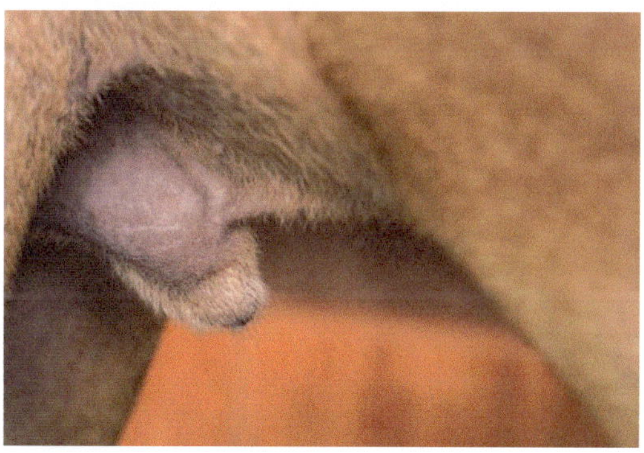

Fig. 18.2 Phimosis secondary to scared preputial hiatus in dog

Incidence of Phimosis

The natural history of non-retractile foreskin and preputial adhesions was extensively documented in the mid-twentieth century, firstly by Gairdner in 1949 [11] and then Oster [12] in 1968. Their combined studies show that in all but a small proportion of boys the foreskin will be retractile once the boys mature into their teenage years. These studies demonstrated that phimosis is present in 8% of 6–7 year olds, 6% of 10–11 year-olds and 1% of 16–17-year old boys. By contrast, preputial adhesions remain much more common throughout childhood and adolescence, by 17 years of age, only 3% will have persisting adhesions.

In contrast, preputial non retractability, previously called physiological phimosis had an incidence which increased from 3.0% in infants aged 1–3 months to 38.4% in children aged 3 years, while the incidence of completely unretractable prepuce decreased from 88.5% in infants aged 1–3 months to 35.0% in children aged 3 years [13].

In 2006, Hsieh et al. [14] examined the foreskin and external genitalia of 2149 Taiwanese schoolboys and showed that 50% of 7 year old boys had phimosis, which decreased to 8% at age 13 years.

Congenital phimosis is recognisable in neonates but may remain undetectable for months, but acquired phimosis may occur at any age.

In human males, the normal non retractability of the prepuce affects 96% of newborns and its incidence decreases with age. About 10% of the boys will still had adherent prepuce at 3 years of age, and only 1% present the disease at 14 years of age [15].

The incidence of true pathologic phimosis has been estimated to be 0.4 cases per 1000 boys per year, the commonly cited incidence statistic for pathological phimosis is 1% of uncircumcised males [16].

A narrow non-retractable prepuce in boys is within the normal range of development and usually causes no problems. The prepuce usually will spontaneously widen until complete retract-

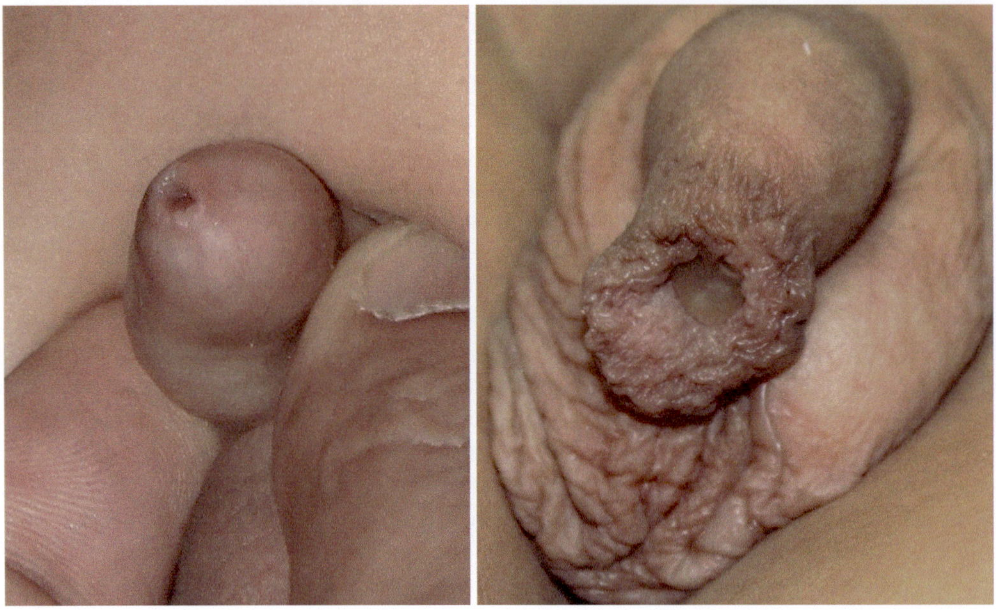

Fig. 18.3 Wide variability of the normal preputial opening, some infants may had a very wide opening, others are not

ability is obtained. About 50–60% of boys at age ten do not have fully retractable foreskins. This is normal. Normally at young age there is a wide variations in the diameter of preputial hiatus, but after puberty, the percentage of boys with full retractability rapidly increases spontaneously (Fig. 18.3).

True pathological phimosis caused by BXO has a relatively stable incidence across all decades of life, with a spike in the third decade of life, and it is relatively rare in children under the age of 5, there is a peak of childhood incidence between 9 and 11 years of age, with 0.6% of boys affected by years of age. Modern studies are questioning this doctrine, reporting varied incidence from 5% to 52% and children younger than 5 years may also have BXO [17] (Fig. 18.4).

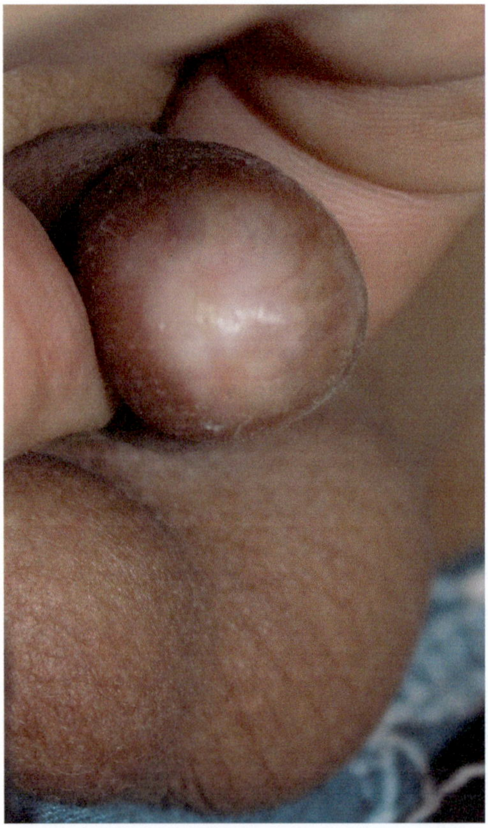

Fig. 18.4 Complete occlusion of the preputial meatus secondary to BXO in 10 months old boy

Pathophysiology

In cases with normally tight preputial opening, attempts of retraction the foreskin results in an apparent constriction ring a few millimetres proximal to the preputial orifice, and paraphimosis will predominate the condition. Preputial ring tearing and bruising supervene any forcible trials

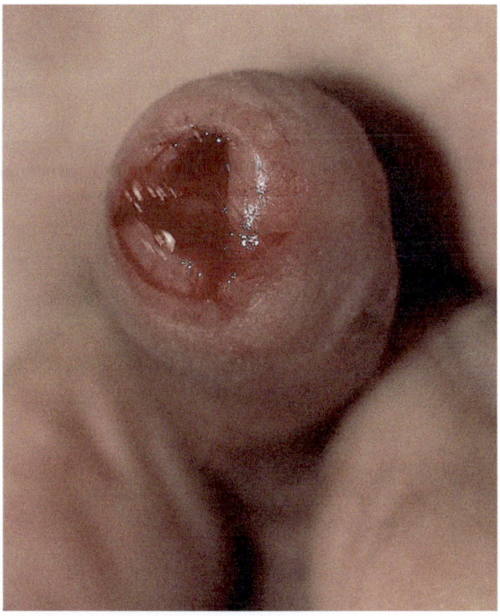

Fig. 18.5 Bleeding and tearing of the preputial ring secondary to forcible trials of retraction

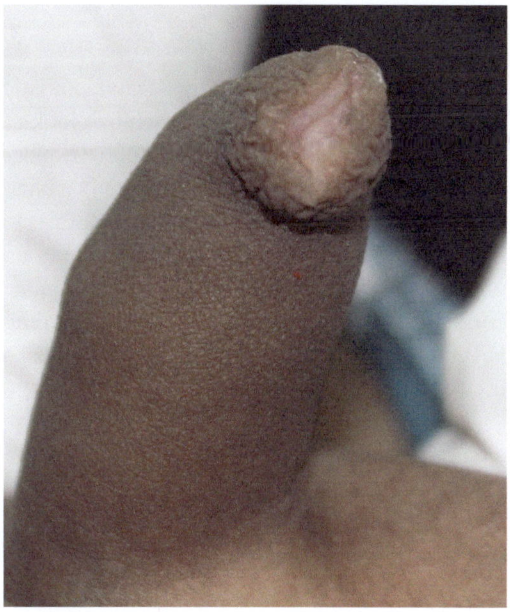

Fig. 18.6 A case of BXO with a sclerotic constricting band 1–2 cm proximal to the distal end of the preputial hiatus

of retracting stenotic preputial ring, and on severe cases bleeding is usually obvious (Fig. 18.4).

The width of the preputial stenotic ring varies and may range from 3 to 12 mm including the inner and outer lamina. The medial lamina is usually affected.

Non appropriated repeated trials without proper use of corticosteroid ointments may end with a long term severe fibrotic scaring with aggravation of the problem.

In contrast, BXO has a sclerotic constricting band of 1–2 cm proximal to the distal end, and there may be glans involvement in a diffuse pattern with whitish discolouration of the perimeatal area and an erythematous area being pathognomonic, in young ages, complete obliteration of the preputial meatus may commences the condition with difficult micturition or even urinary retention (Fig. 18.5).

Non recognised phimosis, specially at the extremes of age, will end with smegma and dirts accumulation at the balanopreputial space, with different grades of balanitis, meatitis, UTI and this long term irritation may explain the recorded association between cancer penis and phimosis (Fig. 18.6).

Classifications of Phimosis

Physiological Phimosis (Preputial Synechiae)

The prepuce firstly appears at the eighth week of gestation as an epithelial ridge, by 16 weeks of gestation the prepuce is complete and encases the glans. At this stage, the epithelial lining of the glans and prepuce are contiguous, and these preputial adhesions are essentially a normal developmental process. Separation begins proximally by the process of desquamation with small spaces forming, which eventually coalesce to form the preputial sac. At birth, the prepuce is non-retractile and remains so for a variable length of time.

Phimosis is a pathological condition, and nothing is physiological, the best term for the previously described term of physiological phimosis is non retractable foreskin. The majority of boys will have an adequately patent preputial hiatus, allowing normal and smooth micturition, with a nonretractable prepuce adherent to the glans up to the age of 10 years [18].

Pathological Phimosis

The pathological process gives characteristic stenosis, scarring and a pallor or whitish look of the preputial opening is typically caused by balanitis xerotica obliterans (BXO), which is a cicatrizing skin condition histologically identical to lichen sclerosis. It is a chronic skin condition with some evidence suggesting an autoimmune etiology. There has been controversy regarding BXO as a precipitant for penile cancer later in life (Chap. 21).

Whether or not BXO is considered a reason to circumcise, it is a significant condition that, if not recognised and treated appropriately, can result in a tight phimosis and lead to meatal or urethral stenosis. Published series of boys under 18 and 15 years, respectively, presenting for circumcision have found BXO in 5–6% [19]. BXO has the following characteristic histological features: hyperkeratosis with follicular plugging, atrophy of the stratum spongiosum with hydropic degeneration of basal cells, hyalinosis, and a band-like chronic inflammatory cell infiltrate with the homogenisation of collagen [20] (Fig. 18.7).

Phimosis in infants and young boys is completely different from adult cases; pathology at younger age group is either congenital or inflammatory, which is secondary to repeated, prolonged or improperly treated posthitis or balanoposthitis, adult who had a previously normal retractable prepuce may develop phimosis secondary to different forms of posthitis, BOX or neoplastic lesions.

Cicatricial Phimosis

It is another phimosis entity, which is specially common in communities practising neonatal circumcision, this sort of phimosis complicating an incomplete circumcision either by Guillotine or Gomco methods, where the excessive remnants of post circumcision untidy scar mingle together in front of the glans penis, and result in a stenotic scared preputial meatus (Fig. 18.8).

In one study a total of 521 infants aged from 2 to 4 months circumcised by Gomco clamp, 15 (3%) developed secondary phimosis [21].

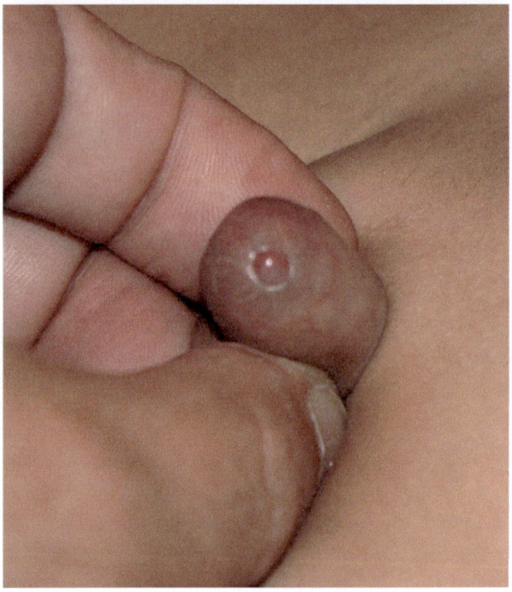

Fig. 18.8 Post circumcision cicatricial phimosis

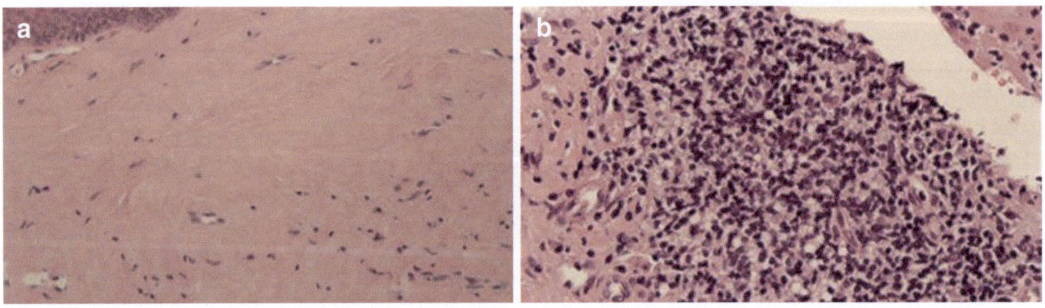

Fig. 18.7 Histopathological features of BXO; (**a**) Mild homogenous collagen bundles in the upper dermis (**b**) Infrabasal inflammatory cells mostly consist of lymphocytes

So phimosis classified into three main categories:

- Congenital primary phimosis.
- Acquired secondary to inflammatory, neoplastic conditions, or other rare pathology.
- Cicatricial following incomplete circumcision.

Grades of Phimosis

Phimosis, whatever its etiology classified according to visibility of the glans into five categories, Atilla et al. [22] also classified phimosis according to the grade of preputial retractability and the appearance of foreskin: (Fig. 18.9) and (Table 18.1).

- Grade 0: Full retraction, prepuce is not tight behind glans, or easy retraction limited only by congenital adhesions to the glans.
- Grade I: Fully retractable prepuce with stenotic ring in the shaft.
- Grade II: Partial retractability with partial exposure of the glans.
- Grade III: Partial retractability with exposure of the meatus only.
- Grade IV: No retractability.

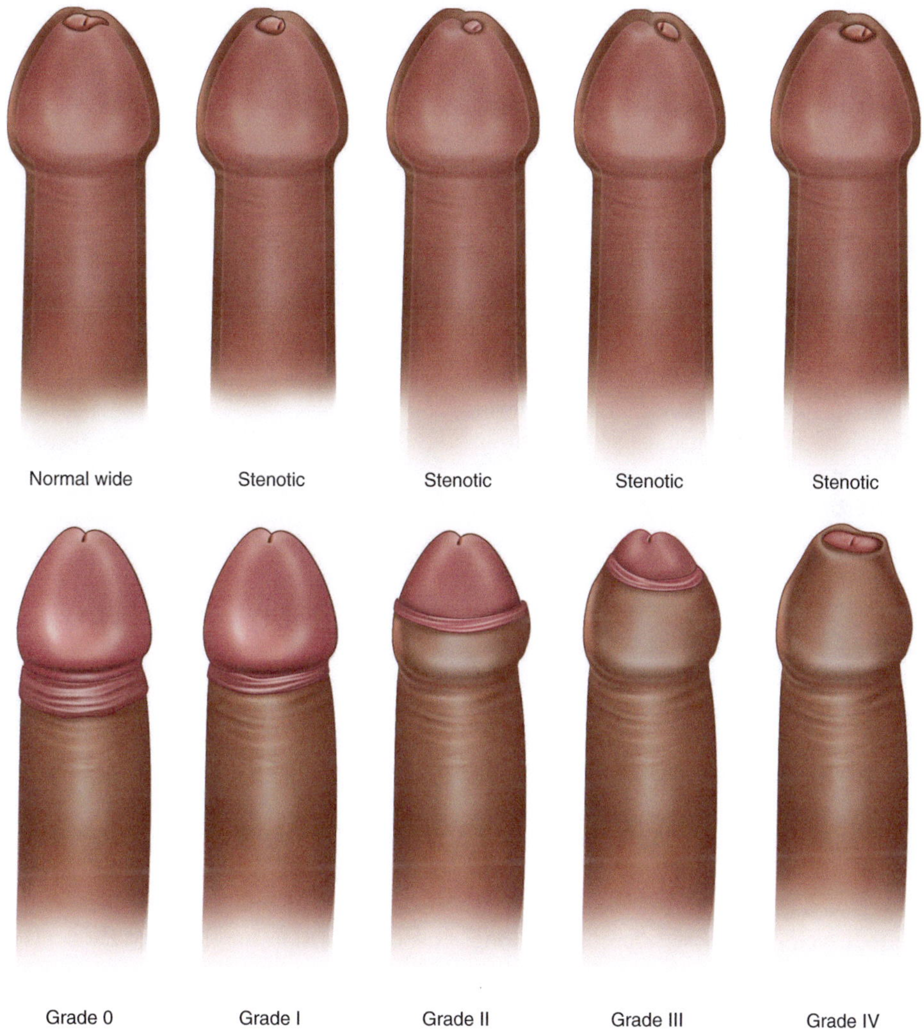

Fig. 18.9 Grades of phimosis

Table 18.1: Classification of phimosis [22]

Grades	(a) Retractability of foreskin	(b) Appearance of foreskin
0	Full retraction	Normal
1	Full retraction of foreskin and tight behind the glans	1 crack in prepuce and skin splitting on gentle retraction
2	Partial exposure of glans	2 small, partially circumferential white scar
3	Partial retraction, meatus just visible	3 balanitis xerotica obliterans or severe scarring
4	Slight retraction, but distance between tip and glans (neither meatus nor glans can be exposed	
5	Absolutely no retraction	

From Atilla MK, Dundaroz R, Odabas O, et al.: A nonsurgical approach to the treatment of phimosis: local nonsteroidal anti-inflammatory ointment application. J Urol. 1997;158:196–197

Etiology of Phimosis

Congenital Phimosis

Normally the neonatal preputial meatus are widely variable (Chap. 5) (Fig. 18.3), and the follow up of a small pinhole preputial meatus will reveal an adequate wide opening latter on, but sometimes a baby delivered with severely stenotic preputial opening; either as an isolated deformaty or in association with other genitourinary anomalies, if a narrow meatus exposed to repeated attacks of posthitis or balanoposthitis with different pathogens; either bacterial or fungal, we will have a manifested phimotic prepuce with its sequelae.

Adults with long prepuce are more likely to develop phimosis, and subsequently may develop cancer penis, specially in some geographic regions with high prevalence of this cancer [23] (Fig. 18.10).

Children with akroposthia are commonly vulnerable to develop phimosis, specially during napkins period, as the long prepuce, even with a wide preputial meatus is more liable for ulceration and infection (Fig. 18.11). The issue of long prepuce will be discussed in details (Chap. 11).

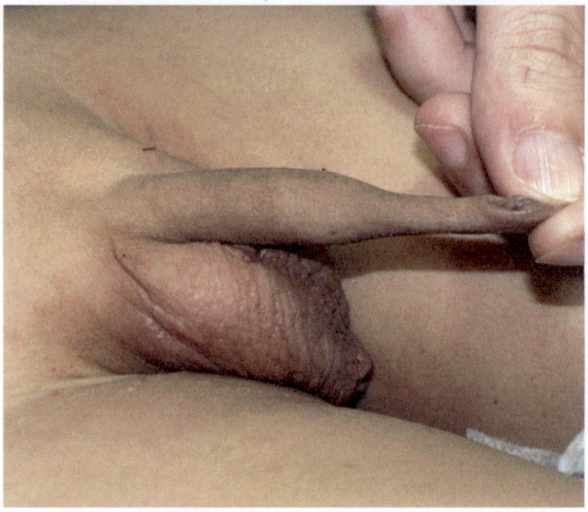

Fig. 18.10 Long prepuce reaching to the mid thigh

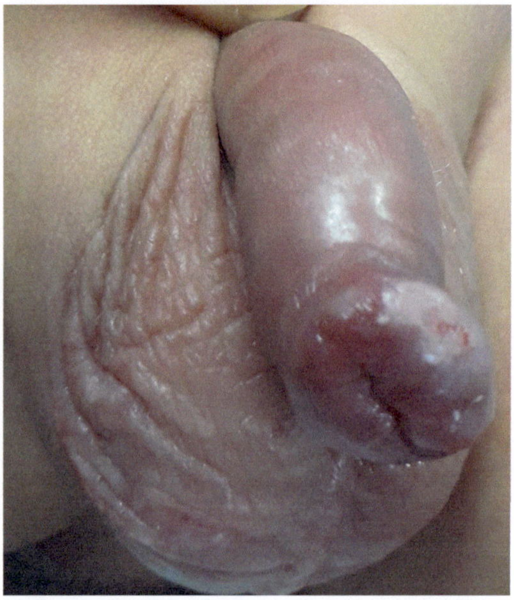

Fig. 18.11 Severe neonatal posthitis at the tip of long (akroposthia) prepuce, expectedly it will end with scaring and phimosis

The buried penis is an abnormality of penoscrotal fusion, in which the penile corpora are also tethered to the deep fascia. It is commonly associated with phimosis, and the appearance of the external skin suggests that the penis is small or even absent [24].

Many cases of megameatus intact prepuce are presented for the first time with phimosis, specially in those with long prepuce, once the phi-

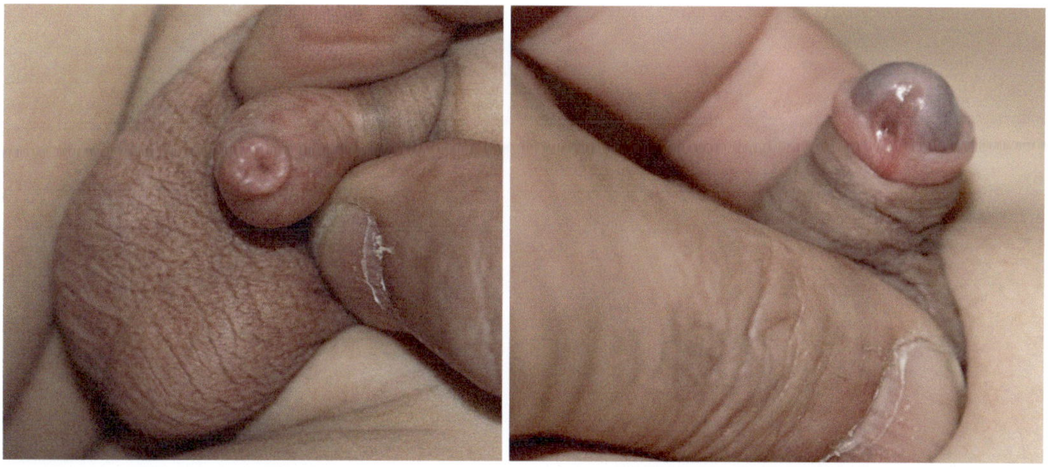

Fig. 18.12 A child 1 year old with marked phimosis, once the prepuce became retractable after conservative measures it revealed a megameatus anomaly

motic prepuce became retractable after sometime of application of topical corticosteroid; will reveal an abnormal wide meatus occupying the whole glans (Fig. 18.12).

Acquired Phimosis

Acquired phimosis is attributed to common and rare causes leading to chronic inflammation that can prevent foreskin retraction due to the formation of adhesions. Common causes include eczema, psoriasis, lichen planus, and lichen sclerosis.

In some rare cases the foreskin involved along a systemic diseases and eventually end with phimosis, in such cases prepuce shows the manifestations of the main disease and phimosis is a self limited; phimotic cases are seen along the angioneurotic oedema (Fig. 18.13), Henoch-Schonlein purpura, and Graft-versus-host-disease, usually phimosis in such cases is a self limited manifestation and regress once the general condition controlled [25] (Fig. 18.14).

Diabetes is a common association with acquired phimosis; in one study diabetes associated with acquired phimosis in almost a third of cases. Therefore it is important that serum glucose levels are analysed when assessing men or toddler with acquired phimosis [26].

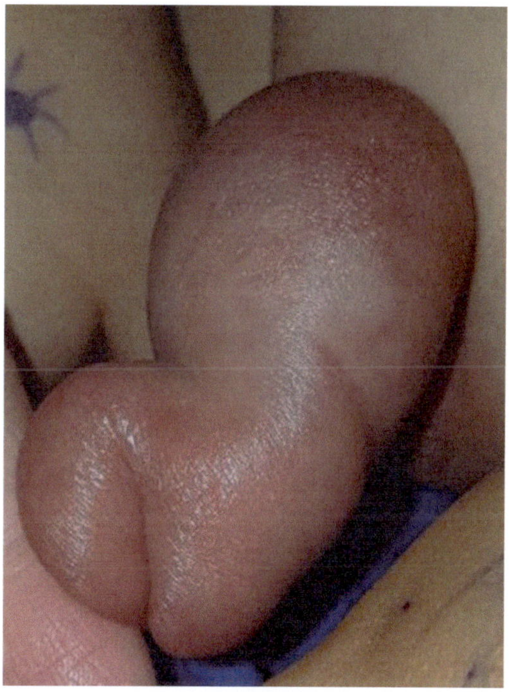

Fig. 18.13 Preputial involvement in a case of angioneurotic oedema, with a subsequent phimosis

Phimosis could be also secondary to local preputial neoplasia or cellulitis, in general, poor hygiene and recurrent balanitis, posthitis or balanoposthitis are the most common conditions followed by phimosis (Fig. 18.15). If a proper care and attention is specially paid to the prepuce early

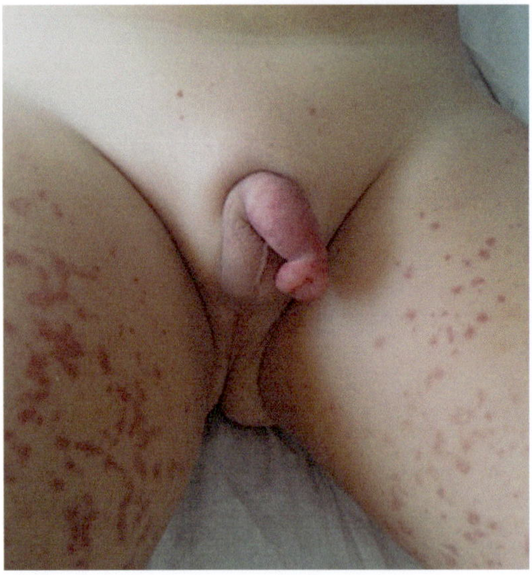

Fig. 18.14 A case of Henoch-Schonlein purpura, with preputial involvement

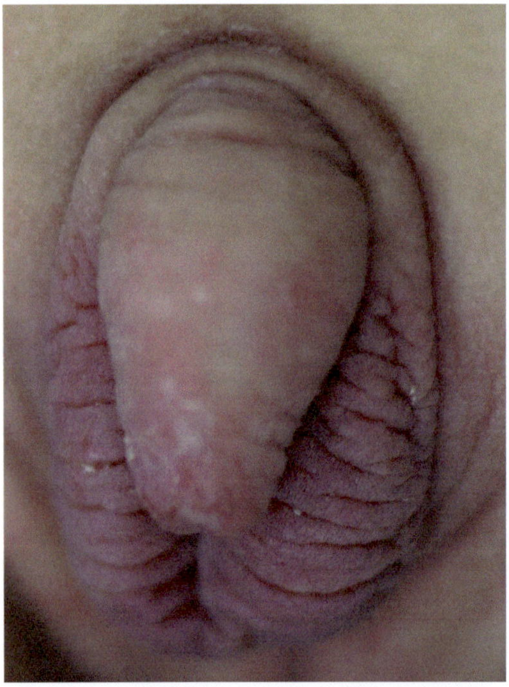

Fig. 18.15 Poor preputial hygiene and candida infection of the prepuce are usually predisposing to phimosis

during such systemic and local diseases, to check its retractability and to clean it properly, many cases could be saved early from the full blown status of phimosis with its complications (Fig. 18.16).

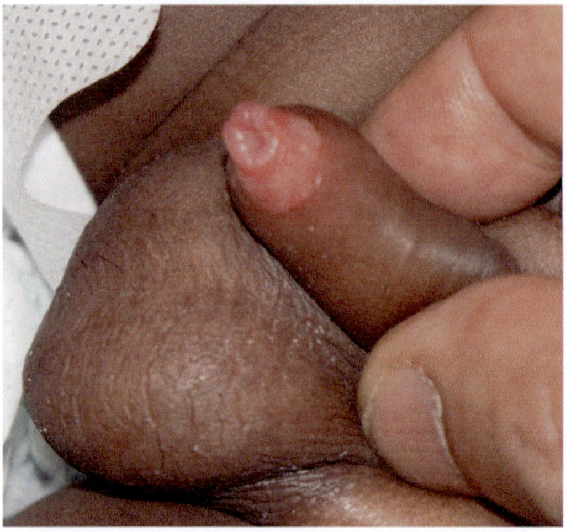

Fig. 18.16 Early preputial involvement in eczema with hypopigmentation, which could be stopped from proceeding to phimosis

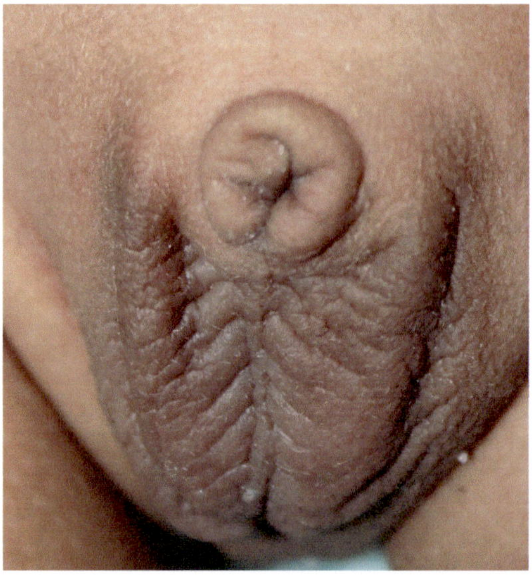

Fig. 18.17 Cicatricial phimosis complicating incomplete circumcision of a small concealed penis

Cases of cicatricial phimosis are commonly following incomplete circumcision, especially if infection supervenes circumcision, and if the preputial remnant not retracted or not cared, cicatricial phimosis is commonly complicating circumcision of the microphallus, concealed and webbed penis (Fig. 18.17).

Diagnosis of Phimosis

Diagnosis of phimosis is mainly clinical (Fig. 18.18). Often non-retractile foreskin is the presenting complaint of a patient, or their parent/guardian, as such it is best to establish whether the process is physiological or pathological, and what is the exact underlying pathology which leads to preputial non retractability, phimosis in older children and adults can vary in severity, with some patients are able to retract their foreskin partially (relative phimosis), and some are completely unable to retract their foreskin even in the flaccid state (full phimosis). Phimosis in adolescents is recognized to be present when the diameter of the preputial orifice is smaller than the diameter of the erect glans.

In pathologic phimosis, there is usually pain, skin irritation, local infections, bleeding, dysuria, poor stream of urine, burning micturition, hematuria, frequent episodes of urinary tract infections, preputial pain, painful erection and intercourse, and weak urinary stream. Occasionally enuresis or urinary retention is noticed. Phimosis interferes with conventional masturbatory practices, so most of the adolescents who had any grade of phimosis will seek for medical advice when phimosis interferes with their masturbation activities [27].

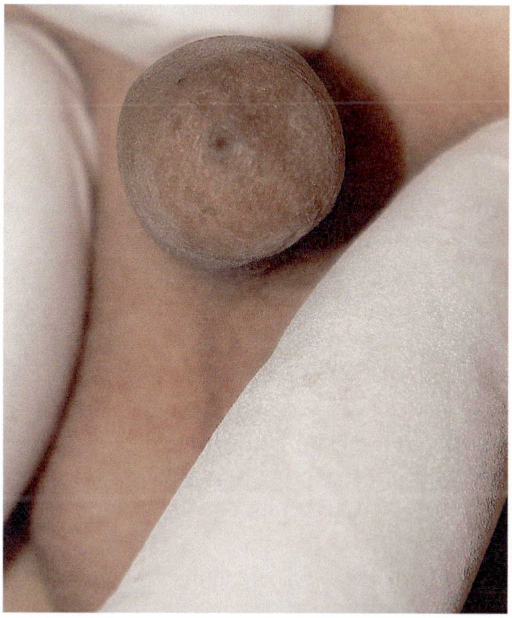

Fig. 18.18 Clinical diagnosis of phimosis; pin hole preputial opening, absent frenular band, and scaring of the preputial skin around the meatus

Ballooning of preputial skin observed during micturition is confirmatory for diagnosis of phimosis, it is a common presentation in childhood when the foreskin is still non-retractile. Typically occurring between 2 and 4 years of age, it is a self-limited phenomenon that resolves once the foreskin becomes more retractile. Parents can be reassured that this does not have any effect on the child's bladder or ability to void. Ballooning is due to inflation of the prepuce during urination by the pressure of urine inside. This can occur if the inner layer of the prepuce is separating or has separated from the glans, which typically happens around 3 years of age, before the prepuce has become fully retractable (Fig. 18.19).

BXO cases has an insidious onset; there may be associated irritation, local infection, dysuria, bleeding and meatal stenosis. The disease can also have a cyclical course with periods of remission. On rare occasions, patients may present with acute urinary retention or nocturnal enuresis from chronic outflow obstruction. Even if urinary infection is present, it is not always attributed to the phimosis [28].

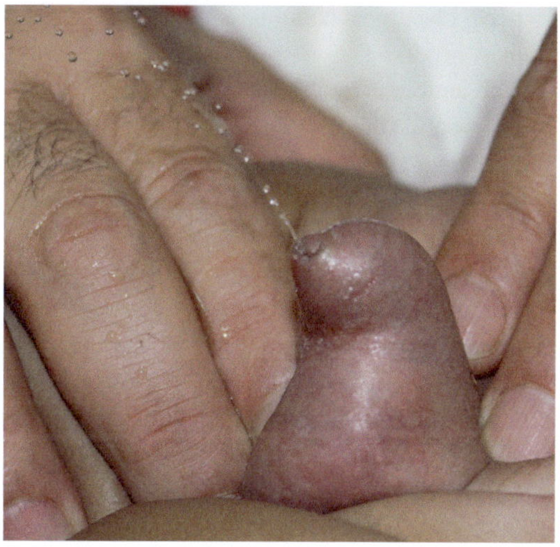

Fig. 18.19 Ballooning and retention of urine secondary to phimosis, in this case ballooning is little proximal than usual, due to partial adhesion between glans and inner prepuce

Investigations

Diagnosis of phimosis is primarily clinical and no laboratory tests or imaging studies are required, these may be only required for associated urinary tract infections or skin infections, also laboratory tests and radiography are not typically required in the assessment of phimosis, and studies have demonstrated no evidence of urinary obstruction from physiological phimosis.

Pathological phimosis treated with surgery should have any surgically excised skin sent for histology to confirm the diagnosis and exclude any evidence of malignancy [29].

Differential Diagnosis

Phimosis and its subtypes have to diagnosed precisely and to be differentiated from other rare conditions:

- Preputial adhesions are a normal physiological feature and resolve spontaneously over time.
- Acute balanoposthitis which is a purulent, pyogenic infection of the prepuce and represents the most severe form of posthitis. These conditions lead to erythema and edema of the prepuce. Dysuria is common, and minor bleeding may occurs. These episodes typically resolve with antibiotic treatment and require no further intervention unless recurrence occurs.
- Congenital megaprepuce is a rare condition, on examination, the outer preputial skin directly meets the abdominal wall dorsally, and the scrotum ventrally with an absence of penile shaft skin. Micturition is always abnormal with the entire preputial sac filled with urine. This can be expressed to leave a more normal appearance; any attempt to treat this condition with a standard circumcision will result in the requirement for revision surgery complicated by the loss of outer preputial skin (Chap. 11).
- Penile pearls, which is a normal findings, also other forms of smegma collection should not be confused as a phimosis, careful removal of these aggregation may reveal a normal retractable preputial ring.

Sequelae and Complications

Enthusiastic forceful attempts to retract foreskin in phimosis and preputial synechia usually lead to microtears, infection, and bleeding with secondary scarring which heals with fibrosis and convert the physiological phimosis to pathological one, or upgrading the degree of phimosis (Fig. 18.5). Paraphimosis is related to manipulation of the foreskin with failure to reduce the prepuce to its natural position (Chap. 19). It presents with pain and edema of both the prepuce and the glans. Paraphimosis does not represent a disease process, and single episodes, once resolved, warrant no surgical intervention. Recurrent episodes are unusual and are an indication for intervention.

Complications related to phimosis can occur throughout life, and their surgical indications depend on the type of lesion present in the foreskin as well as failure of spontaneous resolution or through clinical treatments. Examples of complications related to phimosis are balanoposthitis, difficulty urinating, urinary retention, dysuria, urinary tract infection (UTI), tenesmus, enuresis, priapism, paraphimosis, preputial brake laceration, balloon synechia, and BXO.

Balanoposthitis, recurrent urinary tract infections (UTIs), preputial stone and paraphimosis are the common complications of untreated phimosis (Fig. 18.20).

Different grades of meatitis and subsequently meatal stenosis is the natural sequel of repeated or untreated phimosis (Fig. 18.21). Obstructed flow of urine, secondary to long standing untreated phimosis may lead to residual urine and back pressure changes to upper urinary tract resulting in hydroureter and hydronephrosis.

Fibroepithelial polyp is rarely develop in association with phimosis, and usually manifests as a polypoid or cauliflower-like mass or masses involving the glans penis or prepuce [30].

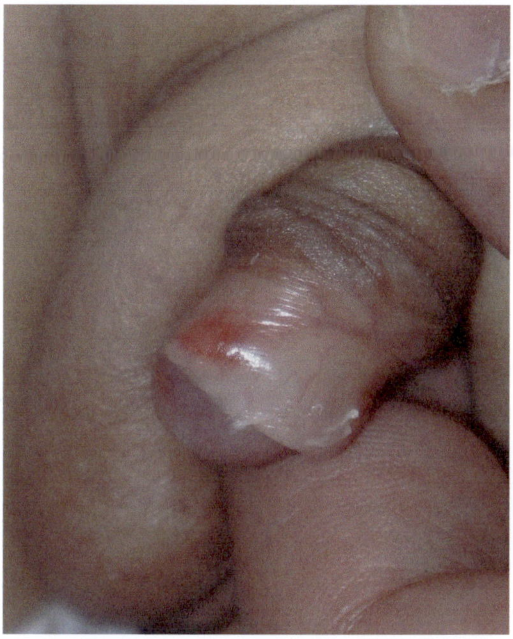

Fig. 18.20 Posthitis secondary to phimosis

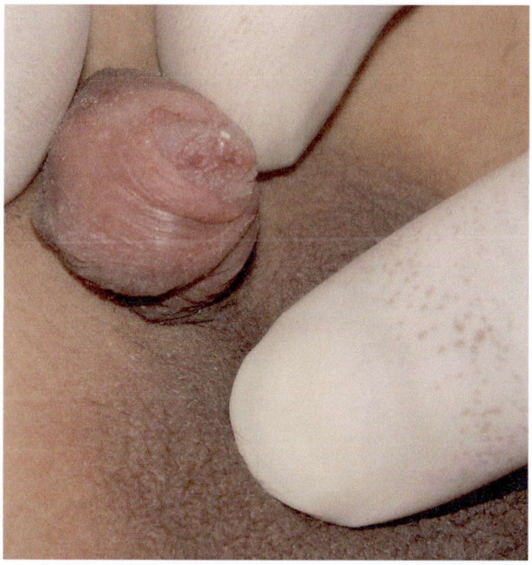

Fig. 18.21 A residual meatitis after medical treatment of phimosis

Phimosis and Cancer Penis

The majority of medical journal or textbook articles produced in the United States on penile cancer have overlooked the lack of supporting, objective, and concrete epidemiological studies and will state that penile cancer is either associated with phimosis or caused by it. On the other hand a Danish population-based evidence study proved that phimosis was confirmed as a strong risk factor for penile squamous cell carcinoma (SCC) [31].

Incidence of cancer penis had a wide range of variation among different ethnic groups and also had a wide geographical variations, so an ethnic-geographic comparison of types of prepuce and penile cancer may be of interest [32].

It may seems difficult to accept that a stenotic small ring at the preputial tip is a precancerous lesion, if we will accept the huge number of researches correlates cancer penis with phimosis; we have to consider a long standing residual secondary irritation in the glans penis which follow untreated phimosis and we have also to take into account some ethnic groups which proved to have a high vulnerability to cancer penis [33].

Preventive circumcision could be necessary only for males harboring long foreskin with recurrent attacks of phimosis in those rural population at high risk to develop cancer penis.

Management of Phimosis

Conservative Measures

Treatment of physiological phimosis is not indicated, reassurance and an explanation of the natural history of the healthy non-retractile foreskin should be given to concerned parents. In some countries with high prevalence of ritual circumcision, this procedure is the preferred treatment for pathological phimosis and represents the only absolute indication for this procedure in children, also BXO remains an absolute indication for circumcision at all ages.

In infancy, application of a mild topical steroid with gentle retraction of prepuce may help in mild phimosis. Betamethasone cream may be applied to the narrowed preputial skin twice daily for 4 weeks. After 2 weeks, the foreskin becomes soft and elastic and is retracted gently and gradually in increments (Fig. 18.22).

For adults a topical 0.1% betamethasone ointment cream applied to the prepuce twice daily for 6 weeks in combination with gentle attempts to retract the foreskin is an effective nonsurgical treatment, and reported to be successful in up to 75–85% of cases of phimosis [34]. Given the low risk associated with short duration topical steroid use, this can be repeated if necessary (Fig. 18.23).

Dorsal Slit

A dorsal slit (often referred to in anthropology as superincision) is a single incision along the upper length of the foreskin from the tip to the corona, exposing the glans without removing any tissue. Dorsal slit has a long history as a treatment for adult phimosis [35].

It is an ancient practice, it has been a traditional custom among a number of peoples, particularly Filipinos and Pacific Islanders, probably for thousands of years [36].

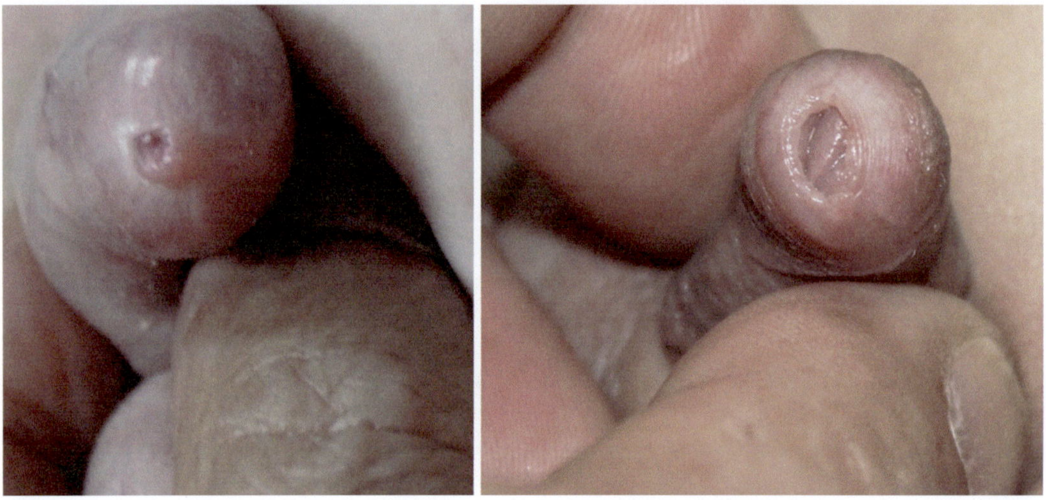

Fig. 18.22 Partial improvement of the phimosis after 2 weeks application of topical corticosteroid, meatus and glans become partially visible

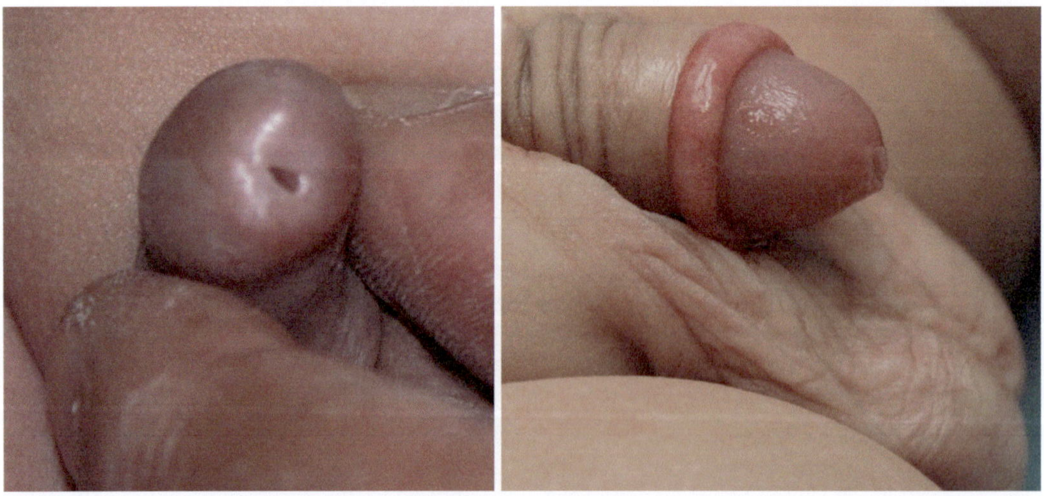

Fig. 18.23 Another case with complete preputial retractability after 4 weeks treatment with local corticosteroid

In Western medicine it was used as an alternative to circumcision to relieve phimosis and paraphimosis, although a perception of poor appearance limited its popularity. While it is a less invasive surgery than circumcision, it is more invasive than preputioplasty since it leaves the incision open. It is still used when circumcision or other measures are considered impractical or undesirable. Compared with circumcision it was relatively easy to perform, did not risk or damage the frenulum, and even before the invention of antibiotics it was less likely to become infected. However, the literature often indicates that despite being a simple operation it was not liked by some or refers to the "untidy apron-like appearance of the prepuce.

Dorsal slit is now rare in Western countries as a treatment for phimosis. Standard guidelines suggest conservative approaches first and, should those fail, either circumcision or preputioplasty to both retain the foreskin and to relieve the phimosis [37].

According to Goodwin, the dorsal slit operation may be reversed by suturing the cut ends together, which restores the tissue to its normal position and recreates the foreskin [38].

In order to maintain the phimotic prepuce intact postoperatively, many authors have suggested their personal techniques. These are reported as variations of Z-plasty, multiple Y-V plasties, lateral preputioplasty, multiple internal foreskin lamina and triple incision plasty [39].

Sutureless preputioplasty (SLP) is a faster, easier, painless and without complications technique, which has excellent cosmetic results, especially in cases of buried penis, where circumcision is contraindicated, SLP was considered as the first choice operation, which can be performed either with local or general anesthesia, a dorsal longitudinal incision in the stenotic ring of the prepuce till the cyclic print in the foreskin circumference will disappear [40].

Dilation

Phimosis can be treated by preputial dilation. A proper sized dilator should be introduced into the narrow preputial opening, this procedure is repeated every 3 days with increase in the size of dilators [41].

Knowing that balloon dilation is helpful in managing the constrictions of blood vessels, oesophagus, urinary tracts and ureters, this method was also applied for treating phimosis in 512 boys in China, by an appropriate balloon catheter under local or topical anesthesia, dilation considered successful if preputial orifice reaches to 3–5 mm greater than the maximal diameter of the glans [42].

Phimosis stretcher kit for curing tight foreskin includes 20 medical grade silicone tunnels for gentle foreskin stretching is available in the market.

Kinesiotherapy

Kinesiotherapy is the treatment of disease by means of passive and active movements, such as massage and exercise. It is an alternatives to circumcision, it is suitable to treat phimosis due to BXO but are designed to achieve a fully retractile foreskin. These treatments can be particularly useful with patients experiencing balanoposthitis.

Postectomy

Is a technique which spares both the prepuce and frenulum while repairing the preputial phimosis, many authors defining its benefits in comparison with circumcision [43].

Experimental Options for Treatment of Phimosis

Prolonged antibiotic therapy, intralesional steroid injection, carbon dioxide laser therapy, and radial preputioplasty alone or with intralesional injection of steroid have all been described as therapies for phimosis, but there are no proper randomised controlled trials of their efficacy and long-term outcomes [24].

Of course the post circumcision cicatricial phimosis have to be treated with a special

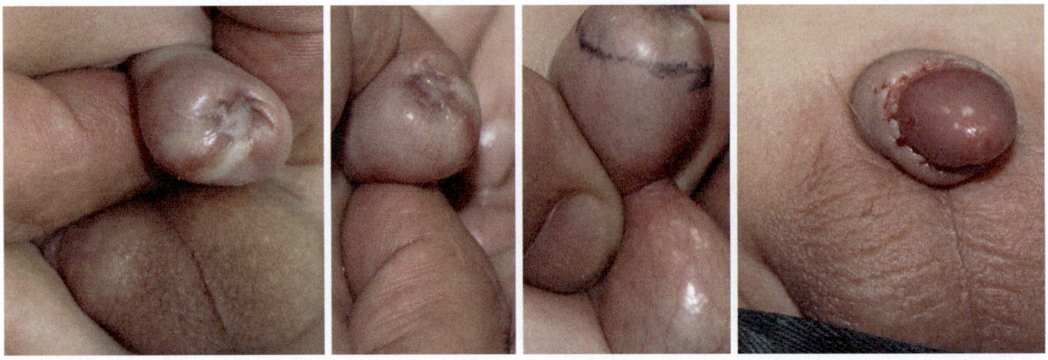

Fig. 18.24 Retrograde dissection of the scared preputial ring to relieve a cicatricial phimosis

technique of retrograde circumcision by dissection to excise the scared stenotic preputial ring (Fig. 18.24).

Conclusion

Preputial non retractability is a manifestation of phimosis, but not all cases of non retractability are necessary to be due to phimosis, incidence of both conditions are variable at different ages.

Phimosis classified to: congenital, acquired and cicatricial (post circumcision).

Aetiology of phimosis are variable at different age groups.

Neonates and even preterms are delivered with smegma of variable amounts before any separation between prepuce and glans so there is no relation between smegma and preputial breakup from glans.

Newer nonsurgical modalities such as topical steroids and adhesiolysis are effective, safe, and cheap for treating phimosis in children. Parents should be made aware of other measures, which alternate circumcision for the treatment of phimosis. If surgery is indeedly needed, conservative plastic surgical techniques should be performed rather than the traditional circumcision.

References

1. Hodges FM. The history of phimosis from antiquity to the present. In: Oenniston GC, Hodges FM, Milos MF, editors. Male and female circumcision: medical, legal and ethical considerations in pediatric practice. New York: Kluwer Academic/Plenum Publishers; 1999.
2. Hsu CC. The development of the prepuce. Taiwan Yi Xue Hui Za Zhi. 1983;82:314–20.
3. Williams N, Chell J, Kapila L. Why are children referred for circumcision? BMJ. 1993;306:28.
4. Celsus AC. De Medicina 7.25.2. In: Spencer WG, editor and translator. Cambridge: Harvard University Press; 1938. vol. 3. p. 422.
5. Dionis P. Cows d'operationsde Chirurgie. Bruxelles: Les Freres t'serstevens; 1708. p. 177.
6. Hunter J. A treatise on the venereal disease. First American ed. Philadelphia: J Webster; 1818. p. 205–8.
7. Rickwood AMK, Hemalatha V, Batcup G, Spitz L. Phimosis in boys. Br J Urol. 1980;52:147–50.
8. Oenniston GC, Hodges FM, Milos MF, editors. Male and female circumcision: medical, legal and ethical considerations in pediatric practice. New York: Kluwer Academic/Plenum Publishers. p. 37–62. https://doi.org/10.1007/978-0-585-39937-9_5. ISBN 978-0-306-46131-6.
9. Hajinasrollah M, Mohitmafi S, Asadian A. Two case reports of unusual phimosis in rhesus monkeys (Macaca Mulatta). J Med Primatol. 2018;48:58. https://doi.org/10.1111/jmp.12367.
10. Papazoglou LG, Kazakos GM. Surgical conditions of the canine penis and prepuce. Compend Contin Educ Pract Vet. 2002;24(3):204–18.
11. Gairdner D. The fate of the foreskin, a study of circumcision. Br Med J. 1949;2(4642):1433–7, illust.
12. Oster J. Further fate of the foreskin. Incidence of preputial adhesions, phimosis, and smegma among Danish schoolboys. Arch Dis Child. 1968;43(228):200–3.
13. Imamura E. Phimosis of infants and young children in Japan. Acta Paediatr Jpn. 1997;39:403–5.
14. Hsieh TF, Chang CH, Chang SS. Foreskin development before adolescence in 2149 schoolboys. Int J Urol. 2006;13:968–70.
15. Favorito LA, Balassiano CM, Rosado JP, Cardoso LEM, Costa WS, Sampaio FJB. Structural analysis of the phimotic prepuce in patients with failed topical

treatment compared with untreated phimosis. Int Braz J Urol. 2012;38(6):802–8.
16. Spilsbury K, Semmens JB, Wisniewski ZS, Holman CD. Circumcision for phimosis and other medical indications in Western Australian boys. Med J Aust. 2003;178(4):155–8.
17. Celis S, Reed F, Murphy F, Adams S, Gillick J, Abdelhafeez AH, Lopez PJ. Balanitis xerotica obliterans in children and adolescents: a literature review and clinical series. J Pediatr Urol. 2014;10(1):34–9.
18. Kumar P, Deb M, Das K. Preputial adhesions – a misunderstood entity. Indian J Pediatr. 2009;76:829–32.
19. Reddy CRRM, Devendranath V, Pratap S. Carcinoma of penis - role of phimosis. Urology. 1984;24(1):85–8. https://doi.org/10.1016/0090-4295(84)90398-4.
20. Johal N, Cuckow P. Phimosis and buried penis. In: Puri P, Höllwarth M, editors. Pediatric surgery, Springer surgery atlas series. Berlin: Springer; 2019.
21. Bromage SJ, Crump A, Pearce I. Phimosis as a presenting feature of diabetes. BJU Int. 2008;101(3):338–40.
22. Atilla MK, Dundaroz R, Odabas O, et al. A nonsurgical approach to the treatment of phimosis: local nonsteroidal anti-inflammatory ointment application. J Urol. 1997;158:196–7.
23. Beaugé M. The causes of adolescent phimosis. Br J Sex Med. 1997;24:26.
24. Shahid SK. Phimosis in children (Review Article). ISRN Urol. 2012;2012:707329. https://doi.org/10.5402/2012/707329.
25. Santander CB, Campos E, Sánchez A, Marcos L, Díaz I. Púrpura de Schönlein-Henoch con afectación peniana. Caso clínico. Arch Argent Pediatr. 2016;114(4):e249–51.
26. Paulson DF. Genitourinary cancer, basic and clinical aspects. In: Cancer treatment research, vol. 6. 1st ed; 1982. p. 32. ISBN 90-247-2480-5.
27. Das S, Tunuguntla HS. Balanitis xerotica obliterans—a review. World J Urol. 2000;18(6):382–7.
28. Yardley IE, Cosgrove C, Lambert AW. Paediatric preputial pathology: are we circumcising enough? Ann R Coll Surg Engl. 2007;89:62–5. https://doi.org/10.1308/003588407X160828.
29. lalock HJ, Vemulakonda V, Ritchey ML, Ribbeck M. Outpatient management of phimosis following newborn circumcision. J Urol. 2003;169(6):2332–6.
30. Turgut M, Yenilmez A, Can C, Bildirici K, Erkul A, Ozyurek Y. Fibroepithelial polyp of glans penis. Urology. 2005;65:593.
31. Madsen BS, van den Brule AJC, Jensen HL, Wohlfahrt J, Frisch M. Risk factors for squamous cell carcinoma of the penis population-based case-control study in Denmark. Cancer Epidemiol Biomark Prev. 2008;17(10):2683.
32. Velazquez EF, Bock A, Soskin A, Codas R, Arbo M, Cubilla AL. Preputial variability and preferential association of long phimotic foreskins with penile cancer. Am J Surg Pathol. 2003;27(7):994–8.
33. Douglawi A, Masterson TA. Updates on the epidemiology and risk factors for penile cancer. Transl Androl Urol. 2017;6:785–90.
34. Ashfield JE, Nickel KR, Siemens DR, Mac Neily AE, Nickel JC. Treatment of phimosis with topical steroids in 194 children. J Urol. 2003;169:1106–8.
35. Kolehmainen M, Taskinen S, Ossi L. Foreskin surgery. Duodecim. 2010;126:75–83.
36. Christianakis E. Sutureless prepuceplasty with wound healing by second intention: an alternative surgical approach in children's phimosis treatment. BMC Urol. 2008;8:6. https://doi.org/10.1186/1471-2490-8-6.
37. Yachia D. Text atlas of penile surgery. London: Informa Healthcare; 2007. ISBN 1-84184-517-5. p. 16.
38. Goodwin WE. Uncircumcision: a technique for plastic reconstruction of a prepuce after circumcision. J Urol. 1990;144(5):1203–5. https://doi.org/10.1016/s0022-5347(17)39693-3.
39. Wåhlin N. "Triple incision plasty". A convenient procedure for preputial relief. Scand J Urol Nephrol. 1992;26(2):107–10.
40. Christianaki E. Sutureless prepuceplasty with wound healing by second intention: an alternative surgical approach in children's phimosis treatment. BMC Urol. 2008;8:6. https://doi.org/10.1186/1471-2490-8-6.
41. Kumar R, Pareek R. A holistic approach to phimosis in children. J Ayurveda Integr Med Sci. 2018;1:66–9. https://doi.org/10.21760/jaims.v3i01.11641.
42. Ying H, Zhou X-H. Balloon dilation treatment of phimosis in boys. Chin Med J. 1991;104(6):491–3.
43. Cicia S, Florio G. Postectomy for phimosis: 5-year-experience. Chir Ital. 2000;52(6):733–6.

19 Paraphimosis

Introduction

Paraphimosis is defined as inability to replace the retracted prepuce. If phimosis is inability to retract the foreskin over the glans, paraphimosis is the reverse of it. The word paraphimosis is derived from two Greek words, 'para' (meaning 'beyond' or 'resembling') and 'phimosis' (meaning 'muzzling' or 'restriction'). Occasionally it is also spelt as 'paraphymosis', as the Greek word phyma (meaning swelling) refers to the characteristic preputial swelling of this condition [1, 2]. Colloquially it is referred to as 'nuptial night tragedy' because it is common among newlywed males who, in exited state, indulge in hasty penetrative intercourse without being aware of their pre-existing phimosis. Scientific literature on paraphimosis is largely anecdotal, most of them being restricted to isolated case series and there are hardly any randomized controlled studies [3–6].

History of Paraphimosis

Earliest mention of paraphimosis is found in Sushruta Samhita, an ancient Hindu surgical text written in *circa* 1200 BCE [7]. The then Sanskrit name of paraphimosis was *Avapatika*. Sushruta vividly describes it as follows:

> *When the integuments of prepuce is abnormally and forcibly turned back by such causes as coition under excitation, with a girl (before menstruation and before the rupture of the hymen and consequently with a narrow external orifice of the vagina) or masturbation or pressure or a blow on the penis, or a voluntary retention of a flow of semen or forcible opening of the prepuce, the disease is called Avapatika*

He recommended reduction by gentle compression of glans using clarified butter as lubricant. Unlike Egyptians, Hindus of ancient India did not practice routine circumcision. This explains as to why paraphimosis is described in Sushruta Samhita but not in Edwin Smith papyrus.

Among the Greek scholars Aulus Cornelius Celsus (25 BC–50 AD) used the term 'phymosis' to mean both phimosis and paraphimosis [8]. He advised hot fomentation as relief. It was the Greek physician Antyllus (circa 100 CE) who first used the term paraphimosis [9]. His writings, copied verbatim into the medical encyclopedia of Oribasius (400 CE), reads as follows:

> *There are two kinds of phimosis: in one case, sometimes the foreskin covers the glans and cannot be pulled back; in the other case, the foreskin is retracted but cannot be returned over the glans. This second type is specifically called paraphimosis*

John Hunter, the great English surgeon and founder of Royal College of Surgeons, held that paraphimosis was a sexually transmitted disease because most of his patients had had associated chancroid, syphilis or gonorrhea. A similar notion had existed ever since the times of the great Galen. Interestingly, none of the ancient surgeons considered paraphimosis as a complication of phimosis.

M. A. B. Fahmy, *Normal and Abnormal Prepuce*, https://doi.org/10.1007/978-3-030-37621-5_19

Pathophysiology

Ability to retract the prepuce over the glans as well as replacing it back depends upon two factors namely the elastic compliance of preputial orifice and the tumescence of glans [10]. When any one or both of them are compromised, difficulty arises in retraction of foreskin as well as restoring it to original position. Thus paraphimosis may occur either as a complication of phimosis (uncommon) or independently in a previously normal prepuce (common). This author prefers to call the former as '*compound paraphimosis*', while the later as '*simple paraphimosis*' [10].

When the preputial orifice is cicatrized and stenosed, it is impossible—even with force—to retract it over a flaccid penis. Thus, penile erection is a pre-requisite of compound paraphimosis. On the other hand, simple paraphimosis results when the compliant foreskin is retracted and negligently left at the coronal sulcus for prolonged period. In both the types, the circumferentially narrow skin of preputial orifice, known as the *preputial band* or constricting paraphimotic band, is stuck at the corona. The inner layer of prepuce is distal to the band while the outer prepuce is proximal to it. Circumferential compression of the preputial band produces a gentle strangulating effect on the glans and the inner prepuce. As the venous return of the glans is hampered it engorges immediately. Tumescent glans prevents spontaneous return of the retracted prepuce. Prolonged impaction impedes lymphatic drainage of inner prepuce and causes it to swell up. Increased tissue pressure of edema worsens the strangulation effect thereby setting a vicious cycle. Vascular congestion of glans in turn precipitates edema of erectile tissue. The combination of preputial band constriction, preputial edema, glans tumescence and glans edema makes reduction of the retracted prepuce increasingly difficult over time. The pace of events occurs much faster in compound paraphimosis than in the simple paraphimosis [10].

As the outer layer of prepuce and penile shaft are proximal to the strangulating preputial band, they remain remarkably normal for a very long period. Onset of infection and inflammation in the edematous ischemic tissue still worsen the situation. It is theoretically possible that in due course, arterial supply to the glans may be compromised leading to necrosis of the penile tip; however, it seldom appears to happen. Rather more practically, capillary ischemia and venous micro infarcts leads to erosions and micro-ulceration of both the glans and the swollen inner prepuce. Frequently, the preputial band is the first to undergo ischemic ulceration. Extraordinary delay in treatment leads to fibroblast infiltration of the edematous inner prepuce, thereby converting it into rubbery tumor like mass [11].

Classification

In 1864 Thompson [12] described two different types of paraphimosis: (1) Primary paraphimosis is a complication of phimosis wherein the preputial swelling is caused by paraphimosis; (2) Secondary paraphimosis occurs as a complication of preputial edema (due to venereal diseases) wherein the preputial swelling was the cause of paraphimosis. In fact, both of them can be included under the compound paraphimosis described above. Rangarajan and Jayakar [11] classified paraphimosis into acute and chronic based on the time delay of seeking medical help and presence of pain. In fact, simple and compound paraphimosis are equivalent but not identical to that of chronic and acute types respectively. However, as the time of presentation depends not only on biological factors but also on socioeconomic factors, the classification of acute and chronic is scientifically imprecise. Some authors have also classified it as 'painful' *versus* 'painless' [13]; others classified it as '*intact-prepuce paraphimosis*' versus '*post-circumcision paraphimosis*'.

Grading System

Kumar and Javle [1] graded the severity of paraphimosis based on the pathogenic sequence (Table 19.1).

Table 19.1 Kumar–Javle's Grading of paraphimosis

Grade	Description	n (%)	Recommended Treatment
I	A rim of preputial edema of inner prepuce with no engorgement of the glans	6 (13)	Simple reduction
II	Tumescence of glans in addition to preputial edema	37 (82)	Puncture technique
III	Associated skin changes in the form of erosion, non-pitting edema and cheese-cutting of the shaft by the tight band	2 (5)	Surgical division of preputial band

Table 19.2 Raveenthiran's grading of paraphimosis

Grade	Description[a]	Recommended treatment[b]
I	TG present but no PE or GE	Manual reduction
II	TG and PE present but no GE	Manual reduction with adjuvant maneuvers
III	TG, PE, and GE present but no ulceration	Manual reduction by hybrid methods
IV	Presence of glanular or preputial ulcers or erosion	Surgical reduction or circumcision
V-a	Partial or complete gangrene of glans	Circumcision + Glans repair
V-b	Superadded infection or edema extending proximal to constricting band	Surgical reduction or circumcision
V-c	Chronic fibrosis of prepuce causing rubbery mass	Circumcision

TG tumescence of glans, *GE* glans edema, *PE* preputial edema

[a]Glans will be swollen in both TG and GE. They can be differentiated by the color of glans: bluish pink in TG and pale pink in GE

[b]Simple reduction with or without adjuncts is the technique of choice and all other methods are recommended only upon the failure of simple reduction

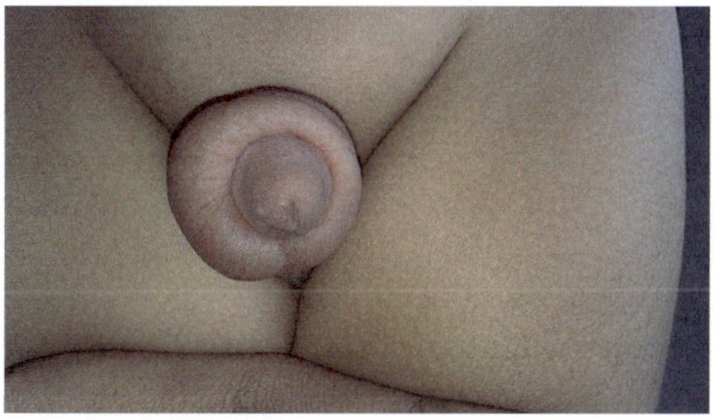

Fig. 19.1 Grade-2 paraphimosis showing the characteristic doughnut like swelling of the inner prepuce around the glans

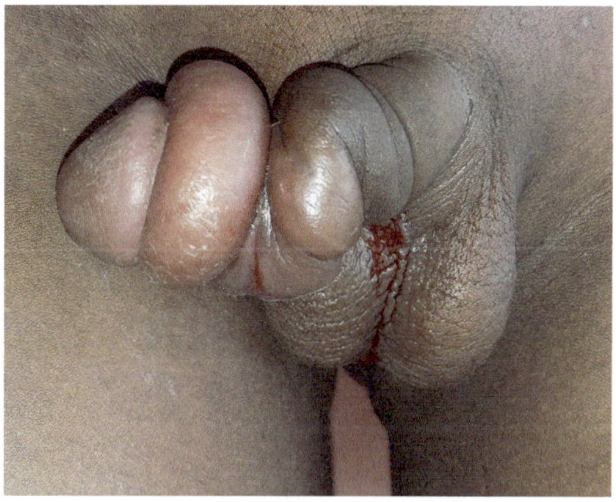

Fig. 19.2 Grade-5 paraphimosis showing extension of edema proximal to the constricting preputial band

Kumar assumed glanular tumescence to occur at a later stage. In fact, it is the first change to occur in response to gentle strangulation of the glans by the preputial band. Further, Kumar's grading system does not accomodate gangrene of the glans or chronic fibrosis of the prepuce. The present author has expanded the grading system (Table 19.2) and found it useful in therapeutic decision making (Figs. 19.1 and 19.2).

Epidemiology

Incidence

The exact incidence of paraphimosis in community is not known. Kumar and Javle in 2001 reported 37 patients from India over a period of

63 months and eight patients from UK over a span of 20 months [1]. Rangarajan and Jayakar from South India reported 68 patients between 1997 and 2005 [11]. Cletsoway from California described 13 patients during 1953–57 [14]. Thus, a busy hospital is likely to see 5–6 new cases every year and this trend appears to remain constant irrespective of the geographical location and chronology of time period. Herzog and Alvarez estimated the frequency of paraphimosis among uncircumcised boys to be 0.2% [15]. The present author personally collected 84 cases over a period of 25 years. From these discussions, contrary to popular perception, paraphimosis appears to be a rare disease.

Notwithstanding the forgoing description, high frequency of paraphimosis has also been reported in some series. For example, Kaker et al. from Pakistan reported 45 pediatric cases over a period of 9 months (Feb 2016–Oct 2016) [16]. Similarly, in 2013 Jadhavs from Pune reported 100 patients over a period of 2 years [17]. It is difficult to calculate the actual frequency of paraphimosis from these data because the denominator—the total number of patients seen during the study period—is missing in all these papers. Burstein and Paquin from Canada reported 46 patients between October 2013 and September 2016 [18]. They cite an annual footfall of 84,000 patients in their emergency department. Thus the calculated incidence of paraphimosis is 1 in 5400 emergency admissions.

Sex Predilection

Paraphimosis is exclusively a male disorder. However, the term "female paraphimosis" has also been rarely used imprecisely to mean female urethral prolapse [19] or edema of the clitoral hood [20].

Age Distribution

In pediatric age group paraphimosis has bimodal distribution; [10] the first and larger peak occurs between 3 and 6 years and the second and smaller peak occurs in adolescence (Fig. 19.3). The first peak corresponds to Freud's phallic phase of personality development during which period children are said to derive pleasure by genital manipulation or massage. The peri-pubertal peak may be explained by the increased frequency of masturbation and sexual misadventures such as self-experimentations [10]. Jadhavs who

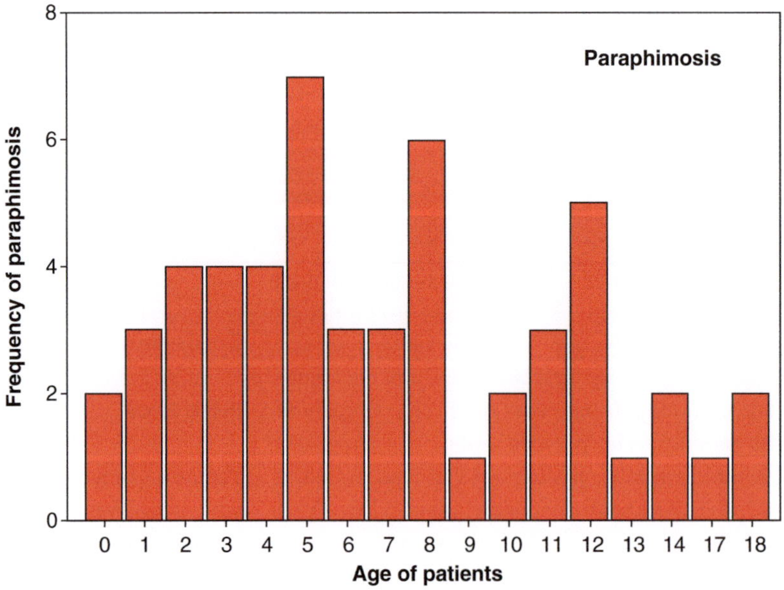

Fig. 19.3 Age distribution of pediatric paraphimosis, (Raveenthiran [10])

extended the study to adult population have also noted a similar bimodal presentation [17]. In their study the first peak occurred between 6 and 12 years of age while the second peak occurred during the sexually active age of 21–60 years. It is perplexing as to why adolescents who are more curious of sexual activities are least affected in this study. It is generally agreed that the incidence of compound paraphimosis decreases with increasing age after adolescence while that of simple paraphimosis remains a constant throughout all age groups.

Geographic Distribution

Since circumcision is preventive of paraphimosis, one may expect it to be uncommon in countries where routine male circumcision is practiced. Paraphimosis defies this simple logic and it has been reported in large numbers from USA [14] and Islamic countries such as Pakistan [16] where neonatal circumcision is widely practiced for hygiene and religious reasons respectively. Inadequate or incomplete removal of the foreskin is the cause of post-circumcision paraphimosis. Similarly there is no difference in the incidence of paraphimosis between temperate and tropical countries [10].

Etiology

Etiology differs according to the age of patient and the type of paraphimosis. As noted earlier, compound paraphimosis cannot occur in the absence of stiff penile erection. Vigorous sexual acts such as penetrative intercourse [21, 22] and masturbation [23] account for majority of compound paraphimosis. In Rangarajan's series 63 of the 68 patients (93%) were newlywed and developed this during maiden intercourse [11]. *Wining*, a form of erotic dancing, wherein the dancers keep rubbing their genitals for several hours has also been described to cause paraphimosis [24]. In a peculiar case, paraphimosis was a corroborative forensic evidence of rape (forced intercourse) [25]. Lichen sclerosis of the prepuce predisposes to paraphimosis by causing phimosis [26].

Table 19.3 Etiology of paraphimosis

Cause	Frequency (%)
Self retraction	30
Retraction by a parent or care taker	10
Masturbation	18
Sexual intercourse	32
Iatrogenic	5
Unknown	5

Data Source: Jadhav and Jadhav [17]

Simple paraphimosis occurs due to self-retraction by a curious child or parental retraction during bathing [17]. It may also occur in children due to spontaneous nocturnal erection or due to vigorous scratching of genitals as in the case of genital scabies or tinea cruris [10]. Although iatrogenic failure to replace the retracted prepuce following catheterization or cystoscopy is often incriminated in the literature, it is extremely rare accounting for only 5% of all paraphimosis (Table 19.3). Adults may develop simple paraphimosis when they fall asleep after coitus without returning the retracted foreskin.

Rarely swelling of the glans penis and edema of prepuce causes the foreskin to roll back and mimic paraphimosis. They are called pseudo-paraphimosis and their etiology is discussed in the section of differential diagnosis [27]. It is possible that some of the pseudo-paraphimosis are actually secondary paraphimosis (i.e. true paraphimosis precipitated by another unrelated disease). Surprisingly, child abuse has never been reported to cause paraphimosis.

Clinical Features

Clinical features of paraphimosis considerably differ between the two subtypes (Table 19.4). A doughnut-like swelling of the inner prepuce around the corona of glans is characteristic but not unique of paraphimosis; it may also be seen in pseudo-paraphimosis. Contrary to popular perception, paraphimosis—especially the simple variety—is often painless. Children often project the

Table 19.4 Clinical features of Simple and compound paraphimosis

Clinical features	Simple paraphimosis	Compound paraphimosis
Common age	All age groups	Sexually active age
Predisposing penile erection	May or may not present	Pre-requisite
Pre-existing phimosis	No	Yes
Pain	Chronic, dull discomfort	Acute excruciating
Presentation	As late as 3–25 days	Early within 1 or 2 days
Ischemia	Often restricted to the preputial band	May involve inner prepuce and glans
Ischemic ulceration	Extremely rare	Not uncommon
Preputial swelling	Slow onset and mild	Rapid onset and severe
Glans edema	Absent until very late	Quick to set in
Urine retention	Extremely rare	Not uncommon
Treatment	Simple reduction	Special maneuver or surgical operation necessary

unpleasant glans sensation as pain [10]. Compound paraphimosis which is highly painful usually presents within 24 h while procrastination the rule in simple paraphimosis. In the series of Jadhavs only 4% presented within few hours; 20% presented within 24 h, 68% between 2 and 4 days, 6% between 5 and 6 days and 2% beyond 6 days [17]. The longest reported delay was 25 days! [11]. Social embarrassment associated with the genital tragedy is the principal cause of delay. Senile dementia, lack of proper caretaker, inadequate transport facilities and economic constraints are also responsible for delayed presentation. It is the type of paraphimosis rather than the delay in presentation that is associated with complications such as retention of urine and ischemic ulceration of the glans [10]. This assertion is supported by the fact that those who presented after a delay of 15 days and 25 days were free of voiding problems or penile gangrene [11, 17]. In my personal experience grade-1 lesion is seen in 2% of patients, grade-2 in 72%, grade-3 in 6%, grade-4 in 17% and grade-5b in 2% and grade-5c in 1% [10].

Differential Diagnosis

Occasionally, swelling of the prepuce or the glans causes the foreskin to roll back and mimic paraphimosis. These are better called as secondary paraphimosis or pseudo-paraphimosis [27] and should be considered in the differential diagnosis of true paraphimosis (Fig. 19.4). Glanular hemangioma has been incriminated as the cause of paraphimosis in a 1-year-old boy [28]. Preputio-glanular edema of genital piercing [29], chancroid [30], viral urethritis, syphilitic balanitis of Follmann [31, 32], angioedema, insect- or ant-bite allergy, contact allergy due to topical application of aphrodisiac such as celandine juice [33] and use of auto-erotic devices such as metal rings [34] are known to cause pseudo-paraphimosis. Professional strippers [24] and prostate cancer patients [35], who self-apply penile tourniquet either to sustain erection or to relieve referred pain respectively, are at increased risk of pseudo-paraphimosis. Bizarre etiologies such as plasmodium infection [36] and spinal cord injury (tetraplegia) [37] have been reported; however, they lack satisfactory explanation of pathogenic mechanism. Occasionally, penile paraffinoma (self-injection of substances like paraffin with a mistaken idea of penile augmentation) has been reported to mimic paraphimosis [38]. Coital and non-coital injuries of penis may also result in preputial edema mimicking paraphimosis [39].

Treatment of Paraphimosis

Paraphimosis is a clinical diagnosis and hence laboratory investigations or imaging are unnecessary. Perhaps, for medico-legal reasons, clinical photography is desirable in those who present with ischemic necrosis. The aim of paraphimosis treatment is to restore anatomical normalcy of prepuce by simple manual reduction; [40] when this is impossible, the foreskin is sacrificed to relieve symptoms. Table 19.5 summarizes various therapeutic options available to treat paraphimosis. If the paraphimosis is due to catheterization, removal of the catheter will facilitate reduction.

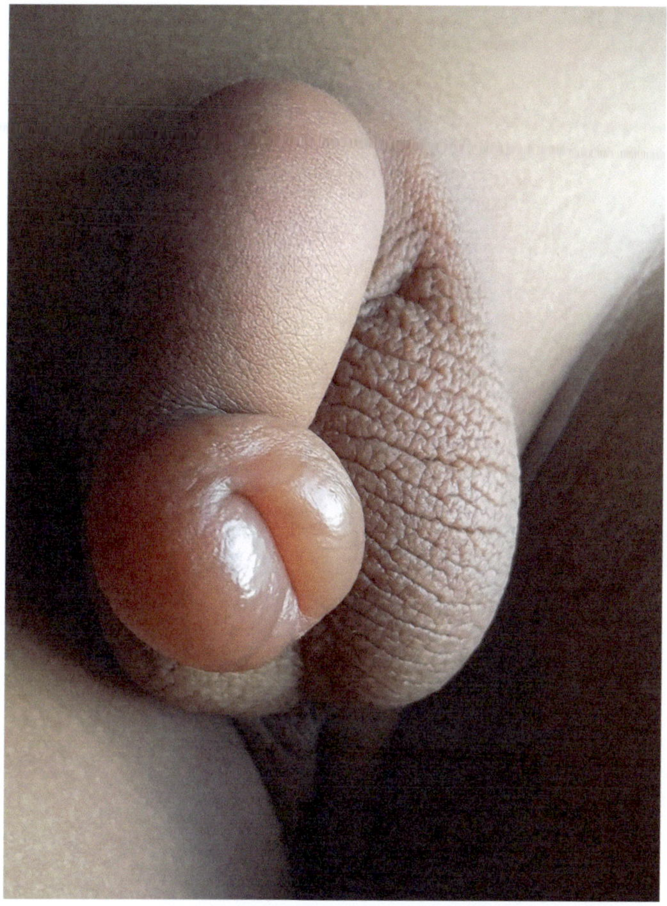

Fig. 19.4 Pseudoparaphimosis

Anesthesia for Paraphimosis Reduction

Reduction of paraphimosis is a painful procedure and hence requires some form of anesthesia. Topical anesthetics, penile nerve block, procedural sedation, spinal or caudal analgesia and general anesthesia have been used. In a non-randomized study Burstein and Paquin [18] compared paraphimosis reduction using topical LET gel (LET: Lidocaine 4%, Epinephrine 0.1%, Tetracaine 0.5%) versus procedural sedation with ketamine (1–2 mg/kg). They found both of them equally good; however minor adverse events were more frequent with procedural sedation. Topical application of eutectic mixture of 2.5% lidocaine and 2.5% prilocaine (EMLA) has also been reported [41]. Alternatively, Flores and Herring used ultrasound guided dorsal penile nerve block [42]. I prefer penile ring-block using 2% lignocaine in older children and procedural sedation with ketamine or propofol in uncooperative young infants [10].

Simple Manual Reduction Techniques

In *thumb-thrusting technique* the shaft of penis is held by palmar grasp in the non-dominant hand and the glans is pushed backward using the thumb of dominant hand. The *3-finger (squeeze) technique* is similar to thumb-thrusting technique except that the glans is squeezed using the first three fingers of dominant hand while reducing it. Toogood described a *6-finger technique* (Fig. 19.5) wherein the preputial doughnut is held between the index and middle fingers of both hands attempting to roll it forward while the

Table 19.5 Summary of various techniques used in the treatment of paraphimosis

Technique
1. Simple manual reduction
• Thumb-thrusting technique
• 3-finger (squeeze) technique
• Toogood's technique (6-finger technique)
• Keyes' technique
2. Adjuvants of manual reduction
(a) Techniques to dissipate preputial edema
Mechanical adjuvants
• Hamdy-Hastie puncture technique[a]
• Southey tube drainage (Barry technique)
• Ganti's turban technique (compression dressing)
• Colorado technique
Enzymatic adjuvants
• Williams-Nicholas-Ratliff method (Hyaluronidase injection)
Osmotic adjuvants
• Topical application of hygroscopic agents
– Granulated sugar
– Mannitol
– 50% dextrose
– Glycerin magnesium sulphate
• Houghton's ice-glove technique
• EMLA glove technique
(b) Techniques of reducing glanular tumescence
• Raveenthiran's glans aspiration technique
3. Instrument assisted reductions
• Bond's fingernail pinch technique
• Turner's dorsal band traction technique
• Skoglund-Chapman's Babcock clamp technique
4. Surgical reduction
• Dorsal slitting of preputial band
• Langer's ventral slitting of preputial band
• Schenck's preputioplasty
5. Cletsoway-Lewis's primary circumcision

[a]This technique is also variously known as Dundee technique, Perth technique, Arbroath-Dundee-Perth technique, needle technique or puncture method

glans is simultaneously pushed backward using both the thumbs [2]. Among them, the Toogood's technique is the most popular method. All these techniques are equally successful in simple paraphimosis especially in stage 1 and 2.

In *Keyes' technique* the constricting band of prepuce is still further retracted proximally and the edematous swelling is squeezed before attempting reduction [43]. Wrinkles of the inner prepuce are then smoothened out by applying liberal amount of Vaseline. These maneuvers are believed to facilitate dissipation of edema and reduction of constricting band. Although Keyes recommended lubrication, others found it slippery and messy. I prefer to have firm grip of the preputial doughnut by wrapped a shawl of dry gauze around it.

Adjuvants of Manual Reduction

When simple manual reduction is difficult, it is facilitated by a variety of adjuvant techniques. They can be broadly divided into techniques of dissipating preputial edema and techniques of causing detumescence of the engorged glans. Preputial edema may be dissipated by mechanical, osmotic or enzymatic methods.

1. *Mechanical adjuvants*

   The most popular of all mechanical adjuvants is the *puncture technique* [44–46]. It was originally described by Hamdy-Hastie from Sheffield [44]. Following a spat of priority claims, it was decided to be called as Arbroath-Dundee-Perth technique or simply the 'needle- or puncture-technique' [47]. The swollen inner prepuce is punctured at multiple places (usually 6–20) allowing edema fluid to seep out. Frequently, squeezing of edematous prepuce is necessary to expel the fluid. The size of needle used was 21G in Sheffield, 25G in Perth and 26G in Oxford [44–46]. Although this technique is invasive, antibiotic prophylaxis is not usually necessary. Critics maintain that it is the manual pressure of squeezing rather than the punctures that is responsible for reduction of edema [48]. It is also said to be ineffective in delayed cases [49].

   In *Barry's technique*, instead of making punctures, multiple Southey's needles are inserted into the edematous prepuce and left in situ for the edema fluid to drip [50]. This method has never gained popularity as it is scary to the young patient as well as his caretakers.

   In *Ganti's technique*, edema can also be reduced by applying constant pressure over the preputial doughnut using a 2-in. wide elastic bandage [51]. The bandage is firmly applied in the distal-to-proximal direction and left in situ for 5–7 min to have the edema reduced. *Colorado technique* [3] is a modification of

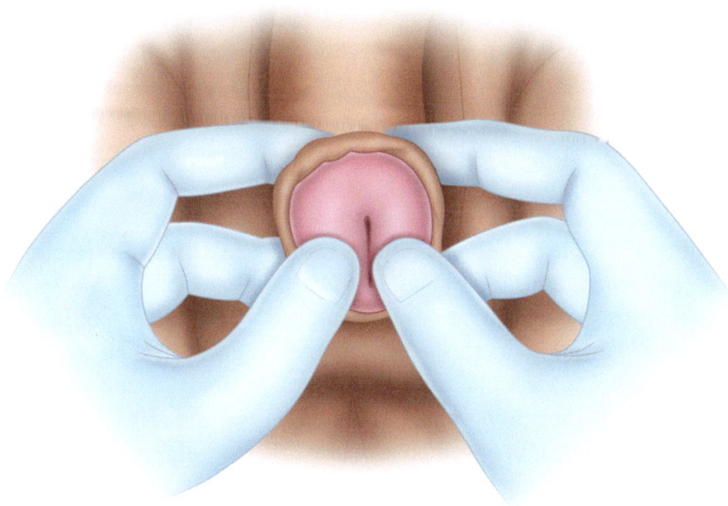

Fig. 19.5 Toogood's 6-finger technique of reducing paraphimosis

Ganti's method, in which elastic adhesive plaster is used instead of elastic bandage and the duration of compression is 20 min instead of 7 min. As the bandage appears like a headgear of the penis, these methods are also called as *turban technique* [52]. In some cases, spontaneous reduction of paraphimosis is said to occur with turban technique without the need for further manual reduction.

2. *Enzymatic adjuvants*: Williams and Nichols [53] first reported the *use of hyaluronidase* in reducing paraphimosis; Ratliff and Engel popularized it [54, 55]. This enzyme digests the ground substance (hyaluronic acid) and facilitates interstitial dispersion of fluid. About 0.5–1 mL of reconstituted enzyme in normal saline is injected into the edematous preputial doughnut at two or three places and it is gently massaged to reduce edema. Most of the authors used 1:150 dilutions [53–55], while Doyle used 1:1000 dilutions [56]. This method enjoyed wide popularity without anyone questioning as to where the fluid would percolate if the preputial band is tightly strangulating proximally. Litzky correctly observed that multiple punctures of the injecting needle rather than hyaluronidase is responsible for reduction of edema [57].
3. *Osmotic adjuvants*: Several hygroscopic materials have been applied over the glans and preputial doughnut aiming to draw out edema fluid under osmotic gradient. This is the most commonly used method in veterinary practice to reduce paraphimosis in horses and dogs. The lists of hygroscopic agents include gauze soaked in 50% dextrose solution [58] or 20% mannitol [59], paste of glycerin magnesium sulphate [60] and granulated sugar [61, 62]. Although they are obviously less frightening, it is often impractical to tie down the child for 20–30 min for the osmotic reduction to occur.
4. *Houghton's iced glove method* [63]: In this technique, a rubber surgical glove is filled with ice cold water and its cuff end is knotted preventing leakage. The affected penis is thrust into the glove by invaginating its thumb. Thus the penis will be inside the glove but without being in actual contact with iced water. In such a position the glove is kept pressed against the pubis until the edema is reduced. It is not known as to whether the low temperature of ice or the compression of gloves that causes the desired effect. Vasospasm induced by ice may reduce venous congestion of glans thereby facilitating reduction. At the same time it is not safe to have vasospasm of penile end artery and risk ischemic gangrene [48]. Further, ice cold temperature is uncomfortable to the patient.
5. *EMLA glove technique* [41]: Thumb of a surgical rubber glove is cut and filled with EMLA cream. EMLA filled sleeve is then applied to the penis. Osmotic effect of EMLA,

compression effect of the rubber sleeve and lubrication effect of the cream probably act additively and cause reduction of edema.

6. *Raveenthiran's aspiration technique* [64]: Unlike the aforesaid methods, this technique aims to facilitate simple reduction by reducing tumescence of the glans. This is achieved by thrusting a 20G hypodermic needle into the glans and aspirating blood (Fig. 19.6). It is important that the needle be inserted parallel to urethra to avoid injury. Spontaneous refilling of corporal space while aspiration is prevented by applying a proximal tourniquet. This technique is useful in compound paraphimosis presenting within 48 h.

Instrumental Reduction

Bond vividly described the cause of failures in paraphimosis reduction by drawing analogy of trying to push a rigid glass tube through a slightly smaller-sized India rubber tube [65]. Edges of the rubber tube would buckle inward preventing easy passage of the glass tube; insertion will be made easy if the edges are seized and drawn out. Bond compared the infolding rubber edge with the tight preputial band. *Bond's technique* involve pinching the preputial band between the finger nails of both hands and drawing it apart dilating the ring while simultaneously pulling it forward over the glans. Sometimes a second operator is required to push down the glans. *Dorsal band traction technique* of Turner is a modification of Bond's method wherein Adson forceps are used instead of finger nails to hold the preputial band [66]. According to the age of patient, either one pair of forceps at 12-o'clock position or two pairs of forceps at 3 and 9-o'clock are used. *Skoglund-Chapman's modification* involves using of four Babcock clamps to pinch the preputial band at each quadrant [67]. In all these techniques it is essential to grasp sufficient bulk of tissue to prevent lacerations during reduction. In small children there will insufficient space to apply four Babcock clamps.

Surgical Reduction

When simple or instrumental reduction fails, surgical division of the constricting preputial band brings in success. In fact, small unintended tears of the friable preputial band occurring during forced reduction is actually responsible for many a success of manual techniques. Traditionally the preputial band is incised across at the 12-o' clock position to avoid bleeding from frenular artery. This *Dorsal slit technique* often leaves behind an unsightly foreskin necessitating circumcision [68]. *Langer-Winthrop's ventral slitting* of preputial band at 6-o' clock position is intended to avoid this cosmetic disfigurement; [69] it works in flaccid penis but loses its relevance with the onset of erection. *Schenck's preputioplasty* involves Heinecke's principle of horizontally suturing the vertical incision of the preputial band thereby widening it [43]. It is easier said than to do delicate suturing in edematous prepuce.

Circumcision

Emergency circumcision is the last resort when everything else fails. It is generally avoided as sutures tend to cut through the edematous tissue and hence the cosmetic outcome is inferior to elective circumcision. Contrary to this view, Cletsoway and Lewis recommended circumcision as the preferred primary modality of treatment in all cases [14]. Even after successful reduction elective cir-

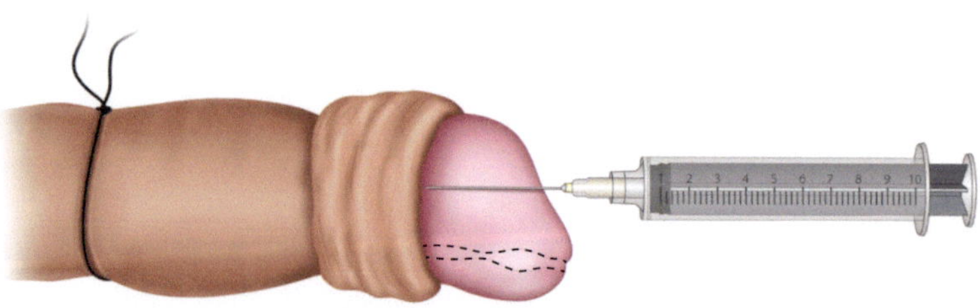

Fig. 19.6 Raveenthiran's glans aspiration technique of paraphimosis reduction

cumcision is recommended by some authors to prevent recurrence. Laceration of preputial band during reduction, underlying phimosis and sloughing (or ulceration) of entangled prepuce are definite indications of elective circumcision.

Comparison of Various Techniques

Most of the literature on paraphimosis are anecdotal and are at the best short series. Personal bias is evident with each author describing a new method. Chance occurrence of treatment success could not be excluded due to extremely small numbers in each series. A systematic review revealed only three out of 33 papers were suitable for analysis. On comparing Houghton's iced-glove, puncture technique and osmotic reduction by granulated sugar, none of them were found to be superior to each other [4].

Complications

Exact frequency of various complications in paraphimosis is not known. Pathogenic mechanism, cause-effect relationship and optimal treatment of many complications are not well established.

Preputial Lacerations

The commonest complication is perhaps unintended tearing of preputial band during forceful reduction [10]. In fact, success of several manual reductions can be attributed to such incidental lacerations. If the laceration heals spontaneously, it leaves behind a narrow preputial orifice (phimosis) thereby predisposing to further episodes of paraphimosis; if it is severe, it causes grotesque swelling of prepuce. Thus, preputial lacerations invariably necessitate elective circumcision.

Acute Retention of Urine

The cause-effect relationship between acute retention of urine and paraphimosis is not clear. On one hand paraphimosis could be the iatrogenic effect of catheterization for acute retention of urine; on the other hand, tightly strangulating paraphimosis could be the cause of retention. Frequently children present after a delay of several days and they do not suffer any voiding difficulty. From these it appears that a small fraction of compound paraphimosis may present with distended bladder. Reduction of paraphimosis often relieves retention.

Recurrence of Paraphimosis

All paraphimosis patients were previously subjected to elective circumcision even after successful manual reduction. It is logical to assume recurrence of paraphimosis when the underlying causes such as phimosis remain uncorrected [37]. However, in actual practice recurrent paraphimosis is extremely rare. Simple paraphimosis do not recur after successful reduction as the prepuce is normal. Compound paraphimosis, although has the potential to recur, are often irreducible and they end up with emergency circumcision during the first episode. A second episode of paraphimosis definitely calls for circumcision but the same can be avoided with first episode especially if the paraphimosis is of simple type [10].

Gangrene of Glans

Necrosis of the glans may be ischemic [13, 21, 23, 70–72] or infective [73]. This is the most feared complication of paraphimosis that is often alluded to in many papers. But a review of literature reveals only seven cases being reported in the world literature over the last two centuries and none of them were in pediatric-adolescent age group (Table 19.6). The youngest was 25 years and five of them (71%) were above 60 years of age. Most of them had had serious co-morbidities such as peripheral vascular disease that could have independently caused glans necrosis. Interestingly, there was no correlation between the occurrence of gangrene and the duration of paraphimosis which ranged from 12 h to 2 weeks. This is corroborated by another report of a patient who presented with healthy glans despite a delay of 25 days [11]. In most of the cases only a part of

Table 19.6 Gangrene of the glans penis in paraphimosis

Sr.no	Author	Age (year)	Duration	Precipitators	Co-morbidities	Status of glans	Intervention	Outcome
1	Ahmed and Mallick [73]	85	2 weeks	Catheterization	Alzheimer, BHP, urinary incontinence	Fournier gangrene	Surgical debridement, antibiotics	Died
2	Hollowood and Sibley [13]	80	?	?	Diabetic neuropathy	Urethrocutaneous fistula	Partial glans amputation	Recovered
3	Palmisano et al. [70]	83	2 days	Catheterization	Pneumonia, UTI	Partial discoloration	Topical hyaluronic acid	Complete recovery in 6 weeks
4	Raman et al. [21]	60	2 days	Coitus	–	Black discoloration	Excision of necrotic patch (?)	Recovered
5	Sato et al. [23]	25	1 week	Masturbation	Schizophrenia	Black scab over glans, necrosis of prepuce, ventral glans necrosis urethrocutaneous fistula	Circumcision	Partial recovery in 30 days
6	Sokhal et al. [72]	34	7 days	Catheterization	Chronic voiding dysfunction	Fever, dry gangrene of glans, sloughing of penile skin	Debridement, glansectomy	Recovered
7	Williams et al. [71]	70	12 h	Self retraction for washing	Tobacco abuse, peripheral vascular disease, erectile dysfunction	Swollen, blue	Dorsal slitting of preputial band	Glans regained colour immediately

glans had necrosed. From the foregoing discussion it appears that paraphimosis per se may not be the cause of gangrene; rather it appears to be a precipitator of necrosis in synchrony with another chronic underlying disorder. Except one death, all the other patients have recovered and even the glans morphology had been partially restored.

Urethro-Cutaneous Fistula

Three cases of urethrocutaneous fistula as a complication of neglected paraphimosis have been described in the literature [13, 23, 74]. In all of them fistula was attributed to ischemic necrosis of the ventral glans; but the diagnosis of paraphimosis was not established beyond doubt. Retrospective critical analysis suggests that they could be secondary or pseudoparaphimosis.

Mortality and Outcome

Outcome of paraphimosis is generally excellent. There are only two reports of death in paraphimosis: one was due to chloroform related complication reported in the last century [75] and the other was a 85-year-old man who died of Fournier gangrene complicating paraphimosis [73]. There are no data on the long-term effect of paraphimosis on sexual function.

References

1. Kumar V, Javle P. Modified puncture technique for reduction of paraphymosis. Ann R Coll Surg Engl. 2001;83:126–7.
2. Toogood J. On the treatment of paraphymosis. Prov Med Surg J. 1842;3:312–3.
3. Pohlman GD, Phillips JM, Wilcox DT. Simple method of paraphimosis reduction revisited: point of technique and review of the literature. J Pediatr Urol. 2013;9:104–7.
4. Mackway-Jones K, Teece S. Best evidence topic reports. Ice, pins, or sugar to reduce paraphimosis. Emerg Med J. 2004;21:77–8.
5. Chung CH. Emergency management of paraphimosis. Hong Kong J Emerg Med. 2003;10:253–7.
6. Choe JM. Paraphimosis. Current treatment options. Am Fam Physician. 2000;62:2623–6.
7. Bhishagratna KL. (Tr) The Sushruta Samhita: an English translation based on original Sanskrit text. Calcutta: Bhaduri publications; 1907.
8. Hodges FM. Phimosis in antiquity. World J Urol. 1999;17:133–6.
9. Hodges FM. The history of phimosis from antiquity to the present. In: Denniston GC, Hodges FM, Milos MF, editors. Male and female circumcision medical, legal, and ethical considerations in pediatric practice. New York: Kluwer Academic; 1999. p. 37–62.
10. Raveenthiran V. On the rationale of paraphimosis treatment based on a new system of classification. Proceedings of 7th annual conference of Indian Association of Pediatric Surgeons (Tamilnadu - Pondicherry chapter), Vellore, 11-12 July 2008.
11. Rangarajan M, Jayakar SM. Paraphimosis revisited: is chronic paraphimosis a predominantly third world condition? Trop Dr. 2008;38:40–2.
12. Thompson J. Paraphimosis. Br Med J. 1864;2:363–4.
13. Hollowood AD, Sibley GN. Non-painful paraphimosis causing partial amputation. Br J Urol. 1997;80:958.
14. Cletsoway RW, Lewis EL. Treatment of paraphimosis. U S Armed Forces Med J. 1957;8:361–4.
15. Herzog LW, Alvarez SR. The frequency of foreskin problems in uncircumcised children. Am J Dis Child. 1986;140:254–6.
16. Kakar M, Rehman M, Shah A. Emergency treatment of paraphimosis by multiple needle puncture technique in children. Pak J Med Health Sci. 2017;11:401–2.
17. Jadhav SE, Jadhav SS. Clinical study of proportion of predisposing events and causes of paraphimosis. Indian J Appl Res. 2013;3:373–4.
18. Burstein B, Paquin R. Comparison of outcomes for pediatric paraphimosis reduction using topical anesthetic versus intravenous procedural sedation. Am J Emerg Med. 2017;35:1391–5.
19. Salim S, Taylor A, Carter C. Female paraphimosis? Management of a large female urethral caruncle, trialling manual reduction. J Obstet Gynaecol. 2014;34:282–3.
20. Willan RJ. Paraphimosis of the clitoris. Br Med J. 1928;2:1130–1.
21. Raman SR, Kate V, Ananthakrishnan N. Coital paraphimosis causing penile necrosis. Emerg Med J. 2008;25:454.
22. Berk DR, Lee R. Paraphimosis in a middle-aged adult after intercourse. Am Fam Physician. 2004;69:807–8.
23. Sato Y, Takagi S, Uchida K, et al. Long-term follow-up of penile glans necrosis due to paraphimosis. IJU Case Rep. 2019;2:171–3.
24. Ramdass MJ, Naraynsingh V, Kuruvilla T, Maharaj D. Case report. Paraphimosis due to erotic dancing. Tropical Med Int Health. 2000;5:906–7.
25. Saini OP, Suman A, Buri S, Saini PK, Mathur PN, Gahlot RK. Paraphimosis – a case report and medicolegal importance. J Indian Acad Forensic Med. 2008;30:82–3.
26. Roh D, Jin H, You HS, et al. Balanopreputial adhesion and paraphimosis due to lichen sclerosus. Ann Dermatol. 2018;30:384–6.

27. Ng KL, Mahadevan DT, Htun TH, Razack AH, Dublin N. Pseudoparaphimosis: a hairy affair. Med J Malaysia. 2011;66:268–9.
28. Yigiter M, Arda IS, Hiçsönmez A. An unusual cause of paraphimosis: hemangioma of the glans penis. J Pediatr Surg. 2008;43:e31–3.
29. Jones SA, Flynn RJ. An unusual (and somewhat piercing) cause of paraphimosis. Br J Urol. 1996;78:803–4.
30. Harvey K, Bishop L, Silver D, Jones T. A case of chancroid. Med J Aust. 1977;26:956–7.
31. Nadimi AE, Carver CM. Syphilis presenting with paraphimosis: painless no longer. J Am Acad Dermatol. 2016;74(5):AB154.
32. Mainetti C, Scolari F, Lautenschlager S. The clinical spectrum of syphilitic balanitis of Follmann: report of five cases and a review of the literature. J Eur Acad Dermatol Venereol. 2016;30:1810–3.
33. Farina LA, Alonso MV, Horjales M, Zungri ER. Contact-derived allergic balanoposthitis and paraphimosis through topical application of celandine juice. Actas Urol Esp. 1999;23:554–5.
34. Low LS, Holmes M. The GEM ring cutter: an effective, simple treatment of penile strangulation caused by metal rings. Urol Case Rep. 2018;19:39–41.
35. Wimsey S, Thiruchelvam N, Keoghane SR. A key cause of paraphimosis. Int Urol Nephrol. 2006;38:111–3.
36. Gozal D. Paraphimosis apparently associated with Plasmodium falciparum infection. Trans R Soc Trop Med Hyg. 1991;85:443.
37. Ghosh S. Recurrent paraphimosis in a tetraplegic patient admitted for inpatient rehabilitation. Turk J Phys Med Rehab. 2014;60(Supp. 1):S78–80.
38. Downey AP, Osman NI, Mangera A, Inman RD, Reid SV, Chapple CR. Penile Paraffinoma. Eur Urol Focus. 2019;5:894–8.
39. Verma S. Coital penile trauma with severe paraphimosis. J Eur Acad Dermatol Venereol. 2005;19:134–5.
40. Vunda A, Lacroix LE, Schneider F, Manzano S, Gervaix A. Reduction of paraphimosis in boys. N Engl J Med. 2013;368:e16 (Video).
41. Khan A, Riaz A, Rogawski KM. Reduction of paraphimosis in children: the EMLA glove technique. Ann R Coll Surg Engl. 2014;96:168.
42. Flores S, Herring AA. Ultrasound-guided dorsal penile nerve block for ED paraphimosis reduction. Am J Emerg Med. 2015;33(863):e3–5.
43. Schenck GF. The treatment of paraphimosis. Am J Surg. 1930;8:329.
44. Hamdy FC, Hastie KJ. Treatment for paraphimosis: the 'puncture' technique. Br J Surg. 1990;77:1186.
45. Waters TC, Sripathi V. Reduction of paraphimosis. Br J Urol. 1990;66:666.
46. Reynard JM, Barua JM. Reduction of paraphimosis the simple way - the Dundee technique. BJU Int. 1999;83:859–60.
47. King PA. Reduction of paraphimosis the simple way - the Dundee technique. BJU Int. 2001;88:305.
48. Saxena A. Reduction of paraphimosis. Br J Urol. 1992;69:220.
49. Kamat N. Reduction of paraphimosis the simple way - the Dundee technique. BJU Int. 1999;84:890–1.
50. Barry CN. A simple method for reduction of paraphimosis. J Urol. 1954;71(4):450.
51. Ganti SU, Sayegh N, Addonizio JC. Simple method for reduction of paraphimosis. Urology. 1985;25:77.
52. Olson C. Emergency treatment of paraphimosis. Can Fam Physician. 1998;44:1253–4.
53. Williams TH, Nichols RK. Method of treating paraphimosis. J Med Assoc Alabama. 1952;21:233–4.
54. Ratliff RK. Hyaluronidase in the treatment of paraphimosis. J Am Med Assoc. 1954;155:746.
55. Engel WJ. Hyaluronidase as an aid to correction of paraphimosis: report of a case. Cleve Clin Q. 1954;21:24–6.
56. Doyle JO. Hyaluronidase in treatment of sequela of paraphimosis. Br Med J. 1954;2:1401.
57. Litzky GM. Reduction of paraphimosis with hyaluronidase. Urology. 1997;50:160.
58. Coutts AG. Treatment of paraphimosis. Br J Surg. 1991;78:252.
59. Anand A, Kapoor S. Mannitol for paraphimosis reduction. Urol Int. 2013;90:106–8.
60. Kamat N. Reduction of paraphimosis the simple way. BJU Int. 1999;84:890–1.
61. Kerwat R, Shandall A, Stephenson B. Reduction of paraphimosis with granulated sugar. Br J Urol. 1998;82:755.
62. Gonzalez Fernandez M, Sousa Escandon MA, Parra Muntaner L. Sugar: treatment of choice in irreducible paraphimosis. Actas Urol Esp. 2001;25:393–5.
63. Houghton GR. The "iced-glove" method of treatment of paraphimosis. Br J Surg. 1973;60:876–7.
64. Raveenthiran V. Reduction of paraphimosis: a technique based on pathophysiology. Br J Surg. 1996;83:1247.
65. Bond CJ. Note on the treatment of paraphimosis. Lancet. 1883;2:1180–1.
66. Turner CD, Kim HL, Cromie WJ. Dorsal band traction for reduction of paraphimosis. Urology. 1999;54:917–8.
67. Skoglund RW Jr, Chapman WH. Reduction of paraphimosis. J Urol. 1970;104:137.
68. Fuenfer MM, Najmaldin A. Emergency reduction of paraphimosis. Eur J Pediatr Surg. 1994;4:370–1.
69. Langer JC, Winthrop AL. Ventral slit for phimosis and paraphimosis in children. Pediatr Surg Int. 1995;10:209–10.
70. Palmisano F, Gadda F, Spinelli MG, Montanari E. Glans penis necrosis following paraphimosis: a rare case with brief literature review. Urol Case Rep. 2017;16:57–8.
71. Williams JC, Morrison PM, Richardson JR. Paraphimosis in elderly men. Am J Emerg Med. 1995;13:351–3.
72. Sokhal AK, Saini DK, Sankhwar S. Para phimosis leading to glans gangrene - a devastating preventable complication. Balkan Med J. 2017;34:180–1.
73. Ahmed J, Mallick IH. Paraphimosis leading to Fournier's Gangrene. J Coll Physicians Surg Pak. 2009;19:203.
74. Chitale AM, Gulati J, Manekar AA, Thakre SB. A rare case of ventral urethrocutaneous fistula post paraphimosis treatment. Indian. J Appl Res. 2018;8:50–1.
75. Eddowes A. Reduction of paraphimosis. Br Med J. 1877;2:324.

20 Posthitis and Balanoposthitis

Abbreviations

C. albicans	Candida albicans
MC	Male circumcision
STI	Sexually transmitted infection

Nomenclature and Definition

The word balanitis is from the Greek βάλανος balanos "acorn" and posthos greek for foreskin.

Balanitis refers to inflammation of the glans penis that often spreads along the shaft, isolated balanitis may occur in the circumcised population. The same term is also applicable for female; if the clitoris is inflamed.

Posthitis refers to inflammation restricted to the foreskin only.

Balanoposthitis is an inflammation of the glans penis and prepuce.

Balanitis is the most common inflammatory disease of the penis, and it is mainly affecting the circumcised men (Fig. 20.1). In uncircumcised penis, the prepuce is affected sooner or later by the inflammatory process to convert balanitis into a full blown picture of balanoposthitis, but in many occasions the only adjacent part of the inner prepuce is affected by the infection, which may resolve with the inception of the treatment (Fig. 20.2).

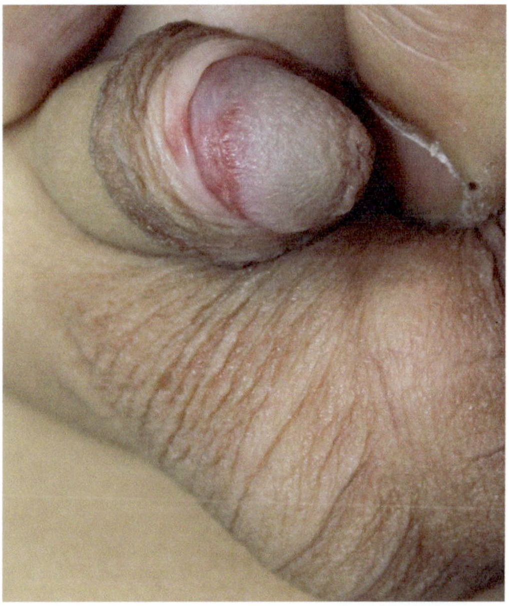

Fig. 20.1 A case balanitis in uncircumcised boy with minimal affection of the inner prepuce

In few cases, specially in young children, who are still in napkin, the brunt of glandular inflammation may extend from the glans to the urinary meatus and present with a different grades of meatitis (Fig. 20.3).

M. A. B. Fahmy, *Normal and Abnormal Prepuce*, https://doi.org/10.1007/978-3-030-37621-5_20

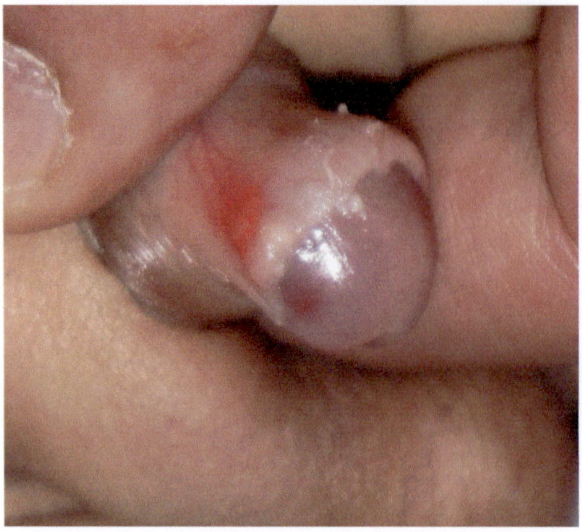

Fig. 20.2 Balanitis and preputial adhesion with an early affection of the inner prepuce

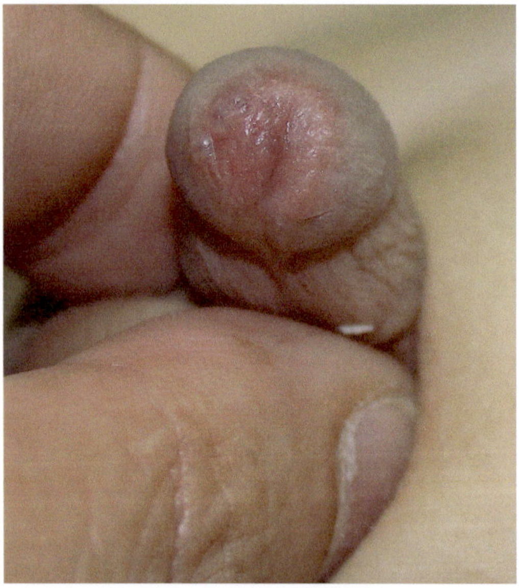

Fig. 20.3 Balanitis around the urinary meatus and severe meatitis, a minute vesicles are apparent around the urinary opening

Clinical Presentation

Balanitis usually presents with mild burning, pruritis, itching, swelling, erythematous patches, and plaques or bullae involving the glans penis, satellite eroded pustules and moist curd-like accumulations may be detectable (Fig. 20.3). Balanitis has worse clinical presentation in diabetic and immunocompromised patients, with a fulminating edema or ulcers in severe cases. Urinary manifestations may supervene the presentation if the infection spreaded to the meatus.

Etiology

Poor hygiene is the most common cause. Irritant balanitis can result from exposure to medications, such as some common antibiotics, and to allergens, including latex condoms, propylene glycol in some lubricants, some spermicides, and corticosteroids. Ammonia, released from urine by bacterial hydrolysis of urea, can induce inflammation of the glans and foreskin. Another common irritant responsible for contact balanitis is the frequent washing with soaps containing topical allergens or irritants [1].

Microbiology of Balanitis

Various bacterial species and yeasts under the foreskin have the potential to cause penile inflammatory conditions. C. albicans is the most frequent fungus isolate from the penis. Fungi are a normal flora, but overgrowth can occurs in certain conditions, especially in diabetic patients with phimosis. Candida colonization was seen in 16% of men visiting a sexually transmitted infection (STI) clinics in UK [2]. Symptomatic infection due to C. albicans is more common in uncircumcised males. Bacterial superinfection with Streptococci or Staphylococci increases pain (Fig. 20.4).

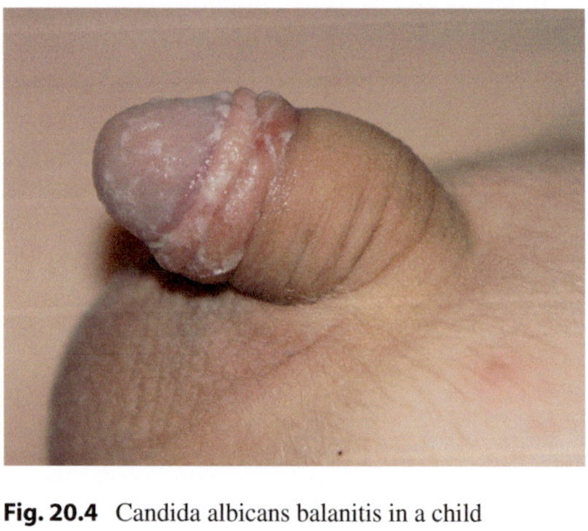

Fig. 20.4 Candida albicans balanitis in a child

Chlamydia trachomatis, genital mycoplasmas, and bacterial STIs such as Neisseria gonorrhoeae, Haemophilus ducreyi, and others can be associated with balanitis and balanoposthitis. N. gonorrhoeae produces an endotoxin which is likely responsible for edema and erythema of the foreskin. Gardnerella vaginalis is responsible for symptomatic anaerobic-related balanitis in men; presentation in such cases includes a subpreputial "fishy" smelling discharge similar to the odour from bacterial vaginosis in women. The prevalence of G. vaginalis was 15% and 25% among heterosexual attendees at STI clinics in London and Alabama, respectively [3].

Other causes of balanitis and balanoposthitis include viral STIs, such as high-risk type of human papillomavirus (HPV), and parasitic infections such as Trichomonas vaginalis and protozoa, all are more common in uncircumcised men [4] (Fig. 20.5).

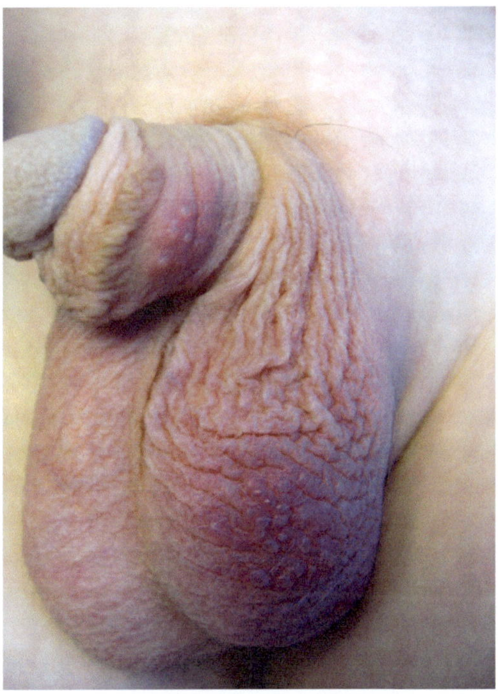

Fig. 20.5 Multiple monomorphous vesicles on an erythematous base on the penile shaft and scrotum that are characteristic of genital herpes

Balanitis in Boys

Approximately 4% of boys get balanitis, most commonly during the preschool years. Balanitis is especially common in uncircumcised boys aged under 5 years with phimosis (25%) compared with those without phimosis (6%) [5].

Post-Male Circumcision Balanitis

I think post-neonatal MC balanitis is an underestimated complication, especially in developing countries, as most of the babies are not followed up properly by the physicians after this procedure, and if they are any followup, this is usually done once in the first week. It is proposed that the naked glans is more liable to different forms of infections after removal of the prepuce (Fig. 20.6), especially if the napkins are not changed frequently and the proper care for the circumcision wound is not followed by the mothers, and also concomitant gastroenteritis and diarrhoea, which are still not uncommon in developing countries, may aggravate the condition and predispose to different forms of balanitis that may progresses to urinary meatus and results in meatitis, UTI, meatal ulcers or stenosis. Post-MC balanitis could be bacterial or fungal.

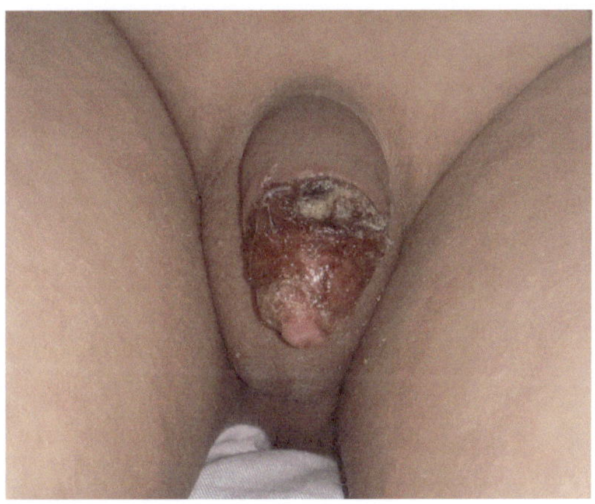

Fig. 20.6 Post MC balanitis with extensive incrustation over the bared glans

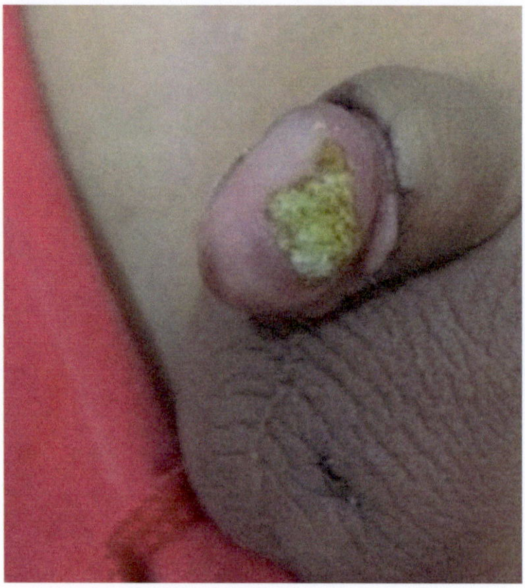

Fig. 20.7 Pseudomonas aeruginosa balanitis developed few days after circumcision

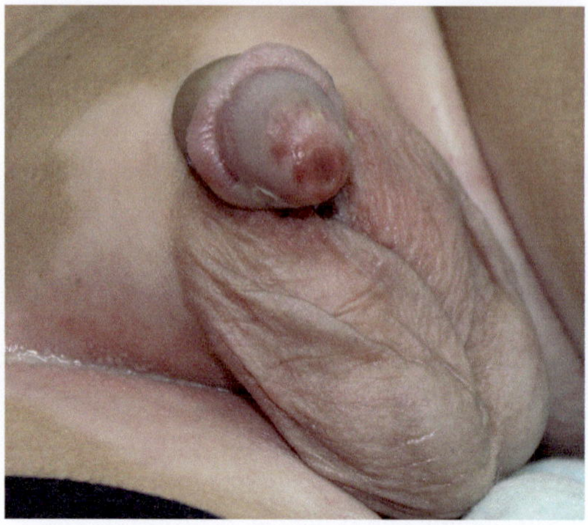

Fig. 20.8 Balanitis and meatitis complicating severe napkin dermatitis

Most of the studies dealing with the incidence of balanitis and the nature of isolated organisms are mainly recruited to promote circumcision, but I think it is not the issue of presence or forfeiture of prepuce, but it is level of hygiene; as we diagnosed many cases with severe balanitis induced by different pathogens after circumcision [6] (Fig. 20.7).

In developing countries, with the lack of proper hygiene, there is a peak of incidence of balanitis at the age between 6 months and 2 years, where different forms of napkin dermatitis affecting the genitalia, and end with different forms and grades of balanitis, which marked by maceration and erosion, yet also whitish patches and desquamation [7] (Fig. 20.8).

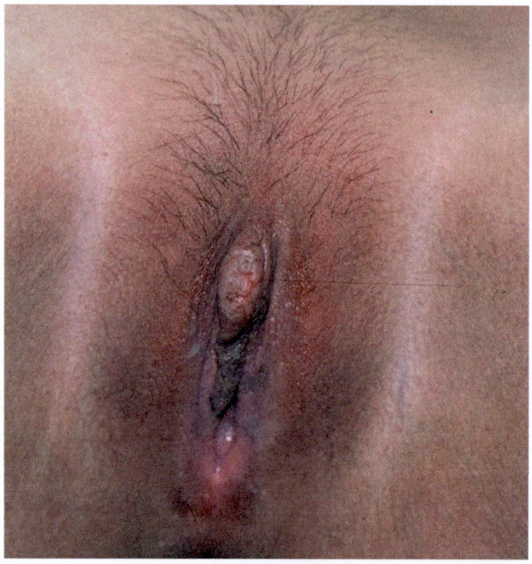

Fig. 20.9 Vulvovaginitis with clitorial affection (balanitis) in adolescent girl

Female Balanitis

Women can also develop balanitis, as the term balanitis is also used to describe an inflammation of the clitorial glans. In adults, clitoral phimosis may complicate repeated attacks of untreated balanitis. In some women with clitorodynia (a localized type of vulvodynia), the skin adhesions to the glans clitoris can give rise to a closed compartment syndrome with accumulation of skin secretions and initiation of balanitis, leading to chronic vulvar pain [8].

In young girls balanitis is not rare, but commonly undiagnosed or unreported, balanitis may be an aspect of the broad term of vulvovaginitis; which may be again secondary to napkin dermatitis, or improper hygiene, candida is the common causative organism [9] (Fig. 20.9).

Balanitis in Adult Males

Lack of penile hygiene has been consistently associated with balanitis in men. Other causes include exposure to certain medications, allergens, and chemical irritants. A 3-year prospective review of men aged 16–95 years (mean age 47 years) at a multi-specialty penile dermatology clinic in Edinburgh, UK, diagnosed nonspecific balanitis in 22% of patients [10]. Acquired phimosis, diabetes, and immunocompromised patient either due diseases or drugs are more liable to develop balanitis.

Treatment of Balanitis

Topical antifungals, if applied consistently until symptoms disappear, may be effective in treatment of fungal sexually acquired balanitis, systemic antifungal may be indicated for severe or recurrent cases. Recurrence is frequent, however, especially in patients with risk factors such as phimosis or diabetes. Treatment of the partner is important to reduce the risk of relapse. Proper antibiotics according to culture and sensitivity is mandatory, local measures with frequent dressing and topical ointment may be also helpful. Prevention entails good hygiene and some authors recommend circumcision during childhood [10].

Posthitis

Isolated inflammation of the prepuce without glandular affection is rare, or may be underestimated and occasionally reported, it is more common in children with different pathogens, but candida is the most common one.

Prepuce may be affected along the whole genital area and buttocks in severe cases of napkin dermatitis, and the symptoms of posthitis in the form of burning micturition and itching will predominate the condition (Fig. 20.10).

Defective prepuce, with incomplete preputial ring may be liable for inflammations as mentioned in cases of microposthia (Chap. 10) (Fig. 20.11).

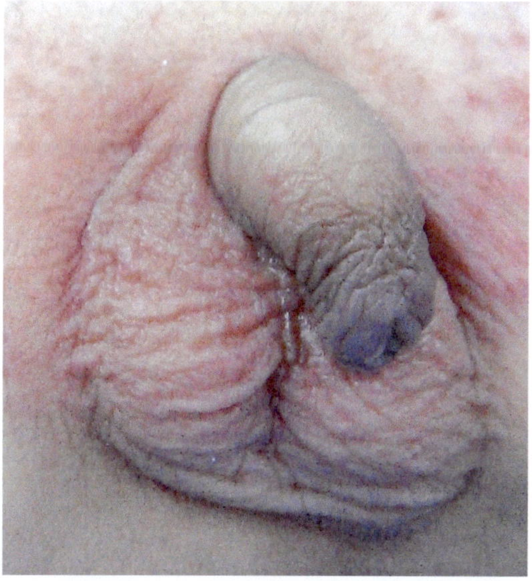

Fig. 20.10 Posthitis secondary to involvement of the prepuce along napkin dermatitis

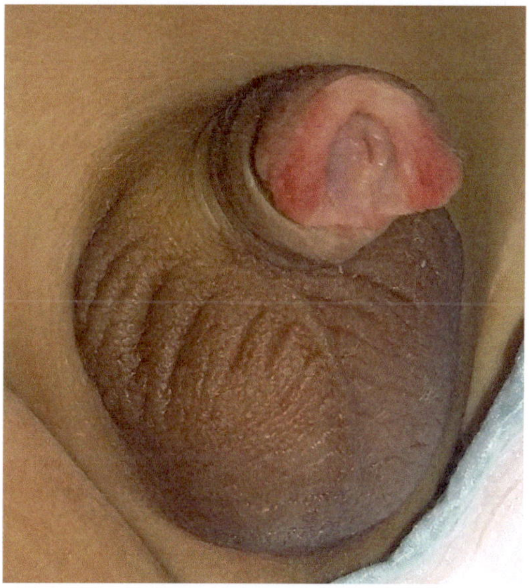

Fig. 20.11 Mild posthitis in a case of microposthia

Posthitis may be only superficial and limited to the preputial ring and tip, and such cases will be definitely complicated with phimosis, if not properly treated. Very rarely a severe infection with an aggressive organisms spread deeply and extend to the whole prepuce and the scrotum, even a Fournier's gangrene may complicates neglected cases, specially those with

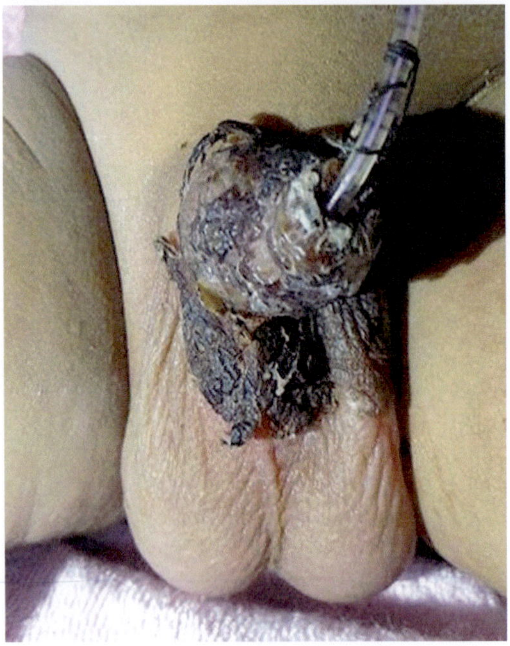

Fig. 20.12 Severe posthitis extended to the scrotum, with extensive incrustation in a 3 years old boy. (This photo provided by Dr. Drpankaj Kumar, Indira Gandhi Institute of Medical Sciences)

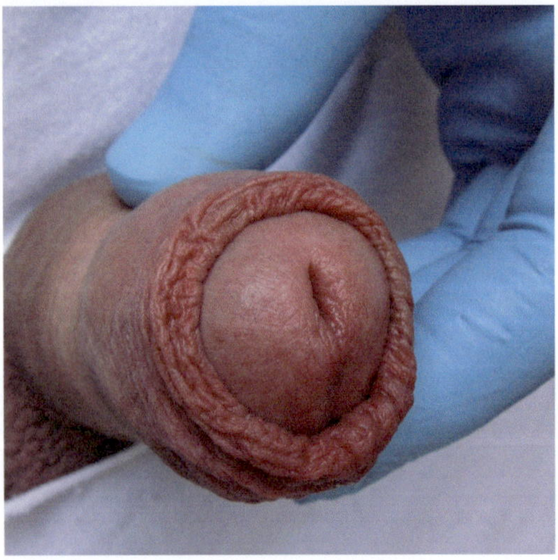

Fig. 20.13 Adult with a wide preputial ring, retractable prepuce and had a mild isolated posthitis

immunocompromisation. Attention should be payed in such cases of severe posthitis to avoid spreading of the infection to the urinary tract (Fig. 20.12). Adults with a healthy retractable prepuce may have a posthitis with different pathogens along other STI (Fig. 20.13).

Balanoposthitis

The International Classification of Diseases, 11th Revision (ICD-11) gave a code: "GB06.0" for Balanoposthitis under the category "GB06": "Certain specified disorders of penis".

Balanoposthitis diagnosed most commonly in uncircumcised men. The prevalence is lower than balanitis. It may present with dramatic swelling and erythema of the distal penis and foreskin associated with discharge, bleeding from the prepuce, dysuria, and occasionally urinary retention.

Etiology: The usual cause of balanoposthitis is poor or exaggerated hygiene. Failure to regularly retract and clean the foreskin; due to either congenital or acquired phimosis, leads to accumulation of smegma, which incites an inflammatory response, and may subsequently result in more phimosis. The accumulation of yeasts and other microorganisms under the foreskin contributes to inflammation of the surrounding penile tissue. The most common cause of balanoposthitis is infection, but contact dermatitis, chemical irritation, fixed drug eruptions, and trauma are other possible causes. Infectious causes commonly include Gram-positive bacteria such as Staphylococcus aureus and Streptococcus pyogenes, and Gram negatives including Neisseria gonorrhea, Chlamydia trachomatis, anaerobes, and fungi [11]. Candida albicans is the most commonly implicated infectious cause and is often associated with diabetes mellitus or immunosuppression. Polymicrobial infections are also common.

Metabolic disorders such as diabetes mellitus or reduced general resistance play a predisposing role. Balanoposthitis occurs less frequently in men with good genital hygiene and in those who are circumcised [12].

In childhood, balanoposthitis presents most commonly between ages 2 and 5 years, which contradicts claims of soiled diapers, as a major cause of penile inflammation, accumulation of smegma with a superimposed infection is the common etiology (Fig. 20.14).

Incidence: Balanoposthitis is a common inflammation occurring in 4–11% of uncircumcised boys. This condition was found in 20% of

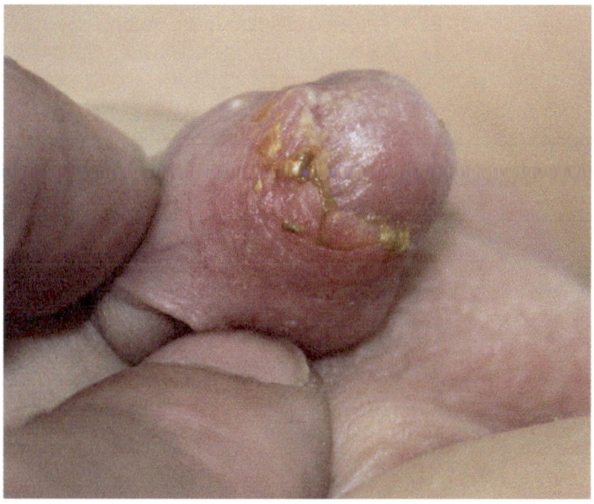

Fig. 20.14 A case of balanoposthitis secondary to aggregation of hard smegma

194 consecutive unselected UK men, all uncircumcised [13].

Regardless of the etiology it is necessary to differentiate acute from chronic balanoposthitis.

Acute Balanoposthitis

This takes its origin from the coronal sulcus. Redness and swelling develop acutely, overlapping onto the glans penis and inner preputial membrane. Especially in cases due to bacterial infections, discharge of serous or seropurulent secretion and secondarily inflammatory phimosis or paraphimosis may occur.

Acute infectious balanoposthitis is never due to a single cause, but develops from many predisposing condition. It occurs suddenly, leading to inflammatory redness and edema and not uncommonly to inflammatory phimosis. Through the marked exudative process the development of a yellowish purulent secretion occurs rapidly [11]. The subjective symptoms (burning) are more severe.

Nonvenereal and venereal types of urethritis must be considered in the etiology. The secretion issuing from the urethra distributes itself in the preputial space and leads to maceration of the epithelium and thus promotes infection. Also the primary lesion of syphilis, soft chancre, or carcinoma in the preputial region can give rise to concomitant balanoposthitis and inflammatory phimosis. Bacteriological investigation is indicated.

Chronic Balanoposthitis

Defective hygiene causes intertrigo as a chronic balanoposthitis diabetica. This is a form of a subacute to chronically progressing inflammatory reaction with a characteristically dusty red color. The aetiology is unclear although infection, contact allergy and contact irritation have been described [12]. Although balanoposthitis may be recurrent, the episodes decrease in frequency in older boys and reflect foreskin maturation.

Chronic diabetes mellitus promotes inflammatory reactions, especially in intertriginous spaces, as a consequence of the elevated glucose concentration of the skin.

Balanoposthitis also can result from specific dermatologic lesions or infectious agents. Various bacterial species and yeasts under the foreskin have the potential to cause penile inflammatory conditions. Candida albicans is the most frequent fungal isolate from the penis. Bacteria, especially Streptococcus spp., by themselves are the second most common cause of infectious balanitis. Less common are Haemophilus parainfluenzae, Klebsiella spp. Chlamydia trachomatis, genital mycoplasmas, and bacterial sexually transmitted infections (STIs) such as Neisseria gonorrhoeae, Haemophilus ducreyi, and others can be associated with balanitis and balanoposthitis. Gardnerella vaginalis is responsible for symptomatic anaerobic-related balanitis in men. Other causes of balanitis and balanoposthitis include viral STIs, such as high-risk human papillomavirus (HPV) types, and parasitic infections such as Trichomonas vaginalis and protozoa, all more common in uncircumcised men [13].

Treatment of Balanoposthitis

Local hygienic measures have been suggested for the treatment of nonspecific balanoposthitis. If the condition is recalcitrant, antifungal and antibiotic creams can be used. Circumcision is suggested as a definitive treatment for the prevention of future occurrence. A study of 476 boys who were circumcised beyond the neonatal period found that balanoposthitis was the reason for performing the surgery in 23% of them [14].

Irritant balanoposthitis usually responds to steroid creams and removal of the offending agent. Patients with recurrent balanoposthitis or those refractory to medical management may require circumcision.

Candidiasis

Genital yeast infection ("candidiasis" or "thrush") is uncommon in healthy individuals, but in immunocompromised individuals, such as those with HIV infection, diabetic and cancer patients. C. albicans can also cause bloodstream infection with serious consequences (Fig. 20.4).

Globally, the annual incidence of C. albicans infection is approximately 400,000, most cases occurring in economically developed regions. Infected individuals are less able to mount a cytokine response to limit the damage caused by the C. albicans peptide toxin candidalysin, which is responsible for the epithelial damage caused when hyphae (filamentous structures of yeast) breach the epidermal barrier of the host cell [15].

Candidiasis of the penis mimics balanitis or balanoposthitis, visible clinically as bright red patches, numerous minute pustules, and erosions. It is common in uncircumcised men in whom heat and retained moisture within the preputial sac create a favorable environment. Diabetes mellitus, lengthy antibiotic treatment, and immunosuppression are other predisposing factors. C. albicans is the most common species and may be identified in the curd-white exudate that often overlies the lesions.

Microscopy of a wet-mount preparation with potassium hydroxide is sufficient for diagnosis. Conversely, positive culture alone is not diagnostic, because fungi may colonize other forms of balanitis [16].

Treatment: Management of candida balanoposthitis includes improved hygiene with gentle foreskin retraction, sitz baths, and cleaning of the foreskin. Antibiotics are indicated for suspected bacterial balanoposthitis. Because Group A beta hemolytic streptococcus is a common bacterial cause of balanoposthitis, first-generation cephalosporins or penicillins have been typically recommended [15]. However, if the patient is sexually active, coverage of gonorrhoea and chlamydia should be considered. Assessment of blood glucose should be considered in patients with candidal balanoposthitis to screen for diabetes mellitus, particularly in patients refractory to treatment or with recurrence. Tight glucose control is important in diabetics with Candidal balanoposthitis, as they are unlikely to respond to treatment if they are hyperglycemic [16].

A Preputial Cavity Abscess

Preputial cavity abscesses with collection of pus between the foreskin and the distal penis are rare and typically occur as a complication of severe balanoposthitis. Inflammation from balanoposthitis can lead to the development of adhesions between the foreskin and glans. This space can fill with debris and bacteria and lead to abscess formation. Inflammatory adhesions can also lead to the development of a phimosis. Little has been published regarding preputial abscesses.

Ultrasound improves the clinical sensitivity of abscess detection, Although there are few articles published in the urology literature describing ultrasound diagnosis of penile abscesses in the corpus cavernosum or periurethral locations. Preputial cavity abscesses should be treated by incision and drainage. Due to the location of the abscess, urologic specialists may be the most appropriate physicians to perform the procedure [17].

References

1. Morris BJ, Krieger JN. Penile inflammatory skin disorders and the preventive role of circumcision. Int J Prev Med. 2017;8:32. https://doi.org/10.4103/ijpvm.IJPVM_377_16.
2. David LM, Walzman M, Rajamanoharan S. Genital colonisation and infection with candida in heterosexual and homosexual males. Sex Transm Infect. 1997;73:394–6.

3. Schwebke JR, Rivers C, Lee J. Prevalence of Gardnerella vaginalis in male sexual partners of women with and without bacterial vaginosis. Sex Transm Dis. 2009;36:92–4.
4. Balci M, Tuncel A, Baran I, Guzel O, Keten T, Aksu N, et al. High-risk oncogenic human papilloma virus infection of the foreskin and microbiology of smegma in prepubertal boys. Urology. 2015;86:368–72.
5. Ladenhauf HN, Ardelean MA, Schimke C, Yankovic F, Schimpl G. Reduced bacterial colonisation of the glans penis after male circumcision in children—a prospective study. J Pediatr Urol. 2013;9(6 Pt B):1137–44.
6. Fahmy MA. Infectious complications of circumcision. In: Complications in male circumcision. St. Louis: Elsevier; 2019. https://doi.org/10.1016/B978-0-323-68127-8.00009-0, Chap. 9.
7. Ginter-Hanselmayer G, Nenoff P. Clinically relevant mycoses dermatomycoses. In: Presterl E, editor. Clinically relevant mycoses. Cham: Springer; 2019. https://doi.org/10.1007/978-3-319-92300-0_10.
8. Aerts L, Rubin RS, Randazzo M, Goldstein SW, Goldstein I. Retrospective study of the prevalence and risk factors of clitoral adhesions: women's health providers should routinely examine the glans clitoris. Sex Med. 2018;6(2):115–22. https://doi.org/10.1016/j.esxm.2018.01.003.
9. Vieira-Baptista P, Bornstein J. Candidiasis, bacterial vaginosis, trichomoniasis and other vaginal conditions affecting the vulva. In: Bornstein J, editor. Vulvar disease. Cham: Springer; 2019. https://doi.org/10.1007/978-3-319-61621-6_24.
10. Birley HD, Walker MM, Luzzi G, et al. Clinical features and management of recurrent balanitis; association with recurrent washing. Genitourin Med. 1993;69:400–3.
11. Kinghorn GR, Jones BM, Chowdhury FH, Geary I. Balanoposthitis associated with Gardnerella vaginalis infection in men. Br J Vener Dis. 1982;58:127–9.
12. Lincopan N, Neves P, Mamizuka EM, Levy CE. Balanoposthitis caused by Pseudomonas aeruginosa co-producing metallo-beta-lactamase and 16S rRNA methylase in children with haematological malignancies. Int J Infect Dis. 2010;14:e344–7.
13. Brown GD, Denning DW, Gow NA, Levitz SM, Netea MG, White TC. Hidden killers: human fungal infections. Sci Transl Med. 2012;4:165rv13.
14. Wiswell TE, Tencer HL, Welch CA, Chamberlain JL. Circumcision in children beyond the neonatal period. Pediatrics. 1993;92:791–3.
15. Wakatsuki A. Clinical experience of streptococcal balanoposthitis in 47 healthy adult males. Hinyokika Kiyo. 2005;51:737–40.
16. Mayser P. Mycotic infections of the penis. Andrologia. 1999;31:13–6.
17. Mahler SA, Manthey DE. Diagnosis of a preputial cavity abscess with bedside ultrasound in the emergency department. J Emerg Med. 2008;35(3):273–6. https://doi.org/10.1016/j.jemermed.2007.03.013.

21 Lichen Sclerosus

Background

Lichen sclerosus (LS) is a chronic inflammatory and atrophic dermatitis of unknown etiology involving the anogenital area of any age group or race [1]. In boys LS is mainly involving the prepuce, glans, and the distal urethra. LS was first reported by Hallopeau in 1887 and in 1892 Darier presented the histological description [2]. Many other names exist for LS: balanitis xerotica obliterans leucoplakia, lichen albus, lichen sclerosus et atrophicus, and kraurosis genitalis [3, 4].

LS was regarded as a disease of the adulthood until a case of a 7 year-old boy was documented in 1962 [5]. In 2000 the pediatric incidence was estimated to be 10–19% in the foreskin of circumcised boys [6]. In a recent review from 2014, the incidence of LS calculated was 35% [7]. A systematic review from 2018 tried to explore the true incidence of LS and a total of 22 articles published from 1980 to 2017 were included. The proportion of LS in those with phimosis had been described in many literature studies, ranging from 2 to 95%. The actual incidence of LS is thought to be clinically underestimated by as much as 50%. The recommendation of the review is to base the diagnosis LS on biopsy for acquired phimosis because clinical findings underestimate the incidence of LS [8].

Send the Prepuce to Histology?

Submission of the prepuce to histological analysis should always be considered, as prognosis differs for LS vs non-LS istology [9, 10] and it has been shown that the diagnosis of LS must be based on biopsy, because clinical findings underestimate the incidence of LS by up to 50%. In another study there was no correlation between histopathologic diagnosis and preoperative symptoms such as dysuria, ballooning, spraying, or penile pain [11]. On the other hand, it has been said that clinical correlation by surgeons has a high degree of accuracy (>90%) [12]. Moreover, the recommendation to perform routine histology is challenged by a study by Alyami et al. In their consecutive small clinical series, the clinical diagnosis correlated with the pathological diagnosis in most cases. They conclude that the clinical suspicion of LS without routine histology will reduces the overall cost to the healthcare system [13].

Etiology

The underlying cause of LS is still unknown, but autoimmunity seems very likely to play a role in the pathogenesis of LS [14].

M. A. B. Fahmy, *Normal and Abnormal Prepuce*, https://doi.org/10.1007/978-3-030-37621-5_21

Genetics and Immunology

Genetic factors may be causative in LS and familial cases have been reported. Newer data show that there seems to be a genetic susceptibility and a link with autoimmune mechanisms [15, 16]. Studies of female and male LS reported significant antibodies to matrix protein I [15, 17]. Immunogenetic studies have demonstrated a significant association with HLA DQ7 [18]. A recent study in boys with LS showed a distinct gene expression profile indicating tissue remodeling in the foreskin with inflammation and fibrosis [19] by over-expression of bone morphogenetic protein 2 and its corresponding receptor, matrix metalloproteinases 1 and 9 and tissue inhibitor of metalloproteinases 1, cytokine chemokine ligands 5 (RANTES) and interleukin 4, and transforming growth factor-β2 and its corresponding receptor.

Infection

Infection as cause of LS is still under discussion. The human papilloma virus, acid fast bacilli, the hepatitis C virus and *Borrelia burgdorferi* have been suggested but not substantiated as infective triggers [1, 20, 21]. A recent study from China aimed to investigate the presence of human papillomavirus and Epstein-Barr virus in male lichen sclerosus patients (adults). HPV had no significant relationship with LS. Patients had a higher EBV infection rate, but the role of EBV in the pathogenesis of LS needs further investigations [22].

Trauma

Mechanical irritation on already scarred or damaged skin ("Koebner phenomenon") is known to occur, so trauma and injury have been suggested as possible triggers of LS [3].

Anatomical Abnormality

Gross anatomical abnormality like phimosis, buried penis or hypospadias has an association with LS [23]. It is speculated that chronic urine pooling on the skin in obesity and phimosis where the urine gets trapped under the skin may amplify and exacerbate whatever fibrotic changes existed initially and may cause LS [24].

Symptoms and Diagnosis

Early symptoms of LS are itching and burning and localised erythematous spots on the foreskin or glans. Edema of the foreskin appears and progresses into sclerosis and chronic inflammation. The typical clinical presentation of LS is a ring-like distal sclerosis of the prepuce with white discoloration or plaque formation [25, 26] (Fig. 21.1). The most common symptoms of LS are obstruction, poor urinary flow, dysuria, hematuria, pain, history of balanitis and urinary tract inflammation [27]. Biopsy of the foreskin after circumcision for pathological phimosis can be carried out, because clinical findings underestimate the incidence of LS in a high percentage of the cases [10]. Histopathology of LS includes nonspecific inflammation and fibrosis, epithelial hyperkeratosis, epidermal atrophy, hydropic degeneration of basal cells, acanthosis, dermo-epidermal cleft, upper dermal edema and

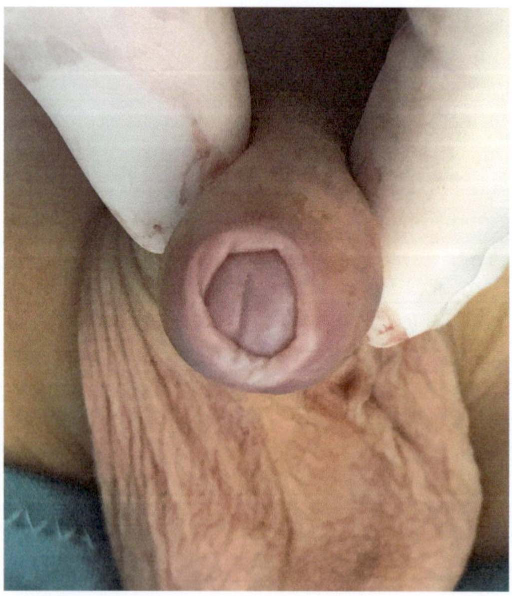

Fig. 21.1 Lichen sclerosus of the forskin. Notice the white scarred ring

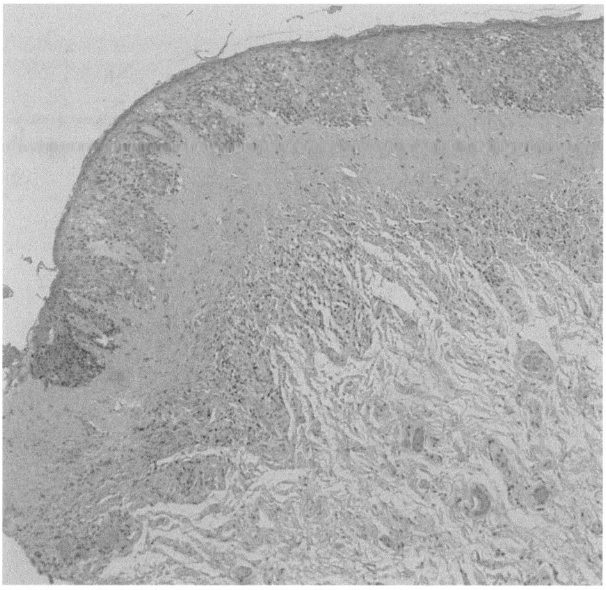

Fig. 21.2 Histology of lichen sclerosus

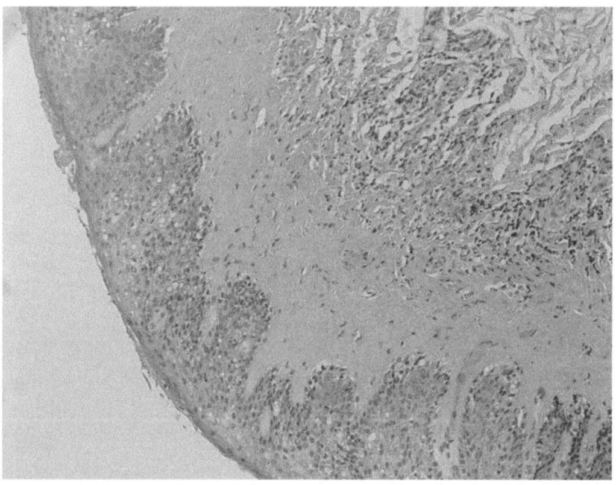

Fig. 21.3 Severe lichen sclerosus involving the glans, meatus and penile skin

homogenization, mid dermal lymphocytic band, and interface dermatitis (Fig. 21.2). Based on these microscopic findings it is even possible to grade LS (early LS, established LS and advanced LS) as it has been proposed by Singh et al. [28, 29]. The inflammatory infiltrate and region of sclerosis is characterized by CD4 and CD8 positive lymphocytes, macrophages and mast cells [3]. However, a recent survey of 23 academic pathologists showed significant disagreement about histology of LS warranting a standardized classification of LS [30].

The glans and penile skin may be involved (Fig. 21.3). Urethral involvement starts at the meatus but may go as proximally as the prostatic urethra [31]. Clinically, the penile urethra feels thickened. Cystourethroscopy may show urethral involvement with areas of pallor of the mucosa or even ulceration. It has not been found in bladder mucosa [31].

Treatment

Early diagnosis and treatment of LS is essential because extensive involvement of penile tissue complicates therapeutic options and worsens prognosis. As already shown, in pediatric populations a high incidence of missed diagnoses of LS has been reported [27, 32, 33].

Medical Treatment

In mild forms of LS with erythema, meatal narrowing and preputial fibrosis, topical application of corticosteroids for 4–8 weeks is indicated and may be repeated in the case of recurrence. In a prospective, placebo-controlled, double-blind, randomized study by Kiss et al. in 2000 it was clearly demonstrated that local corticosteroid treatment is effective in LS when the inflammatory mechanism is active and irreversible tissue damage has not occurred [34, 35]. It has also been reported that pre-circumcision topical steroids may help decrease the rate of later meatal stenosis [9]. Tacrolimus has also been used in the treatment of LS. It is thought to have analogous clinical benefits to corticosteroids with less side effects. In a pediatric prospective phase 2 study the adjuvant topical tacrolimus treatment in boys with LS the safety and tolerability was clearly shown [36–38]. However, long-term follow-up studies are missing. A small prospective trial (20 patients) showed the same benefit of vitamin E in comparison to corticosteroids in the treatment of LS. In histology both showed an increase of IL-13 and cadherin. Nevertheless, larger studies are required to show the clear benefit of vitamin E with less side-effects [39].

Surgical Treatment

Circumcision is the treatment of choice in LS of the foreskin [7]. Since "LS has a predilection for the warm, moist, urine-exposed environment that exists under the foreskin" [31] the effectiveness of circumcision makes sense (Fig. 21.4a, b). In severe cases involving the glans, glandular resurfacing or extensive preputial adhesions, complete excision of the LS tissue and skin grafting is necessary [40]. A recent population based audit from the UK including roughly 8000 patients showed that in 96% of the cases circumcision was performed. In only 4% preputioplasty was performed. Age at surgical intervention was 9 (6–11) years. Of those treated with preputioplasty 22% had subsequent circumcision at a median of 677 (277–1203) days post operation. More children underwent a second operative procedure following preputioplasty than those having had a primary circumcision (27.9% vs. 7.9%, $p < 0.001$) [41].

It is a well-known fact that bleeding after circumcision is more likely in boys with LS [42].

One out of five patients with LS of the foreskin will end up with meatal stenosis needing subsequent surgery [9]. Meatal stenosis is treated by meatoplasty and its modifications [43–45]. Simple meatotomy in LS regularly is followed by re-stenosis [29]. There is no surgical gold standard for the treatment of extensive LS and guidelines are based on retrospective single-center studies and expert opinion [46]. Urethral involvement by LS can be seen in up to 30% of the cases and it varies from meatal stenosis to –rarely- extensive panurethral strictures [47]. Treatment of these stenotic lesions remain a challenge. Radical excision of all affected parts of the skin and urethra is essential. In cases where LS is affecting the urethra urethral reconstruction must be considered. Even then outcome is plagued by a high complication and reoperation rate. Therefore some institutions have shifted from primary extensive surgery towards potent corticosteroids and minimally invasive surgical techniques. Management of recurrence

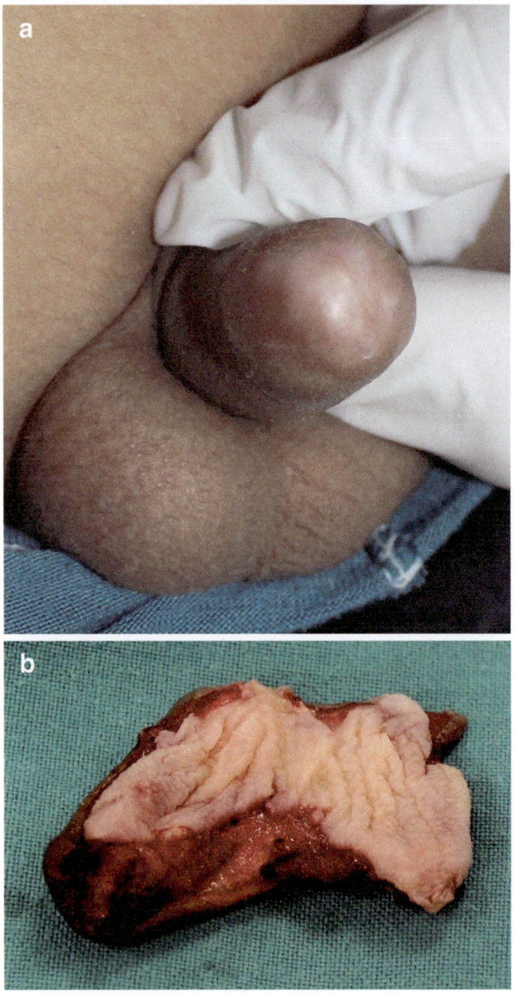

Fig. 21.4 (**a**, **b**) Lichen sclerosus has a predilection for the warm, moist, urine-exposed environment that exists under the foreskin

includes dilation, meatotomy/meatoplasty, and finally different urethroplasty techniques [48]. The tissue of choice is buccal mucosa and the use of genital or non-genital skin cannot be recommended [46, 49, 50]. Complete excision of LS should be carried out and is followed by primary or staged urethroplasty [31, 48, 51, 52]. Other techniques have also been applied successfully, i.e. one-stage dorsal onlay buccal mucosa urethroplasty with excellent cosmetic and functional results has also been described [53, 54].

Prognosis

The natural course of LS is unknown [14]. Long-term follow-up after treatment is mandatory for all patients because of a high recurrence rate [31]. A recent study recommends routine uroflowmetry for a prompt identification of post-voiding dysfunction following circumcision in BXO [55]. In an adult study including 99 patients it was shown that there was an interval of more than 10 years between circumcision due to LS and urethral involvement. Also, progression of LS from meatus to the bulbar urethra was suggested to occur over many years. The authors conclude that reporting circumcision to be "curative" in 96% is possibly erroneous, as most reports do not follow patients up for this long [56]. Even in the pediatric population it has been shown that recurrent symptoms of LS can occur a long time after surgery, and prolonged follow-up is necessary [12]. Approximately 1 out of 5 boys who underwent circumcision due to LS subsequently require meatotomy [9]. After meatotomy, roughly 1 out of 4 patients will restenose and require further surgery [50]. Therefore, appropriate counselling of the patient/parents and their primary caregiver is imperative, as recurrence is common.

LS and Penile Cancer

Penile squamous cell on pre-existing lesions of LS. In patients with LS the risk for the development of SCC is about 2–8% [3, 31, 46]. On the other hand, 30–50% of patients with penile carcinoma had an association with histological features of LS [1, 57, 58]. Therefore, it might be mandatory to arrange long-term follow-up of patients with LS.

References

1. Pugliese JM, Morey AF, Peterson AC. Lichen sclerosus: review of the literature and current recommendations for management. J Urol. 2007;178:2268–76.
2. Funaro D. Lichen sclerosus: a review and practical approach. Dermatol Ther. 2004;17:28–37.
3. Powell JJ, Wojnarowska F. Lichen sclerosus. Lancet. 1999;353:1777–83.
4. Stuhmer A. Balanitis xerotica obliterans (post operationem) und ihre Beziehung zur "Kraurosis glandis et preputil penis". Arch Dermatol Syphil. 1928;156:613–23.
5. Catterall RD, Oates JK. Treatment of balanitis xerotica obliterans with hydrocortisone injections. Br J Vener Dis. 1962;38:75–7.
6. Uemura S, Hutson JM, Woodward AA, Kelly JH, Chow CW. Balanitis xerotica obliterans with urethral stricture after hypospadias repair. Pediatr Surg Int. 2000;16:144–5.
7. Celis S, Reed F, Murphy F, et al. Balanitis xerotica obliterans in children and adolescents: a literature review and clinical series. J Pediatr Urol. 2014;10:34–9.
8. Li J, Deng C, Peng Q. Underestimation of genital lichen sclerosus incidence in boys with phimosis: results from a systematic review. Pediatr Surg Int. 2018;34:1245–50.
9. Homer L, Buchanan KJ, Nasr B, Losty PD, Corbett HJ. Meatal stenosis in boys following circumcision for lichen sclerosus (balanitis xerotica obliterans). J Urol. 2014;192:1784–8.
10. Bochove-Overgaauw DM, Gelders W, De Vylder AM. Routine biopsies in pediatric circumcision: (non) sense? J Pediatr Urol. 2009;5:178–80.
11. Kato T, Mizuno K, Nishio H, et al. Can lichen sclerosus be diagnosed by preputial appearance or symptoms? Res Rep Urol. 2018;10:89–94.
12. Pradhan A, Patel R, Said AJ, Upadhyaya M. 10 years' experience in balanitis xerotica obliterans: a single-institution study. Eur J Pediatr Surg. 2019;29:302–6.
13. Alyami FA, Bateni ZH, Odeh R, Farhat WA, Koyle M. Routine histopathological examination of the foreskin after circumcision for clinically suspected lichen sclerosus in children: is it a waste of resources? Can Urol Assoc J. 2018;12:E231–e233.
14. Mangera A, Osman N, Chapple C. Recent advances in understanding urethral lichen sclerosus. F1000Res. 2016;5:96.
15. Oyama N, Chan I, Neill SM, et al. Autoantibodies to extracellular matrix protein 1 in lichen sclerosus. Lancet. 2003;362:118–23.

16. Marini A, Blecken S, Ruzicka T, Hengge UR. Lichen sclerosus. Hautarzt. 2005;56:550–5.
17. Edmonds EV, Oyama N, Chan I, Francis N, McGrath JA, Bunker CB. Extracellular matrix protein 1 autoantibodies in male genital lichen sclerosus. Br J Dermatol. 2011;165:218–9.
18. Tasker GL, Wojnarowska F. Lichen sclerosus. Clin Exp Dermatol. 2003;28:128–33.
19. Pilatz A, Altinkilic B, Schormann E, et al. Congenital phimosis in patients with and without lichen sclerosus: distinct expression patterns of tissue remodeling associated genes. J Urol. 2013;189:268–74.
20. Lau PW, Cook N, Andrews H, Bracka A, Myint SH. Detection of human papillomavirus types in balanitis xerotica obliterans and other penile conditions. Genitourin Med. 1995;71:228–30.
21. Fujiwara H, Fujiwara K, Hashimoto K, et al. Detection of Borrelia burgdorferi DNA (B garinii or B afzelii) in morphea and lichen sclerosus et atrophicus tissues of German and Japanese but not of US patients. Arch Dermatol. 1997;133:41–4.
22. Zhang Y, Fu Q, Zhang X. The presence of human papillomavirus and Epstein-Barr virus in male Chinese lichen sclerosus patients: a single center study. Asian J Androl. 2016;18:650–3.
23. Bunker CB. Male genital lichen sclerosus and tacrolimus. Br J Dermatol. 2007;157:1079–80.
24. Morey AF. Re: dermatopathology of the foreskin: an institutional experience of over 400 cases. J Urol. 2014;191:1319–21.
25. McKay DL Jr, Fuqua F, Weinberg AG. Balanitis xerotica obliterans in children. J Urol. 1975;114:773–5.
26. Meuli M, Briner J, Hanimann B, Sacher P. Lichen sclerosus et atrophicus causing phimosis in boys: a prospective study with 5-year followup after complete circumcision. J Urol. 1994;152:987–9.
27. Gargollo PC, Kozakewich HP, Bauer SB, et al. Balanitis xerotica obliterans in boys. J Urol. 2005;174:1409–12.
28. Singh L, Sengar M, Goyal S, Mansi M, Khurana N, Mohta A. Childhood phimosis secondary to lichen sclerosus: is there a spatial pattern of histopathological changes? Am J Dermatopathol. 2018;40:824–8.
29. Das S, Tunuguntla HS. Balanitis xerotica obliterans--a review. World J Urol. 2000;18:382–7.
30. Erickson BA, Tesdahl BA, Voznesensky MA, et al. Urethral lichen sclerosus under the microscope: a survey of academic pathologists. Can J Urol. 2018;25:9328–33.
31. Depasquale I, Park AJ, Bracka A. The treatment of balanitis xerotica obliterans. BJU Int. 2000;86:459–65.
32. Schinella RA, Miranda D. Posthitis xerotica obliterans in circumcision specimens. Urology. 1974;3:348–51.
33. Huntley JS, Bourne MC, Munro FD, Wilson-Storey D. Troubles with the foreskin: one hundred consecutive referrals to paediatric surgeons. J R Soc Med. 2003;96:449–51.
34. Kiss A, Csontai A, Pirot L, Nyirady P, Merksz M, Kiraly L. The response of balanitis xerotica obliterans to local steroid application compared with placebo in children. J Urol. 2001;165:219–20.
35. Vincent MV, Mackinnon E. The response of clinical balanitis xerotica obliterans to the application of topical steroid-based creams. J Pediatr Surg. 2005;40:709–12.
36. Ebert AK, Rosch WH, Vogt T. Safety and tolerability of adjuvant topical tacrolimus treatment in boys with lichen sclerosus: a prospective phase 2 study. Eur Urol. 2008;54:932–7.
37. Assmann T, Ruzicka T. New immunosuppressive drugs in dermatology (mycophenolate mofetil, tacrolimus): unapproved uses, dosages, or indications. Clin Dermatol. 2002;20:505.
38. Pandher BS, Rustin MH, Kaisary AV. Treatment of balanitis xerotica obliterans with topical tacrolimus. J Urol. 2003;170:923.
39. Russo T, Curro M, Ferlazzo N, et al. Stable ozonides with vitamin E acetate versus corticosteroid in the treatment of lichen sclerosus in foreskin: evaluation of effects on inflammation. Urol Int. 2019;103:459–65.
40. Campus GV, Ena P, Scuderi N. Surgical treatment of balanitis xerotica obliterans. Plast Reconstr Surg. 1984;73:652–7.
41. Green PA, Bethell GS, Wilkinson DJ, Kenny SE, Corbett HJ. Surgical management of genitourinary lichen sclerosus et atrophicus in boys in England: a 10-year review of practices and outcomes. J Pediatr Urol. 2019;15:45.e41–5.
42. Somov P, Chan BKY, Wilde C, Corbett H. Bleeding after circumcision is more likely in children with lichen sclerosus (balanitis xerotica obliterans). J Pediatr Urol. 2017;13:208.e201–4.
43. Kumar MV, Harris DL. Balanitis xerotica obliterans complicating hypospadias repair. Br J Plast Surg. 1999;52:69–71.
44. Steffens JA, Anheuser P, Treiyer AE, Reisch B, Malone PR. Plastic meatotomy for pure meatal stenosis in patients with lichen sclerosus. BJU Int. 2010;105:568–72.
45. Malone P. A new technique for meatal stenosis in patients with lichen sclerosus. J Urol. 2004;172:949–52.
46. Stewart L, McCammon K, Metro M, Virasoro R. SIU/ICUD consultation on urethral strictures: anterior urethra—lichen sclerosus. Urology. 2014;83:S27–30.
47. Barbagli G, Lazzeri M, Palminteri E, Turini D. Lichen sclerosis of male genitalia involving anterior urethra. Lancet. 1999;354:429.
48. Granieri MA, Peterson AC, Madden-Fuentes RJ. Effect of lichen sclerosis on success of urethroplasty. Urol Clin North Am. 2017;44:77–86.
49. Venn SN, Mundy AR. Urethroplasty for balanitis xerotica obliterans. Br J Urol. 1998;81:735–7.
50. Singh JP, Priyadarshi V, Goel HK, et al. Penile lichen sclerosus: an urologist's nightmare! - a single center experience. Urology annals. 2015;7:303–8.
51. Das SK, Kumar A, Sharma GK, et al. Lingual mucosal graft urethroplasty for anterior urethral strictures. Urology. 2009;73:105–8.

52. Levine LA, Strom KH, Lux MM. Buccal mucosa graft urethroplasty for anterior urethral stricture repair: evaluation of the impact of stricture location and lichen sclerosus on surgical outcome. J Urol. 2007;178:2011–5.
53. Dubey D, Sehgal A, Srivastava A, Mandhani A, Kapoor R, Kumar A. Buccal mucosal urethroplasty for balanitis xerotica obliterans related urethral strictures: the outcome of 1 and 2-stage techniques. J Urol. 2005;173:463–6.
54. Ashraf J, Turner A, Subramaniam R. Single-stage urethroplasty with buccal mucosal inlay graft for stricture caused by balanitis xerotica obliterans in boys: outcomes in the medium term. J Pediatr Urol. 2018;14:66.e61–5.
55. Arena S, Russo T, Impellizzeri P, Parisi S, Perrone P, Romeo C. Utility of uroflowmetry during the follow-up of children affected by balanitis xerotica obliterans (BXO). Archivio italiano di urologia, andrologia : organo ufficiale [di] Societa italiana di ecografia urologica e nefrologica. 2018;90:123–6.
56. Barbagli G, Mirri F, Gallucci M, Sansalone S, Romano G, Lazzeri M. Histological evidence of urethral involvement in male patients with genital lichen sclerosus: a preliminary report. J Urol. 2011;185:2171–6.
57. Perceau G, Derancourt C, Clavel C, et al. Lichen sclerosus is frequently present in penile squamous cell carcinomas but is not always associated with oncogenic human papillomavirus. Br J Dermatol. 2003;148:934–8.
58. Pietrzak P, Hadway P, Corbishley CM, Watkin NA. Is the association between balanitis xerotica obliterans and penile carcinoma underestimated? BJU Int. 2006;98:74–6.

22 Zoon's Balanitis

Abbreviations

SCC Squamous cell carcinoma
ZB Zoon's balanitis

Definition

Zoon's balanitis (ZB) is a chronic inflammatory benign mucositis of the glans penis, the coronal sulcus and sometimes the prepuce, usually affecting middle-aged or elderly uncircumcised men. Its etiopathogenesis still remains hypothetical and speculative.

Historical Background

First described by Zoon, a Dutch dermatologist in 1952 and named "balanitis chronica circumscripta plasmacellularis", but now it is commonly known as Zoon's balanitis [1].

Etiology

The aetiology of ZB is still a matter of debate. It is thought to be due to irritation, partially caused by urine, in the context of a 'dysfunctional prepuce'. Smoking and a poor genital hygiene are associated most cases and were investigated as an etiology of ZB, the mean daily cigarettes consumption and the number of weekly foreskin retractions are significantly associated with increased incidence of ZB [2].

Porter et al. [3] underlined the key role of chronic inflammation suggesting that the presence of "dysfunctional foreskin" may promote a Koebner phenomenon (the appearance of skin lesions on lines of trauma) and the development of ZB.

Clinically

ZB generally presents as a single asymptomatic well-defined shiny orange-red plaque of the glans or the prepuce with multiple pinpoint redder spots, named "cayenne pepper spots". When both glans and opposing prepuce are involved the lesion can acquire a "kissing" aspect (Fig. 22.1).

ZB had not been reported in children, but we have only one case of kissing form of Zoon's balanitis in a 6 years old child, whose diagnosis confirmed histologically and he responded well to local corticosteroid (Fig. 22.2).

Sometimes patients report pruritus, dysuria, pain or a burning sensation. Lesions with analogous features have been described in the vulva, labial and oral mucosa and conjunctiva. Moreover, erosive and vegetative variants of ZB have been described. A uniform nomenclature for these "Zoon-like lesions" does not exist, but the

M. A. B. Fahmy, *Normal and Abnormal Prepuce*, https://doi.org/10.1007/978-3-030-37621-5_22

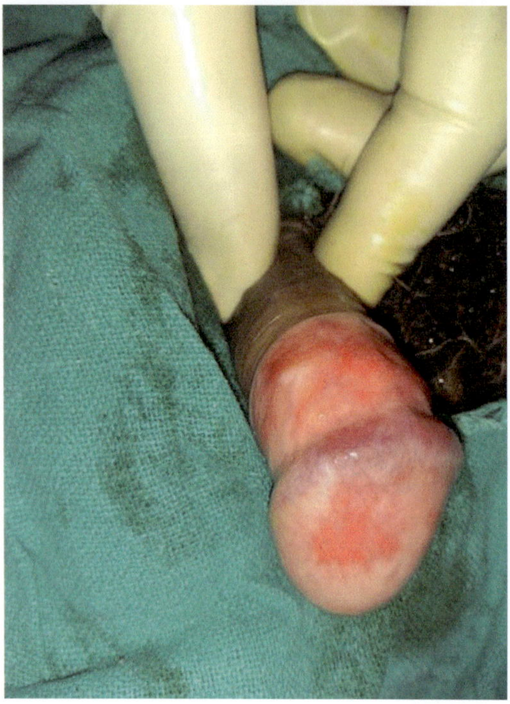

Fig. 22.1 A case of ZB with a well demarcated moist erythematous plaque was present on the glans and shaft of penis [9]

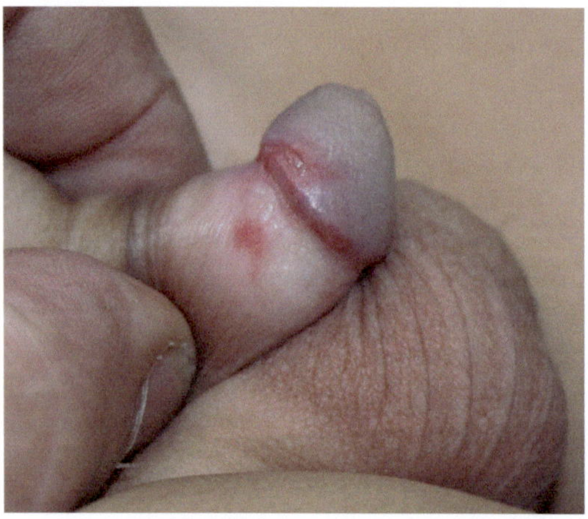

Fig. 22.2 Kissing ZB affecting the glans, coronal sulcus and inner prepuce

term idiopathic lymphoplasmacellular mucositis-dermatitis has been proposed.

The disease is generally considered benign although, but cases of Erythroplasia of Queyrat and one of carcinoma of the penis arising on lesions of ZB have been reported [4].

Clinical and dermatoscopical features allow to differentiate ZB from Erythroplasia of Queyrat and Bowen's disease, but only the histological examination (and, likely, also Reflectance Confocal Microscopy) can confirm the diagnosis and exclude a squamous cell carcinoma in situ [5].

Differential Diagnosis

The differential diagnosis with erythroplasia of Queyrat and lichen sclerosus may be difficult and in those cases a skin biopsy must be performed.

Epidemiology

Even if ZB is classically considered a rare disease, a prevalence of 10% in patients examined in a genitourinary medicine clinic has been reported, which suggests that ZB could be an under diagnosed entity [5].

Complications

Development of SCC in this disease was described since 1999, but there was only one case of SCC in Marcos-Pinto et al. [6] recent series of 30 patients.

Management

The optimal treatment strategies are still a matter of debate. There are some evidences about a transitory efficacy of topical steroids, calcineurin inhibitors, mupirocin, and imiquimod. In Marcos-Pinto et al. series of 30 patients, 79% (26/30) of these patients responded well to corticosteroids.

Carbon dioxide laser and ablative Erbium-YAG laser are curative in some studies [7].

Circumcision have shown a permanent regression of the lesions. The improvement after circumcision suggests a pathogenic role of poor genital hygiene and repeated local infections [8].

References

1. Zoon JJ. Chronic benign circumscript plasmocytic balanoposthitis. Dermatologica. 1952;105:1–7.
2. Piaserico S, Orlando G, Linder MD, Cappozzo P, Zarian H, Iafrate M. A case-control study of risk factors associated with Zoon balanitis in men. J Eur Acad Dermatol Venereol. 2019;33:1591. https://doi.org/10.1111/jdv.15594.
3. Porter WM, Bunker CB. The dysfunctional foreskin. Int J STD AIDS. 2001;12:216–20.
4. Starritt E, Lee S. Erythroplasia of Queyrat of the glans penis on a background of Zoon's plasma cell balanitis. Australas J Dermatol. 2008;49:103–5.
5. Pearce J, Fernando I. The value of a multi-specialty service, including genitourinary medicine, dermatology and urology input, in the management of male genital dermatoses. Int J STD AIDS. 2015;``26(10):716–22.
6. Marcos-Pinto A, Soares-de-Almeida L, Borges-Costa J. Nonvenereal penile dermatoses: a retrospective study. Indian Dermatol Online J. 2018;9(2):96–100. https://doi.org/10.4103/idoj.IDOJ_23_17
7. Retamar RA, Kien MC, Chouela EN. Zoon's balanitis: presentation of 15 patients, five treated with a carbon dioxide laser. Int J Dermatol. 2003;42:305–7.
8. Edwards SK, Bunker CB, Ziller F, van der Meijden WI. 2013 European guideline for the management of balanoposthitis. Int J STD AIDS. 2014;25(9):615–26.
9. Kumar R, Parshad S, Karwasra RK, Arora BK. Erythroplasia of Queyrat with Zoon's balanitis: a diagnostic dilemma. J Dental Med Sci. 2018;17(3):87. https://doi.org/10.9790/0853-1703108789.

23 Preputial Injuries and Trauma

Types

There are specific types of trauma affecting the prepuce; which are zipper injuries and hair tourniquet, but other penile trauma may affect the prepuce like burns, electrical injuries, ring impaction, avulsion injuries, animal bites, penetrating or blunt trauma, which may affect the prepuce due to toilet seat and straddle injuries (Fig. 23.1).

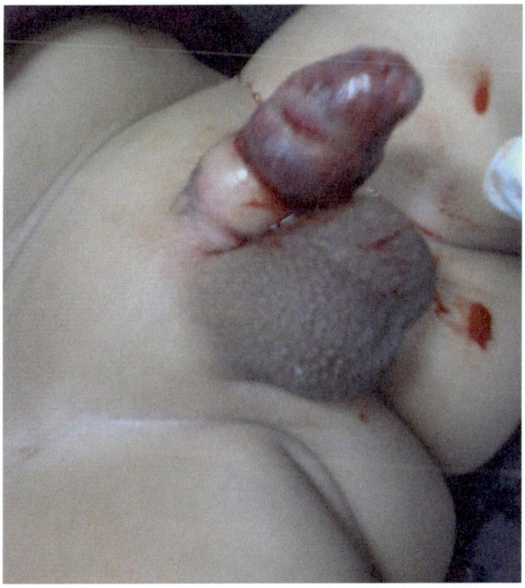

Fig. 23.1 Severe preputial trauma with bleeding in an infant after fall down in a heavy object

Etiology

Iatrogenic preputial and penile injuries occurring during circumcision procedures remain among the most common etiology worldwide [1].

Injuries to the prepuce usually occur in children and adults who are uncircumcised. The pattern of injury vary with geographic location; in Europe; the most common causes of penile injuries was iatrogenic after repair of congenital penile anomalies, from traffic accidents and burns. In Africa the reported cases are mainly after injuries causing penile fractures, genital mutilation from self and attacks from assailants in cases of sexual abuse [2]. According to the National Electronic Injury Surveillance System (NEISS), genital injuries represented 0.6% of all pediatric injuries [3].

Child Abuse

Generally there are fewer studies of boys who have been sexually abused in comparison to girls. The commonest site for injury overall was the prepuce, suggesting that forceful masturbation was responsible in many cases; this is a difficult part of the anatomy to injure accidentally. Hobbs and J Osman reported 86 cases of child sexual abuse; thirty seven of them had an injury to the prepuce, and 29 to the shaft of the penis. Wide range of injuries was encountered in this study

M. A. B. Fahmy, *Normal and Abnormal Prepuce*, https://doi.org/10.1007/978-3-030-37621-5_23

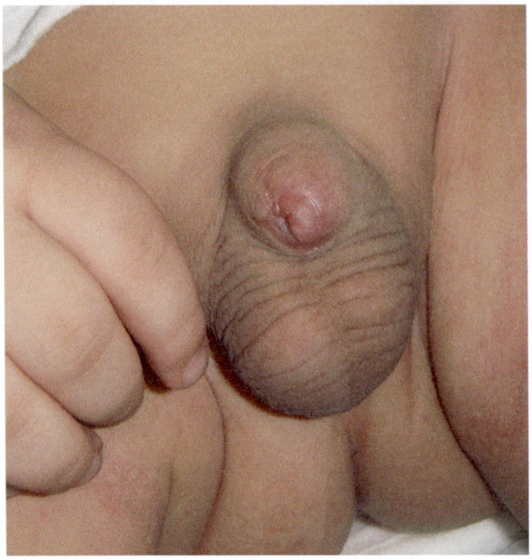

Fig. 23.2 Preputial injury without an obvious history or conspicuous cause

including bruises, burns, lacerations, incised wounds, and scars as well as tears of the foreskin including the frenulum [4].

Sometimes child abuse or cultural and traditional insult could only expected, if a small infant or a child diagnosed to have an unusual trauma to the prepuce (Fig. 23.2).

Predisposing Factors

The penis is usually protected from injuries by its location and mobility, therefore it is prone to injuries when it is erect. In patients with coital injuries, predisposing phimosis or a short frenulum was common. Patients who are particularly at risk of genital self-mutilation are psychotics, schizophrenics with religious delusions and patients with character disorders like transsexuals [5].

Classifications

It is difficult to make a generalized classification of penile and preputial injuries due to the complexity of the injuries. However, a broad classification into blunt and penetrating or avulsion, penetrating and amputating injuries may suffice [6].

The extent of injury may vary from mild to severe and total amputation. Penile injuries can also be classified anatomically into four types according to the structure involved: skin, erectile tissue, urethra, and complex injuries. The severity of these injuries also can be assessed using the American Association for the Surgery of Trauma (AAST) injury score. This organ injury scaling is based on the magnitude of anatomic disruption and is graded as 1 (minimal), 2 (mild), 3 (moderate), 4 (severe), 5 (massive), and 6 (lethal) [7].

Strangulation penile injuries in children are graded by Bhat et al. [8] as follows:

- Grade I. Edema of distal penis. No evidence of skin ulceration or urethral injury.
- Grade II. Injury to skin and constriction of corpus spongiosum, but no evidence of urethral injury. Distal penile edema with decreased penile sensation.
- Grade III. Injury to skin and urethra but no urethral fistula. Loss of distal penile sensations.
- Grade IV. Complete division of corpus spongiosum leading to urethral fistula and constriction of corpora cavernosa with loss of distal penile sensations.
- Grade V. Gangrene, necrosis, or complete amputation of distal penis.

Management

In all cases, the goal of treatment is to reconstruct penile injury, that is functionally and aesthetically acceptable, isolated penile skin lacerations and penile fractures when identified early and treated properly, usually resulted in a good functional outcome. The policy of staged management for the more complex injuries is acceptable, this invariably reduces morbidity and improves outcome. Early and immediate microvascular anastomosis of amputated glans penis also achieves a good result in centers with adequate facilities for managing such cases [9].

Preputial Strangulation Injuries

Hair Tourniquet

It is also known as hair thread tourniquet syndrome, which has been recognized since the 1960s [10]. Since then, sporadic reports have appeared in the literature describing different degrees of strangulation and/ or amputation of the penile structures caused by a hair thread being inadvertently tied around the penis. The patient usually presents acutely and responds well to removal of the tourniquet.

When there is a delay in presentation, partial amputation of the penis, or the glans is often seen, with varying degrees of urethral transection (Fig. 23.3).

Most cases are due to accidental wrapping of the mother's hair around the glans or rarely the prepuce of her child or infant, however, Barton et al. [11], reported a case of hair thread tourniquet syndrome due to child abuse.

The mechanism of injury in hair thread tourniquet is ischemia in the parts distal to the site of tourniquet. Presentation in the acute state is usual, with swelling, erythema, circumferential constriction and distal edema with little discomfort to the child [12].

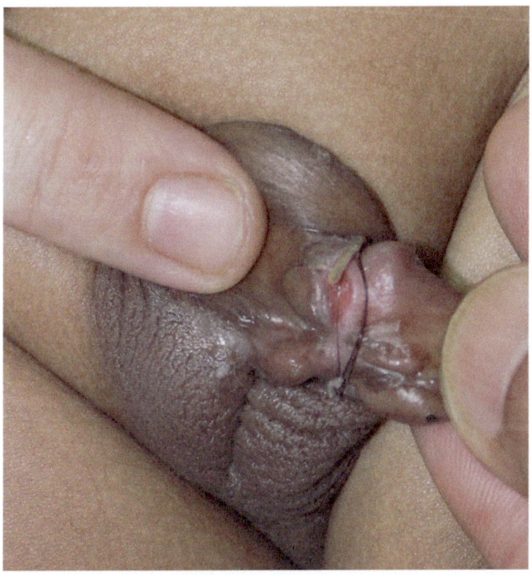

Fig. 23.3 A neglected hair tourniquet with an ulceration at the coronal sulcus

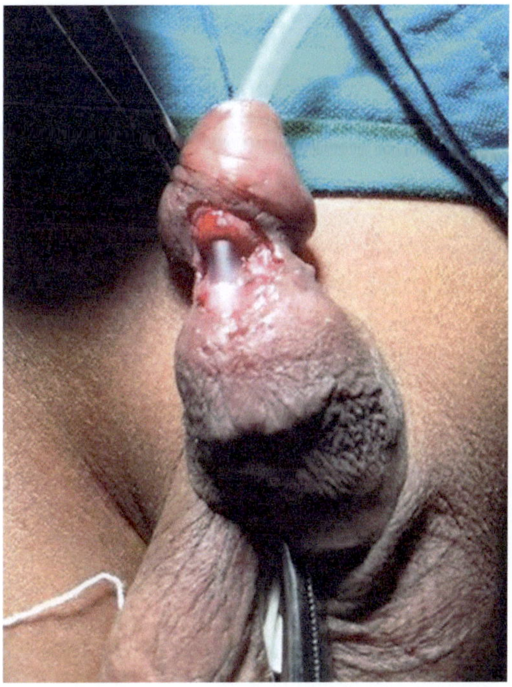

Fig. 23.4 A wide coronal fistula secondary to hair tourniquet syndrome

Injury vary from trivial to more severe with a dreadful functional and psychosocial consequences. Removal of the constricting hair at the early stage prevents complications, which is mainly urethrocutaneous fistula [13] (Fig. 23.4).

Zipper Injuries

Typically this injury will occur in young children who are distracted, had mental disabilities, psychic problems or just not paying attention, less commonly injury will happen in men where the zipper is being closed by someone else as in patients with dementia or other disabilities.

Epidemiology

The majority of cases are in pediatrics and young teenagers. The penile prepuce is often caught between the fastener and zipper usually during the closure. Incidence is quite low at less than half to 1% of all emergency room pediatric cases [14].

Pathophysiology

Typically, the pathophysiology is obvious with direct tissue damage to the prepuce or penile skin from entrapment. This injury may be associated with bleeding, swelling, pain, and direct tissue damage. Rapid extraction from the zipper is usually recommended as the longer the tissue is trapped and being damaged, the greater the degree of edema, scarring and tissue trauma.

The individual often presents in excruciating pain and may be difficult to examine. While most cases only have a partial involvement of the prepuce, in some cases there may be full thickness injury to the preputial skin. Most of the time, patients and caregivers will have tried to extract the foreskin, and this usually causes additional tissue damage and delays their appearance in the emergency room resulting in further pain, swelling and bruising [15].

Management

It is preferable if the zipper can be removed without a formal surgical intervention, but care should be taken to avoid further tissue injury when attempting manipulative removal. Attempt painful manipulation in the emergency room without anesthesia is hazardous, because it is counterproductive and uncomfortable. In children and young teenagers, anesthesia is usually required to remove the prepuce from the zipper.

Intravenous sedation may be adequate because the procedure is generally of short duration. A formal penile block with injected local anesthesia can be performed to provide immediate pain relief and allow for additional manipulation.

Edema around the site of the injury can be reduced by fomentation or by use of a small (narrow) elastic wrap. This will compress the involved area and reduce the edema which will allow for easier manipulation and removal of the zipper [16].

Initial therapy should begin with an attempt to mechanically remove, destroy or separate the zipper to free up the prepuce and other entrapped tissue. First, cut the cloth portion of the zipper with scissors as close as possible to the zipper teeth. This will usually allow the individual teeth of the zipper to fall out and release the entrapped skin. Once the skin is released, there may be bleeding, abrasions, contusions, lacerations and may be an unsuspected injury to the underlying tissue [17].

The central or median fastener portion of the zipper can be cut with various tools. Cutting will destroy part of the zipper mechanism and help in separating the two interlocking strips. This may require the use of significant hand tools such as a hacksaw, bone cutter, or wire cutters.

If not successful, treatment then proceeds to a partial surgical incision and/or removal of part or even all of the prepuce in the emergency department.

In more severe cases, the patient may require formal surgical excision particularly if extraction of the skin by manual manipulation is not possible or there is involvement of penile tissue other than the foreskin [18].

The prognosis is excellent for most children. Skin injuries to the prepuce can be closed primarily with absorbable sutures. If the zipper cannot be extracted from the skin, an excision of the affected skin can be done. This can then be repaired primarily or can be left open with the edges oversewn leaving a dorsal slit-type of a result. A circumcision can be done as a last resort, but it is usually reserved for those cases where a lesser surgery, such as local excision or a dorsal slit, is not feasible. If a circumcision is recommended, it may need to be delayed to allow the initial edema to subside [19].

References

1. Fahmy MAB. Chapter 7 - Prevalence of male circumcision complications. In: Complications in male circumcision. St. Louis: Elsevier; 2019. https://doi.org/10.1016/B978-0-323-68127-8.00007-7.
2. Oranusi CK, Nwofor AME. Traumatic penile injuries: mechanisms and problems of treatment in a tertiary institution in Nigeria. Niger J Clin Pract. 2014;17(6):763–6. https://doi.org/10.4103/1119-3077.144392.

3. Casey JT, Bjurlin MA, Cheng EY, et al. Urology. 2013;82(5):1125–30.
4. Hobbs CJ, Osman J. Genital injuries in boys and abuse. Arch Dis Child. 2007;92(4):328–31. https://doi.org/10.1136/adc.2006.111195.
5. Halis F, Inci M, T Freier M, Gokce A. Self-inflicted strangulation of prepuce in a child. APSP J Case Rep. 2013;4:4.
6. Perovic SV, Djinovic RP, Bumbasirevic MZ, Santucci RA, Djordjevic ML, Kourbatov D. Severe penile injuries: a problem of severity and reconstruction. BJU Int. 2009;104:676–87.
7. Moore EE, Moore FA. American Association for the Surgery of Trauma Organ Injury Scaling: 50th anniversary review article of the Journal of Trauma. J Trauma. 2010;69:1600–1.
8. Bhat AL, Kumar A, Mathur SC, Gangwal KC. Penile strangulation. Br J Urol. 1991;68:618–21.
9. El-Bahnasawy MS, El-Sherbiny MT. Paediatric penile trauma. BJU Int. 2002;90:92–6.
10. Vâquez Rueda F, Núñez Núñez R, Gómez Meleno P, Blesa Sánchez E. The hair thread tourniquet syndrome of the toes and penis. An Esp Pediatr. 1996;44:17–20.
11. Barton DJ, Sloan GM, Nichter LS, Reinisch JF. Hair-thread tourniquet syndrome. Pediatrics. 1988;82:925–8.
12. Okeke LI. Thread embedded into penile tissue over time as an unusual hair thread tourniquet injury to the penis: a case report. J Med Case Rep. 2008;2:230. http://www.jmedicalcasereports.com/content/2/1/230.
13. Oulad Saiad M. Penile injuries in children. Turk J Urol. 2018;44(4):351–6. https://doi.org/10.5152/tud.2018.92231.
14. Yip A, Ng SK, Wong WC, Li MK, Lam KH. Injury to the prepuce. Br J Urol. 1989;63:535–8.
15. Patil MR, Sunilkumar GR, Durgigudi PH. Zipper injuries: extrication technique. Sri Lanka J Child Health. 2018;47(2):149–54.
16. Watson CC. Zipper injuries. Clin Pediatr (Phila). 1971;10(3):188. https://doi.org/10.1177/000992287101000323.
17. Maurice MJ, Cherullo EE. A novel, nonoperative treatment for delayed penile zipper injury. Am J Emerg Med. 2013;31(2):419–20.
18. Oquist M, Buck L, Michel K, Ouellette L, Emery M, Bush C. Comparative analysis of five methods of emergency zipper release by experienced versus novice clinicians. Am J Emerg Med. 2017;35(5):783–4.
19. Djordjevic ML, Bumbasirevic MZ, Krstic Z, Bizic MR, Stojanovic BZ, Miocinovic R, Santucci RA. Severe penile injuries in children and adolescents: reconstruction modalities and outcomes. Urology. 2014;83(2):465–70.

Preputial Implants

24

The first written evidence about penile modifications can be found in the Kama Sutra, enumerating different possibilities of penile enhancement with small round objects strapped around the shaft or by perforating the penis or the glans in order to insert stimulating items. The first scientific report of this kind of implants under the foreskin was issued by Hovorka in 1894. The majority of these (61.9%) having undergone the procedure at the age of 15–24 years. The average number of beads implanted was 2.71. The average time was 6.35 years prior to the day of examination [1].

In 1994, the American Urological Association adopted a policy saying that fat injection procedures to increase penile girth, and procedures that sever the suspensory ligament of the penis to make it longer, have not been shown to be safe and efficacious [2]. The only FDA-cleared permanent silicone penile implant is "Penuma", which is a silicone sleeve inserted under the penile skin which increases both length and girth of a penis in both flaccid and erect states [3].

Types and Varieties

- *Bolitas*: Bolitas is a practice dating back to sixteenth century, and originating in Southeast Asia, where the penis would receive a small incision, and tiny balls are placed underneath the skin. The purpose of the implant is alleged to increase the pleasure of a sexual partner. However, 13.9% stated having the insertions made to make their partners scream and suffer during intercourse. In 1999, a study found that the procedure had occurred to 57% of randomly selected Filipino seaman. In the late twentieth Century, and early twenty-first century these balls were made of plastic [4] (Fig. 24.1). Other potential material which the balls maybe made of include metal, glass, or minerals. The practice also occurs outside of the Filipino mariner community, with implant

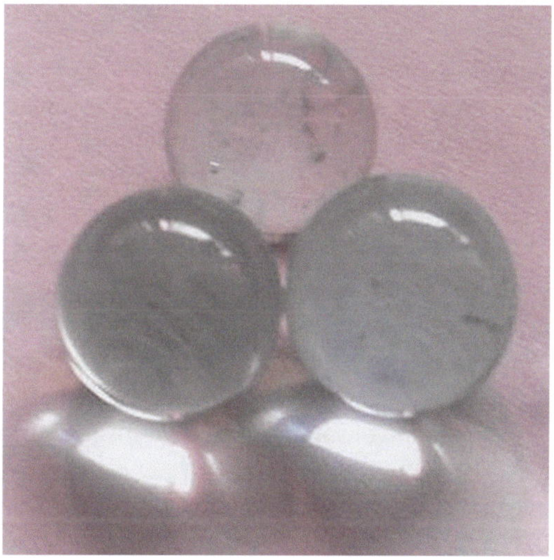

Fig. 24.1 Silicone beads used of penile implants. "A public Domain file, from: Enjoying The Great Life blog: https://ludtohan.blogspot.com/2017/02/bolitas-pinoys-secret-weapon.html"

M. A. B. Fahmy, *Normal and Abnormal Prepuce*, https://doi.org/10.1007/978-3-030-37621-5_24

recipient also documented in Japan and Cuba. In other countries injections of fat, gels, or other fillers to pump up the penis and give it the appearance of large girth is not rare. Furthermore, injected fillers may be absorbed into the body often unevenly, and this left patients with lumpy, misshapen phallus [5].

In the Philippines, this practice is called 'bulleetus' in Sumatra 'persimbraon' in Korea 'chagan ball', in Russia "sputnik" and in Thailand 'mukhsa' or 'tancho' [1].

Patients may take it upon themselves to inject various substances with the aim of maintaining erection or enlarging the penis, but the consequences may not be desirable. Infection is an obvious risk. Mineral oil, petroleum jelly and silicone introduced into the genital skin can elicit lipogranuloma or paraffinoma [6].

- *Penile and preputial beads implant*: Penile prepuce bead implants or genital beading is a form of body modification which involves the implantation of beads under the skin of the prepuce or penile shaft. These are performed primarily for the purpose of physical erotic stimulation and usually intended to enhance the sexual pleasure (for both the wearer and their partner), as well as for aesthetic reasons. Genital beading is more commonly done by men in detention center or jail. The implanted materials for these purposes included plastic, wood, glass, stainless steel and agate. The implanted beads were variable from one to ten item.

  These implants may became a surgical issue and the patients may ask for medical aid to remove the bead implants because of reasons such as (1) infection, (2) uncomfortable sexual intercourse (3) no enhancement on the sexual pleasure, (4) sexual partner dislike.

  The surgery for the infected genital beading should excise the bead combining with the surrounding infected soft tissue.
- *Tancho Nodules and Paraffinomas*: Tancho nodules refer to an unusual custom among some Slavic and Asian populations to implant foreign material under the skin of the penis to improve sexual pleasure. Most beads are derived from the bottoms of Tancho pomade glass jars. The name "tancho-nodules" for glass balls in Thailand derives from a pomade brand ("Tancho"). The nodules are manufactured from the base of the pomades' glass container, which is either been melted or polished to a sphere.
- Paraffinomas (also known as sclerosing lipogranulomas) result from the injection of mineral oil in the penis usually done with the purpose of penile enlargement. This reaction may occur several years after the injection. Histologically, these materials may cause foreign body reaction that may need surgical resection [7]. Other foreign lipidic substances, which may be injected into the penis, and induce the same reaction are vaseline, paraffin, silicone, or wax. Most of the time, the lesion affects exclusively the penis, although in some cases, there is extension to adjacent sites, especially the prepuce and scrotum

Macroscopic

Beyond the more or less distorted aspect of the organ, sometimes suggesting a neoplasia, no specific gross abnormalities are characteristic of this condition. Areas simulating cysts may occasionally be observed.

Microscopic

Penile lipogranuloma is characterized by a prominent inflammatory cell infiltrate and abundant foreign body-type multinucleated giant cells. Sclerosis can sometimes be very prominent, and so the designation of "sclerosing lipogranuloma" is appropriate in these cases [8] (Fig. 24.2).

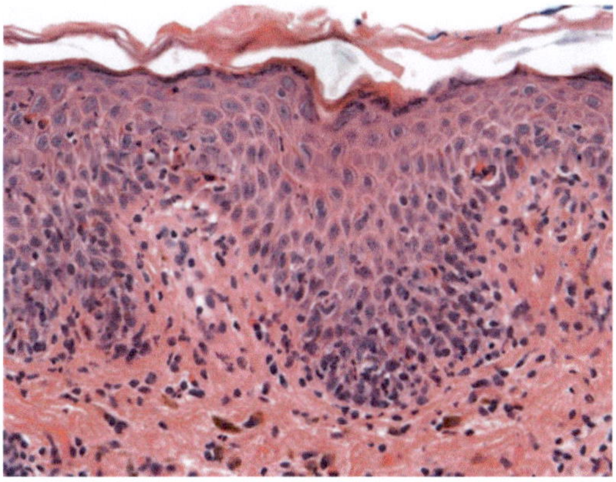

Fig. 24.2 Histology of the lipogranulomas, a fixed drug reaction, with an interface dermatitis, necrotic keratinocytes and a dermal infiltrate with lymphoid cells, eosinophils, and melanophages [7]

The inflammatory cells surround vacuoles and cyst-like spaces of variable size which correspond to the areas of lipidic materials.

Complications

The incidence and severity of early or delayed complications are unknown but are probably underreported. Penile implants bearers had suffered from imminent inflammation, fixed beads pain, or secondary inflammations years after implantation.

The bearers also had a higher risk of acquiring a sexually transmitted disease by sharing instruments used for insertion, open wounds during intercourse, and condom leakage [1].

Partner complications were abrasions, wounds, vaginal bleeding, pain, and dyspareunia. The risk of infection with sexually transmitted diseases is increased, additionally in this group.

Differential Diagnosis

An neoplastic tumor, cyst or a lymphangioma may be considered in differential diagnosis. The vacuole-like spaces of lymphangioma are lined by endothelium, while in the cyst-like areas of lipogranuloma, there is no epithelial lining. Sclerosing liposarcoma should also be ruled out. The presence of foreign body-type giant cells, the more prominent inflammatory infiltrate, and the absence of lipoblasts are indicative of a lipogranuloma.

References

1. Fischer N, Hauser S, Brede O, Fisang C, Müller S. Implantation of artificial penile nodules—a review of literature. J Sex Med. 2010;7:3565–357.
2. Santucci RA, Zehring RD, McClure D. Petroleum jelly lipogranuloma of the penis treated with excision and native skin coverage. Urology. 2000;56:331.
3. Elist JJ, et al. A single-surgeon retrospective and preliminary evaluation of the safety and effectiveness of the Penuma silicone sleeve implant for elective cosmetic correction of the flaccid penis. J Sex Med. 2018;15(9):1216–23. https://doi.org/10.1016/j.jsxm.2018.07.006.
4. Bunker CB. Male genital skin disease. London: Saunders; 2004.
5. Wilcher G. Artificial penile nodules—a forensic pathosociology perspective: four case reports. Med Sci Law. 2006;46:349–56.
6. Al-Mutairi N, Sharma AK, Zaki A, et al. Penile self-injections: an unusual act. Int J Dermatol. 2004;43:680–2.
7. Lin J, Jiang H, Chen J, Wang B, Chang C, Yen M, Huang S, Shi H, Chou M. Penile prepuce bead implants. Urol Sci. 2016;27:S30. https://www.scipedia.com/public/Lin_et_al._2016abcdefa.
8. Matsuda T, Shichiri Y, Hida S, et al. Eosinophilic sclerosing lipogranuloma of the male genitalia not caused by exogenous lipids. J Urol. 1988;140:1021–4.

Preputial Cysts

25

Abbreviations

AH	Apocrine hidrocystoma
EC	Epidermoid cyst
MRC	Median raphe cysts
PEP	Prepucial Epstein pearl
PPP	Pearly penile papule

Classifications Preputial cyst generally divided into two main categories: median raphe (urethroid) cysts and epidermoid (follicular) cysts. Epidermoid cysts are the most common cystic lesions of the penis and occur primarily on the shaft. Median raphe cysts are midline developmental cysts that occur at sites from the external urethral meatus to the anus, including the ventral penis. Occasional examples are seen of true retention cysts of the prepuce, mucoid preputial cyst, and other rare cysts were reported.

Median Raphe Cyst (Urothelial Cyst) (Fig. 25.1)

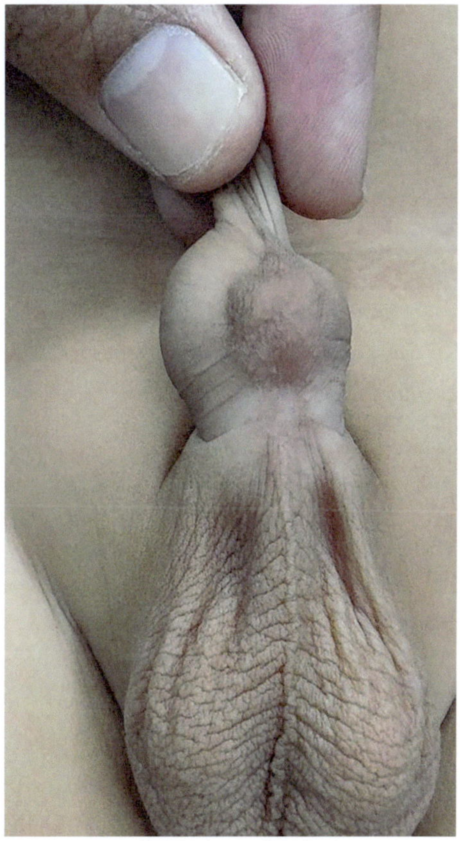

Fig. 25.1 Median raphe cyst, diagnosed in 4 years old boy, at the distal part of the prepuce

Definition

Median Raphe Cysts (MRC) are congenital epidermal cysts formed in the median penile raphe, which corresponds to the midline ectodermal fusion during embryogenesis, it occur only in males. They may be found on the penis, scrotum, or perineum, although penile lesions are certainly more frequent than rare scrotal and perineal counterparts, prepuce is very rarely affected by this cyst. It was described for the first time in detail by Mermet at1895 [1, 2].

M. A. B. Fahmy, *Normal and Abnormal Prepuce*, https://doi.org/10.1007/978-3-030-37621-5_25

Etiology

Although MRC of the penis have been widely reported, their etiopathogenesis is obscure. They are thought to arise from embryologic developmental defects in the closure of the urethral folds and, hence, are always located at the ventral midline of the penis, from near the meatus to the scrotal median raphe, and this also explain why it is not reported in female.

Epidemiology

MRC are not a common condition. A recent extensive literature search has revealed only 200 reported cases, but many cases are probably not reported. Patients present at any age with higher incidence in childhood and lower number of cases seen in the elderly [3].

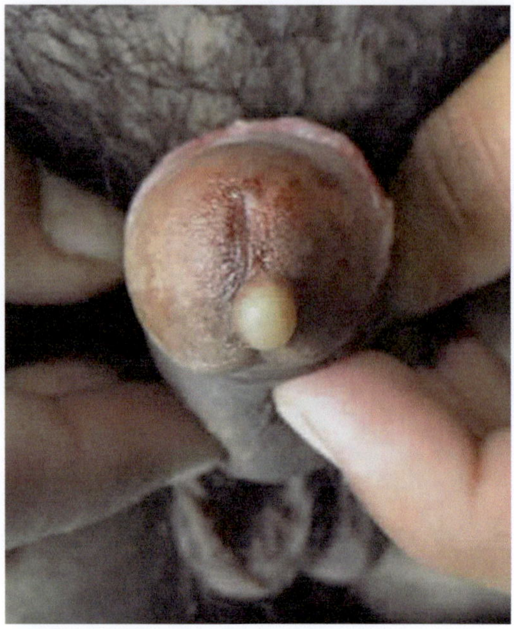

Fig. 25.2 Paraurethral or parameatal cyst

Clinical Appearance

MRC occur as solitary, freely movable nodules on the ventral surface of the penis or the prepuce. In general, the lesion is asymptomatic and does not interfere with urinary or sexual function, unless it acquires a larger size or complicated. Trauma and infection are possible complications.

Clinically, median raphe cysts manifest as unilocular or multilocular painless lesions, although in occasions they can be associated with local discomfort, dysuria, or even dyspareunia. Sometimes they are traumatized and manifest as painful nodules or ulcerated areas.

MRCs usually do not communicate with the urethra, but when located near the urinary meatus, they are referred to as "parameatal cysts" (Fig. 25.2).

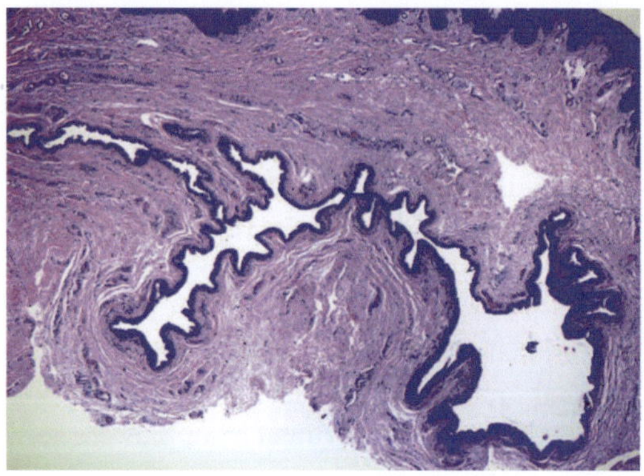

Fig. 25.3 Median raphe cyst, typically lined by pseudostratified columnar epithelium and contain mucinous material (from MacLennan et al. [8])

Clinical Course

Most lesions are present at birth but remain undetectable until adolescence or adulthood. As the patient grows older, the cyst may also progress slowly. In some cases, the cyst may progress rapidly or become symptomatic owing to infections or trauma, which could make diagnosis difficult.

Histologically, median raphe cysts reveal a single cystic space located in the dermis with no urethral communication, lined commonly by one or both of the following types of epithelium: stratified squamous epithelium or pseudostratified columnar epithelium, the latter being the most common [4] (Fig. 25.3), as majority of cysts have only one type of epithelium, while some may have areas of both. Rarely the cyst has transitional epithelial lining in addition to stratified squamous epithelium and pseudostratified columnar epithelium constituting very rare and interesting triple histological lining [5].

Due to the appearance of their epithelial lining, they may be considered as urothelial cysts. There is no epithelial atypias should be present. Ciliated epithelium in some median raphe cyst has been attributed to metaplastic change, similar to that reported to occur in the penile urethra secondary to local irritation [6].

Diagnosis

Is mainly clinical, Videodermatoscopy may be helpful in the differentiation between cysts and canals of the median raphe of the penis, showing in the latter case the presence of a tract connecting cystic lesions [7]. Sometimes if there is a confusion a cystourethrogram may be indicated.

Ultrasound

Epidermoid cysts appear as ovoid or lobulated masses with well-defined margins, relatively echogenic content with hypoechoic foci.

Magnetic Resonance Imaging

In rare occasions, specially if the cyst is huge or shows a suspicion of pelvic extension; an MRI may be indicated. Epidermoid cysts present with well-circumscribed masses without contrast enhancement. T1-weighted images signal intensity is similar or higher compared to muscle, while signal intensity is high on T2-weighted images [8] (Fig. 25.4).

Therapy

Even if these cysts are small and asymptomatic, surgical excision is recommended for treatment and diagnostic confirmation [9].

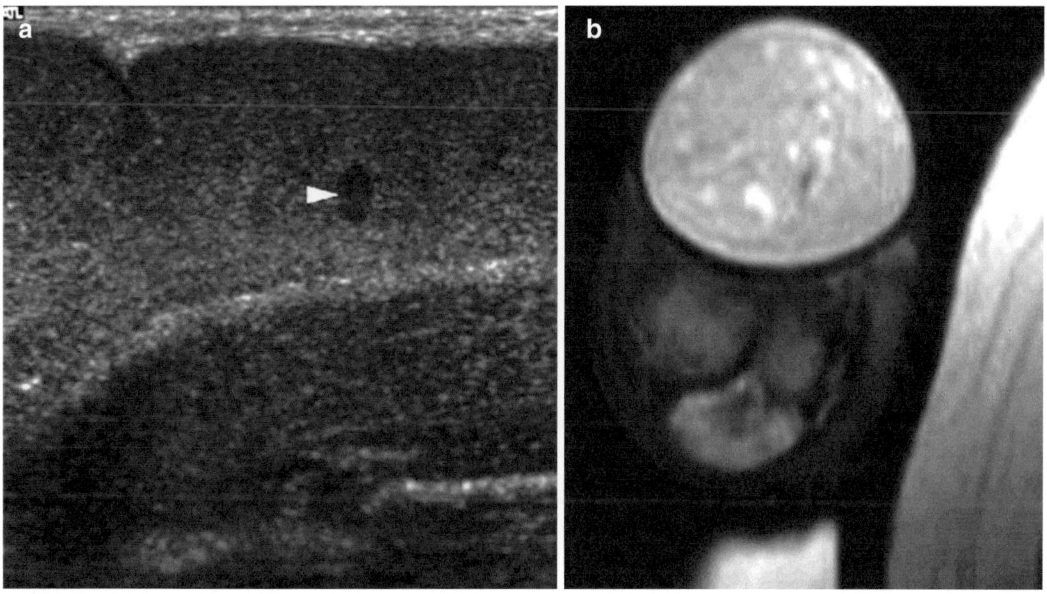

Fig. 25.4 Radiological findings of penile cyst: (**a**) Longitudinal ultrasound scan showing a well-circumscribed dorsal echogenic mass containing a hypoechoic focus (arrowhead). (**b**) Axial T2-weighted MR image showing a high-signal-intensity lesion with irregular low-signal-intensity foci [8]

Epidermoid Cysts

Definition

Epidermoid Cysts (EC) are small bumps that can develop beneath the skin of face, neck, trunk, and sometimes genital area, and rarely it may affect the prepuce. Epidermoid glands arise from the cells that make up the outer layers of skin (epidermal).

Etiology

Some epidermal or follicular cells close to the skin surface may move into deeper parts of the skin while continuing to proliferate. These cells may arrange themselves into round structures, gathering the keratin that they produce and that would normally be released on the top layer of the skin. The keratin becomes soggy and turns into a toothpaste-like substance. Epidermoid/sebaceous cysts may be congenital or acquired. In the etiology of acquired cysts, trauma (damage to a hair follicle, rupture of sebaceous gland) or previous surgery can be considered as causes.

Epidemiology

Penile and preputial EC are uncommon in general, it can affect anyone, but they are most common in young and middle-aged adults, few cases are diagnosed in infants and children.

Clinical Appearance

EC detected in various sizes, they are usually solitary and only rarely multifocal. Commonly these cysts seen in the dorsal surface of the prepuce. They appear as round, usually small, mobile cystic swelling.

In Fig. 25.5 we diagnosed a rare case with two small epidermoid cysts in the dorsum of the prepuce, giving it the look of copra head appearance (Fig. 25.5).

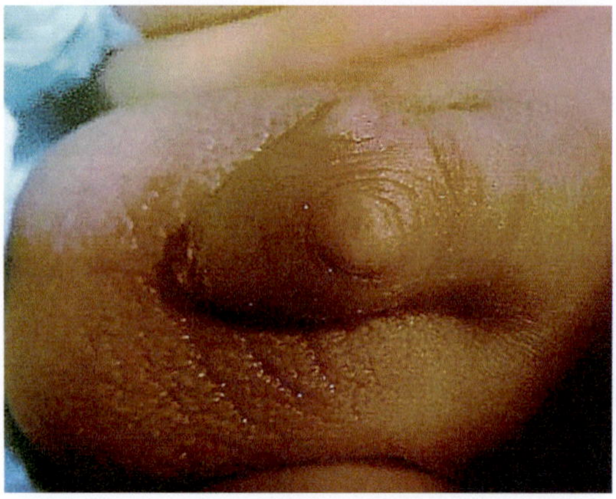

Fig. 25.5 A rare case of two small epidermoid cysts on the dorsum of the prepuce; giving a false impression of copra head appearance, which usually seen in cases of hooded prepuce of hypospadia

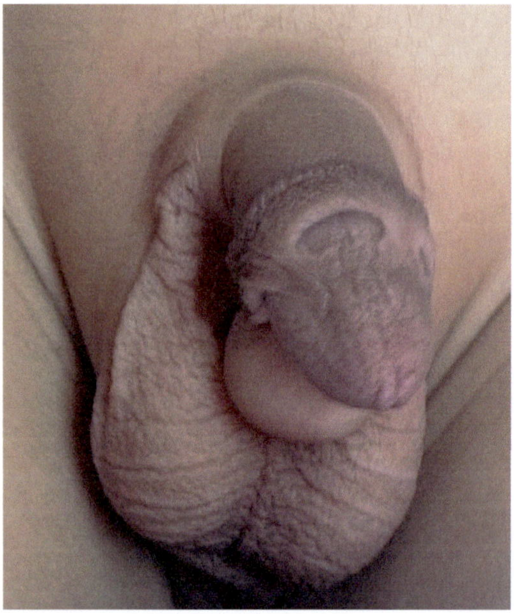

Fig. 25.6 A large epidermoid cyst in the ventral surface of the penis

Large size epidermoid cyst are rare, and if seen in the ventral aspect of the penis or prepuce it may be difficult to differentiate it from MRC, except after histopathological studies (Fig. 25.6). They are usually white or yellow, though people with darker skin may have pigmented cysts. Lesions may be asymptomatic, but rupture may result in significant discomfort [10].

Clinical Course

Epidermoid cysts are benign and do not cause functional problems, unless it is large or complicated. The cysts may became red, inflamed, ruptured and painful if infected.

Diagnosis

It is usually easily made based on the clinical findings, but cysts in the ventral penile surface may be not distinguishable from the MRC except after histological examination (Fig. 25.7).

Therapy

Indications for treatment are secondary cyst infection, pain on intercourse, cosmetic concerns, or obstruction of the urinary tract. A course of antibiotics will usually clear an infection if it occurs. Simple complete excision followed by primary closure has generally been regarded as the best treatment procedure. To minimize scarring, a carbon dioxide laser may be used to vaporize a small epidermoid cyst on a sensitive area [11].

Epidermal Inclusion Cyst

Epidermal inclusion cysts is an acquired cystic lesions of the prepuce or its remnants, which may form after penile surgery, including circumcision, hypospadias repair, and penile girth augmentation surgery.

They are similar to those occurring elsewhere. The exact etiology is unknown, but in some cases, they are associated with hypospadias, phimosis. Usually, they are found in young boys and elderly men, they are considered by some authors as the most common genital cystic lesions [12].

They are preferentially located in the foreskin, but cases can also be seen at the glans, coronal sulcus, near the frenulum, and, less frequently, the shaft of the penis. Most of them do not exceed 1.0 cm in maximum diameter (Fig. 25.8), large sized cysts are reported after hypospadias surgery (Fig. 25.9).

Histologically, epidermal inclusion cysts are lined by a nonatypical keratinized squamous epithelium surrounding the cyst cavity, which is usuallly filled of keratin debris. Keratinization pattern is orthokeratotic with the presence of a more or less evident granular layer. Skin adnexa are absent [13].

Meticulous dissection, with preservation of the prepuce and penile skin and excision of the cyst without rupture is indicated in all inclusion cysts (Fig. 25.9).

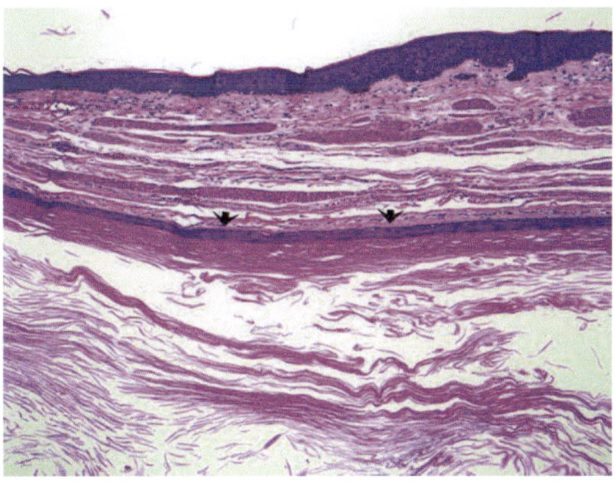

Fig. 25.7 Histology of epidermoid cyst: the skin is at top, and the cyst wall epithelium, consisting of keratinizing squamous epithelium, is shown in the center of the image (arrows). Desquamated keratinous debris, at bottom, occupies the central portion of the cyst

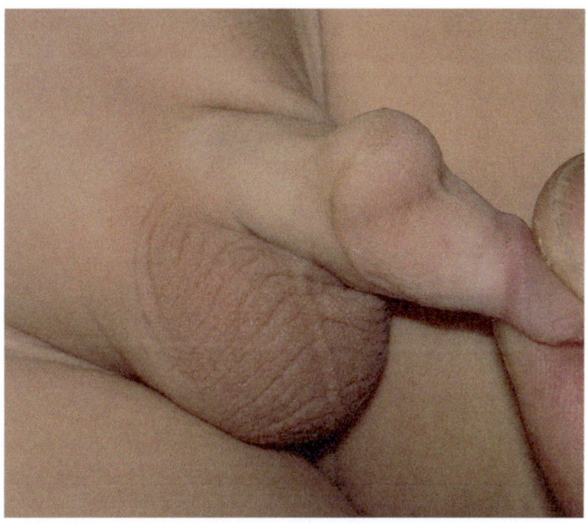

Fig. 25.8 Inclusion epidermoid cyst on the remnant of circumcision extended to the dorsal penile skin

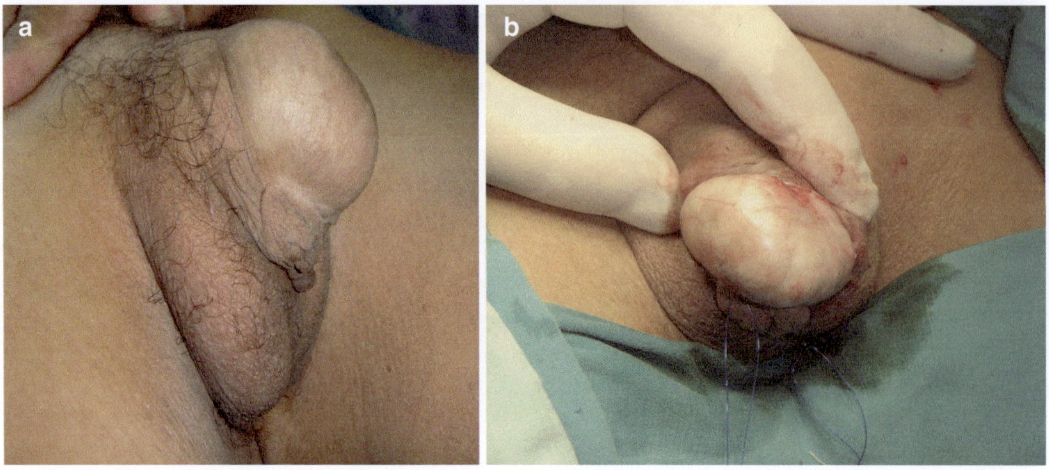

Fig. 25.9 A large inclusion cyst at the dorsum of preputial skin, diagnosed 6 months after hypospadias repair (**a**), (**b**) the cyst wall after dissection of the covering skin

Smegma Cyst

Nomenclatures

There is a great confusion in nomenclature of the smegma cyst with the different conditions of smegma collections, so we will define smegma cyst and other related pathologies:

Smegma Cyst

It is an inclusion cyst of smegma; with a well formed epithelial wall, it lies in-between the preputial layers (Fig. 25.10).

Smegma Aggregations (Smegma Pearls)

Are a collection or aggravation of the smegma without any covering sac, lies in the preputial sac; between the inner prepuce and the glans penis; it may attributes different sizes; and it is easy removable after preputial retraction, it is commonly known as smegma pearls (Fig. 25.11).

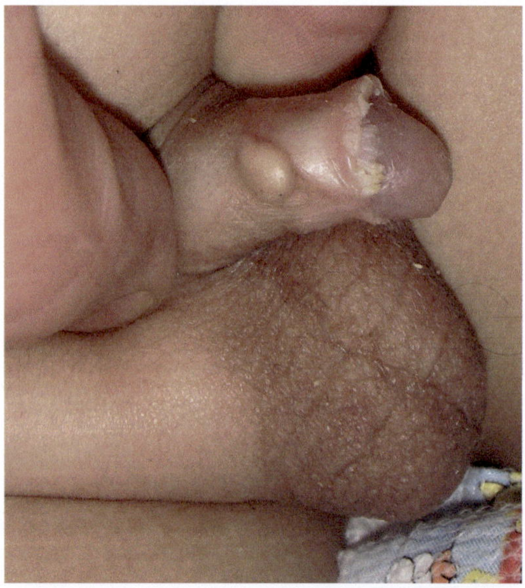

Fig. 25.10 Smegma cyst in between the retracted prepuce

Smegmoliths

It is a hard concretions of smegma in the preputial sac, It looks like a stone, yellowish in colour and consisted of uric acid, and to a lesser extent of calcium phosphate (Fig. 25.12) (Chap. 17).

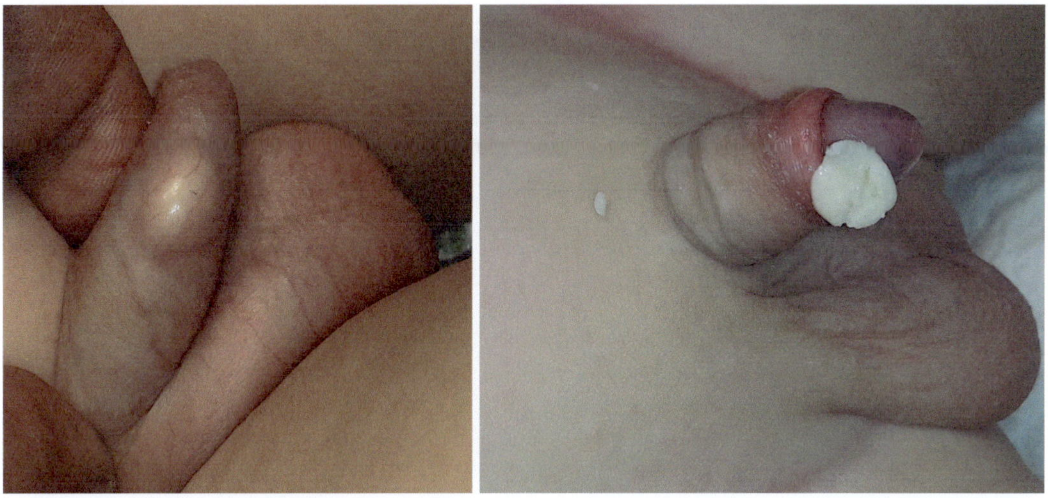

Fig. 25.11 Smegma pearls detectable at the undersurface of unretractable prepuce, it had no surrounding sac

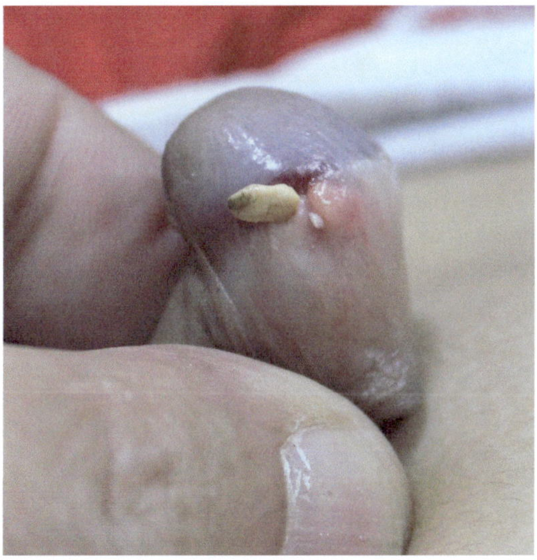

Fig. 25.12 Smegmolith; a hard stony concrete of smegma collection under the prepuce, at the coronal sulcus

Prepucial (Preputial) Epstein Pearl (PEP)

This is a normal physiological papules, situated on the tip of the foreskin, commonly at 6 and 8 O'Clock position. It is a firm 1–2 mm superficial white epidermal inclusion cysts containing laminated keratinized material and epithelial cells. Epstein pearls is mainly described on the hard palate. They are present in neonates as a physiologic finding (Fig. 25.13).

Faridi MM, Adhami have reported incidence of PEP in 7.3/1000 live-born male newborn infants from India [14].

Pearly Penile Papules (PPP)

Is a completely different findings, but had a confusing terminology, which is also known as a Papillae Coronae Glandis, it is detected normally in in up to 50% of men. They present as flesh-coloured, pink, smooth, rounded, 1–3 mm papules, occurring predominantly around the coronal margin of the glans. This is a manifestation without a disease significance at the proximal border of the glans, before its transition into the coronary sulcus, manifested as one or many fringed papillary projection (Chap. 5, Fig. 38).

Smegmoma

Is not a scientific name, sometimes this term is given roughly to any smegma collection under the foreskin; either it is a cyst or just an aggregation [15].

Some authors reported that the most common cystic lesion of the penis and prepuce is the smegma cyst, which sometimes called "smegmoma", and usually seen under the unretractable prepuce, it may appear yellowish due to smegma content [16].

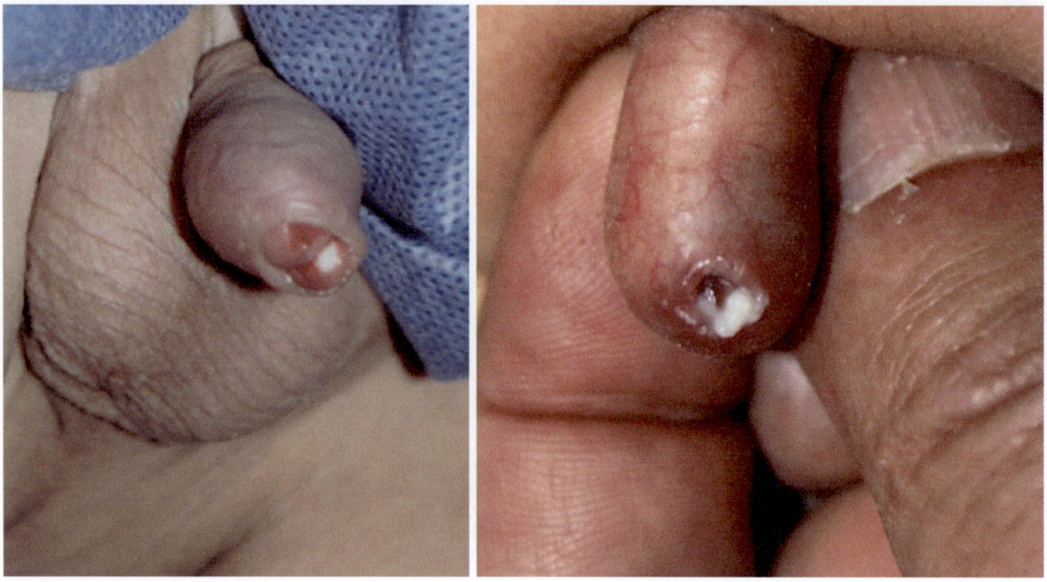

Fig. 25.13 Two cases with a different forms of preputial Epstein pearl (PEP)

The nodule of entrapped smegma, "smegma pearl" is fairly common in young uncircumcised boys. Despite expected spontaneous resolution, parents usually become apprehensive. In spite of the common appreciation of smegma cysts, it has been reported only recently [17].

The lesions appeared as pearly white lumps, ranging in size from 0.5 to 2 cm. They were round to ovoid in shape, with a doughy sensation and were located between the base of the glans and the distal junction of the attachment of the preputial membrane with the glans. The majority of the lesions were located on the ventral aspect of the glans, adjacent to the frenulum. The urethral meatus was clear from the attachment and a thin inner preputial membrane seemed to be delicately attached with the mucosa of the glans (preputial adhesion) [17]. The prepuce in all cases was partially retractable, stopping after one-third to one-half the course of retraction but allowing partial inspection of the subpreputial space. On application of gentle pressure over the lesion with both thumbs and index fingers, the contents of the lumps tend to pop out, consisting of cheese-like whitish material (Fig. 25.11).

Etiology

There is no clear explanation why some boys developing a smegma aggregation to be manifested as pearls papule under the prepuce or over the glans penis, infrequent wash and cleaning of smegma in uncircumcised boy may be implicated as a cause of formation of such cyst.

Diagnosis

Smegma cyst present with one or more yellowish lumps on the penis that are often diagnosed by the general practitioner as sebaceous cysts or lipoma of the penile shaft, invariably, on outpatient assessment, these prove to be collections of retained smegma trapped by surrounding preputial adhesions, lipoma and sebaceous cyst are extremely rare in penis. Preputial cyst are generally asymptomatic, but it may result in abnormal micturition, urine retention and difficult sexual intercourse [18]. Some differential diagnoses include dermoid cyst, teratoma, and urethral diverticulum.

Management

Parents reassurance is essentially required, as the smegma is released when the adhesions lyse spontaneously over time, such patients may be better served with a circumcision or preputioplasty. Localised cysts can be enucleated easily either with scarification or preservation with reconstruction of the remnant prepuce according to family wishes.

Preputial calculi (Smegmoliths) usually occur in adults, they develop secondary to a severe obstructive phimosis, or poor penile hygiene with inspissated smegma. Treating the underlying cause with a dorsal preputial slit or a formal circumcision prevents recurrent calculi.

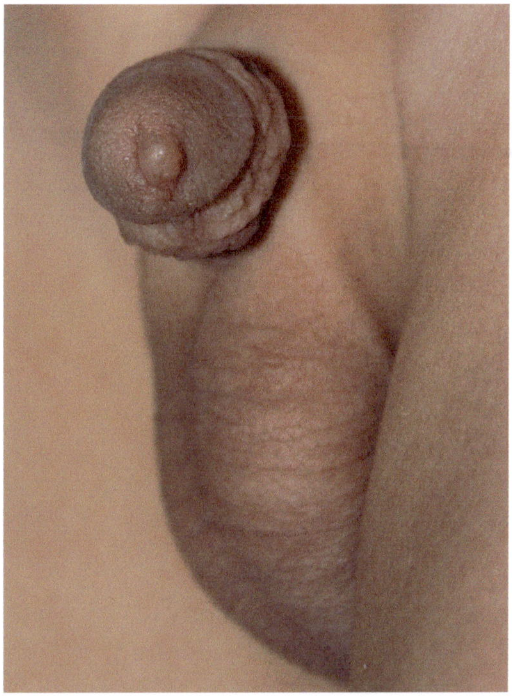

Fig. 25.14 A small perimeatal mucoid cyst

Other Rare Cysts

Mucoid Cysts or Mucinous Cyst

These are rare lesions that are present at birth or develop during childhood as small, flesh-coloured, mobile cystic papules or nodules with no punctum, commonly on the ventral glans or foreskin, rarely in the perineum. When these cysts locate in the glans near the meatus; it have been described as paraurethral or perimeatal cysts. It is considered as a retention mucoid cysts. Sometimes the histological features suggest that they arise from ectopic urethral tissue during embryological development and are lined by a stratified columnar epithelium with mucinous cells [19] (Fig. 25.14).

Mucoid cysts can be asymptomatic, become infected or interfere with intercourse [20] (Fig. 25.15).

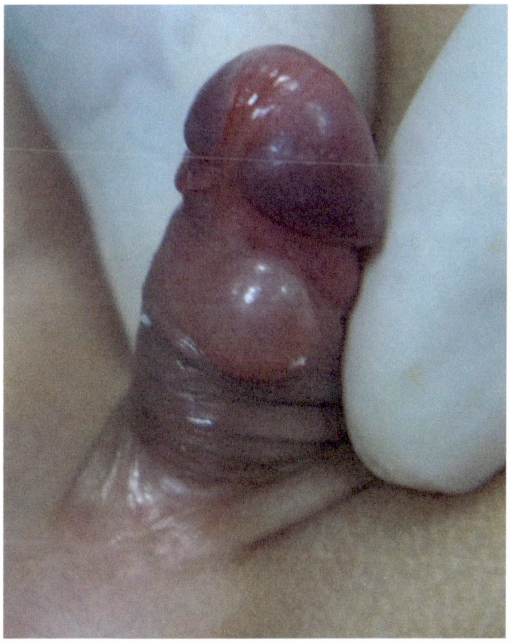

Fig. 25.15 Mucoid preputial cyst on the ventral surface of the inner prepuce in a 3 years old boy

Dermoid cysts have been occasionally reported in the prepuce, and their aspect is identical to that observed elsewhere in the body. The clinical aspect is similar to other penile cysts.

It is very rarely to have a neonate with a small retention cyst at the tip of the prepuce; which is very difficult to distinguishes it from the preputial Epstein pearl, except after careful examination and, mucoid cyst is usually compressible

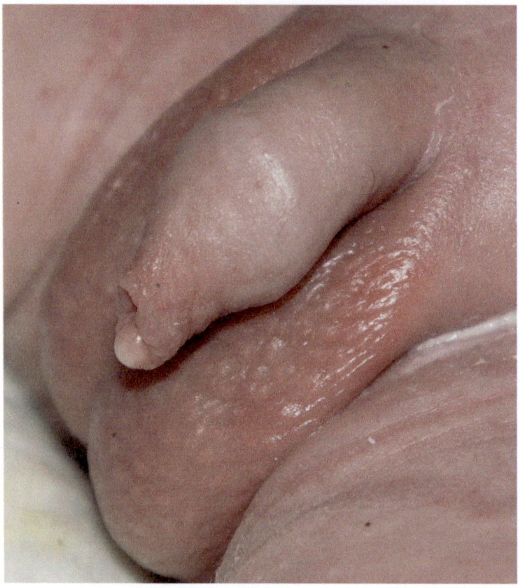

Fig. 25.16 A small mucoid cyst at the tip of the prepuce in a neonate

(Fig. 25.16). Histologically, the cyst is lined by a stratified squamous epithelium with adnexal structures such as sebaceous glands and hair follicles [21].

Dermoid cyst affecting the penis, presenting with pain, swelling and suppuration from abscess formation, has been reported.

Apocrine Hidrocystoma of the Foreskin

Apocrine hidrocystoma (AH) is an uncommon benign cystic tumor that arises from the apocrine secretory coil, most often found on the face or scalp. The tumor occurs in any age group and is prevalent in adults between 30 and 70 years of age. This lesion is usually solitary and equally prevalent among males and females.

The tumor rarely occurs on the genitalia. Only nine cases of this cyst have been reported on the penis [22].

The lesion may involves the foreskin followed by the shaft. The average maximum diameter was 1.6 cm (range 0.3–3 cm). The majority (70%) of tumors are unilocular. Their color may vary from skin coloured to blue, or even brown or pigmented.

AH of the foreskin is rare and may present as an asymptomatic swelling. The condition needs to be differentiated from other congenital or acquired cystic lesions of the penis. Although the lesion may have a proliferative character, recurrence or malignant transformation has not been described. Treatment should include complete excision [23].

Lymphatic cysts can also be observed at the penis but they are exceedingly rare. The histological picture is identical to similar cysts elsewhere.

References

1. Kirkham N. Tumors and cysts of the epidermis. In: Elder D, Elenitsas R, Jasorsky C, Jonhson B, editors. Lever's histopathology of lever. 8th ed. Philadelphia: Lippincott-Raven; 1997. p. 685–746.
2. Fahmy M. Preputial cysts. In: Congenital anomalies of the penis. Cham: Springer; 2017. https://doi.org/10.1007/978-3-319-43310-3_7.
3. Singh TV, Ahmad DB, Kumar MC. Penile median raphe cysts: serial retrospective analysis. Int J Sci Res. 2018;7(9).
4. Shao IH, Chen TD, Shao HT, Chen HW. Male median raphe cysts: serial retrospective analysis and histopathological classification. Diagn Pathol. 2012;7:121.
5. Bertolotto M, et al. Congenital and acquired nonneoplastic disorders of the penis and scrotum. In: Dogra V, MacLennan G, editors. Genitourinary radiology: male genital tract, adrenal and retroperitoneum. London: Springer; 2013.
6. Cardoso R, Freitas JD, Reis JP, Tellechea O. Median raphe cyst of the penis. Dermatol Online J. 2005;11:37.
7. Lacarrubba F, Tedeschi A, Francesconi L, Micali G. Canal versus cysts of the penile median raphe: advancing diagnostic methods using videodermatoscopy. Pediatr Dermatol. 2010;27:667–9.
8. Rattan J, Rattan S, Gupta DK. Epidermoid cyst of the penis with extension into the pelvis. J Urol. 1997;158:593.
9. Micali G, Lacarrubba F. Augmented diagnostic capability using videodermatoscopy on selected infectious and non-infectious penile growths. Int J Dermatol. 2011;50:1501–5.
10. Singh S, Kaur T. Epidermoid cyst of penis. Indian J Dermatol Venereol Leprol. 2011;77:627.
11. Suwa M, Takeda M, Bilim V, Takahashi K. Epidermoid cyst of the penis: a case report and review of the literature. Int J Urol. 2000;7:431–3.

12. Ealai PA, Yadav VK, Vanjare HA, Gibikote S. Penile epidermal inclusion cyst: a rare location. BMJ Case Rep. 2015;2015:bcr2015212137.
13. Saini P, Mansoor MN, Jalali S, Sharma A. Penile epidermal inclusion cyst. Indian J Pediatr. 2010;77(7):815–6.
14. Faridi MM, Adhami S. Prepucial Epstein pearls. Indian J Pediatr. 1989;56(5):653–5.
15. Fahmy M. Smegmoma "Smegma collection in health and disease". In: Congenital anomalies of the penis. Cham: Springer; 2017. https://doi.org/10.1007/978-3-319-43310-3_36.
16. Oaster J. Further fate of the foreskin: incidence of preputial adhesions, phimosis, and smegma among Danish schoolboys. Arch Dis Child. 1968;43:200.
17. Sonthalia S, Singal A. Smegma pearls in young uncircumcised boys. Pediatr Dermatol. 2016;33(3):e186–9. https://doi.org/10.1111/pde.12832.
18. Rajaian S, Masih D, Kekre NS. Preputial cyst in an adult causing difficulty in coitus. ANZ J Surg. 2011;81:946–7. https://doi.org/10.1111/j.1445-2197.2011.05908.x.
19. de Mendonça RR, et al. Mucoid cyst of the penis: case report and literature review. Can Urol Assoc J. 2010;4(6):E155–7.
20. Cole LA, Helwig EB. Mucoid cysts of the penile skin. J Urol. 1976;115:397–400.
21. Tomasini C, Aloi F, Puiatti P, Caliendo V. Dermoid cyst of the penis. Dermatology. 1997;194:188–90.
22. Anzai S, Goto M, Fujiwara S, Da T. Apocrine hidrocystoma: a case report and analysis of 167 Japanese cases. Int J Dermatol. 2005;44(8):702–3.
23. Val D, Val-Bernal J. Apocrine hidrocystoma of the foreskin. A case report and review of the literature. Rom J Morphol Embryol. 2017;58(2):651–3.

26 Preputial Stone

Nomenclature

Smegmoliths, Smegma stone, Preputial calculi.

Smegmoliths or smegma stones is a hard accumulation of concretions of smegma in the preputial sac, it looks like a stone, usually yellowish in colour and consisted of uric acid, and to a lesser extent of calcium phosphate. They develop because of gradual accumulation of smegma causing chronic balanoposthitis and present with penile irritation and discharge (Fig. 26.1).

Smegma pearls are benign soft collections of smegma in the subpreputial space common in young uncircumcised boys that tend to collect if the prepuce is not retracted regularly to clean the glans and coronal sulcus (Chap. 25).

Incidence

Preputial calculi are so rare to diagnose, or it may be occasionally reported, literature search could find only 14 cases that are reported. Almost all the cases occur in uncircumcised males with phimosis. Although they can occur in any age, but few cases reported in children and women.

Preputial Stones in Animal

Some geldings and occasionally, stallions may also form a "smegma bean" or stones, which is a hardened ball of smegma inside the sheath or even the urethra that, in extreme cases, can interfere with urine flow. Although a gelding retains the same beneficial microorganisms in the sheath as a stallion, they seem to accumulate smegma and other debris at a higher rate, probably because geldings rarely fully extrude the penis, and thus dirt and smegma build up in the folds of skin [1].

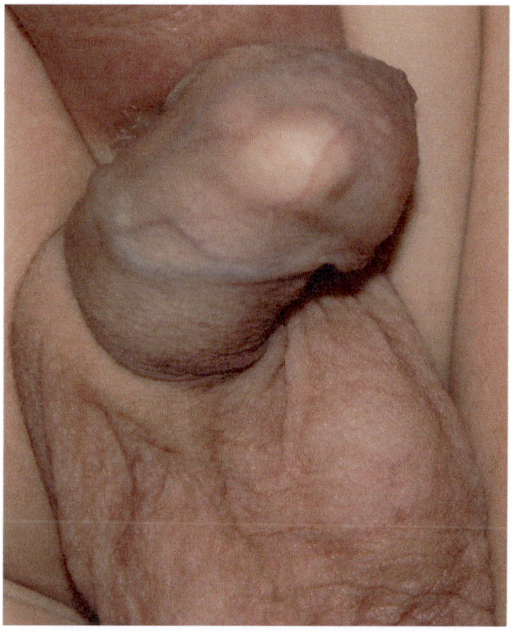

Fig. 26.1 A single subpreputial smegma stone

M. A. B. Fahmy, *Normal and Abnormal Prepuce*, https://doi.org/10.1007/978-3-030-37621-5_26

Clinically

The preputial calculi are easily diagnosed by clinical examination as they are freely mobile within the preputial sac, but it is expected that many patients harbouring these calculi may be not aware about their problems; specially the neurologically impaired patients. It is commonly a single stone, but multiplicity is not rare (Fig. 26.2).

Presentation is commonly in the form of urinary retention or drippling preceded by preputial ballooning with a history of preputial non retractability. Some cases may manifest as strangury, poor flow, prolonged voiding time, haematuria, and foul smelling discharge from prepuce.

Inguinal lymphadenopathy may result secondary to inflammatory process in case of severe infection.

Urinary tart infection is the common presentation in complicated cases, other rare presentations is skin ulcer with preputial perforation [2], and there is one case reported with a coexisting penile malignancy with preputial calculi [3].

Kaan [4] reported a case of retained, hardened smegma in a woman, forty-three years old. The smegma concretion was irregular in contour with sharp edges, and another case was reported recently [5].

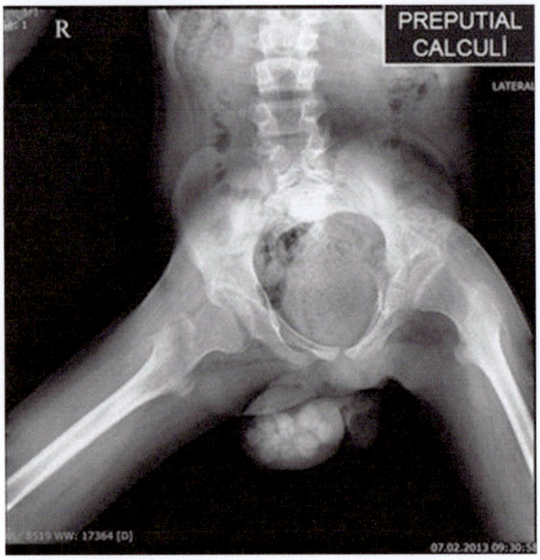

Fig. 26.3 A plain X ray showing a multiple stone in the preputial sac [2]

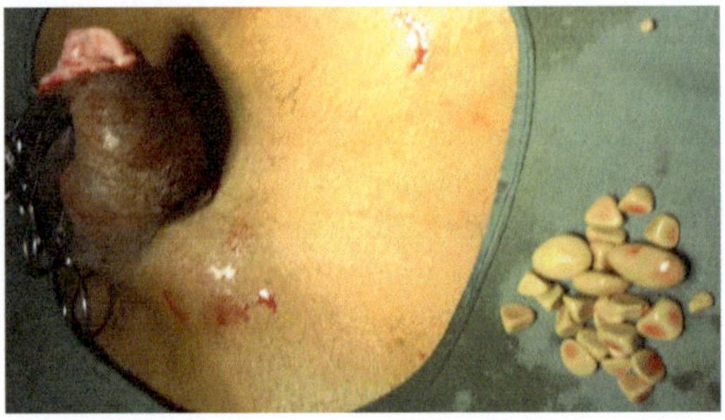

Fig. 26.4 Multiple faceted preputial calculi extracted from the preputial sac [6]

Investigations

A plain radiography is a useful to confirm the diagnose, as most of the preputial calculi are a radiopaque lesions (Fig. 26.3). Once the diagnosis is confirmed, it is important to evaluate the rest of the urinary tract to disclose the presence of calculi from proximal urinary tract which may migrate to the narrowed passage such as the urethra and to some extent down to the phimotic prepuce. Metabolic evaluation can provide clues to the etiology of calculi especially in a situation wherein the calculi are found in the other parts of urinary tract other than the prepuce.

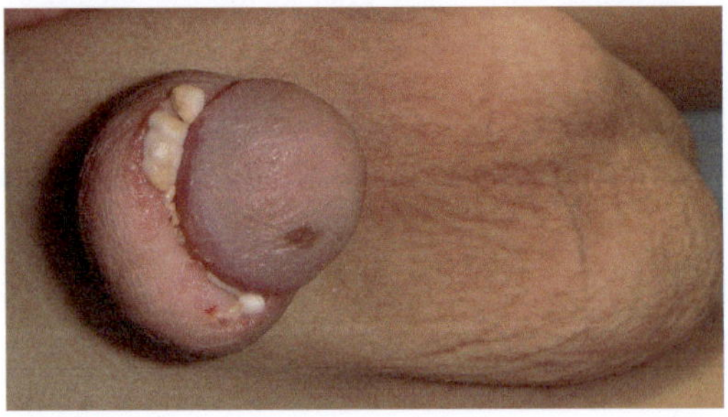

Fig. 26.2 Multiple small smegmoliths at the coronal sulcus

Pathogenesis

Prepuce may had a single calculus or a multiple calculi; Bhat G S [6] reported an elderly male, with azotaemia who had a 25 calculi in his prepuce (Fig. 26.4).

Preputial calculi may be primary formed over a hard smegma, or it could be secondary from the upper urinary tract expelled in urine and impacted at the stenotic preputial ring or a phimotic preputial meatus.

Preputial calculi arise from many possible mechanisms:

1. Inspissated smegma alone forming a concrete
2. Combination of smegma and urinary salts.
3. Concentration of urinary salts alone.
4. Struvite composition secondary to infection.
5. Trapped stones during migration from the proximal urinary tract calculi.

Stone analyses often reveal calcium oxalate, calcium phosphate and in few cases, triple phosphate as well. Culture of the subpreputial space most often reveals infection with Escherichia coli, Enterococcus sp., and Citrobacter sp. E. coli acting upon urea makes ammonia which combines with the fat in the smegma and forms ammonia soaps [7]. Urinary salts and epithelial debris are deposited around this nucleus which increases the size and the density of the stone.

Stone composition varies in the published reports, but stones are most commonly composed of ammonium magnesium phosphate; however, other materials, including urate, calcium phosphate, and calcium oxalate, may be encountered as well.

Predisposing Factors

- Phimosis is a common pathology with the most reported cases, but only one case of multiple preputial calculi is reported after balanitis xerotica obliterans [8].
- UTI: Unsolved inflammatory process will lead to chronic inflammation and ultimately cause scarring of the prepuce.
- Bad preputial hygiene, with smegma collection, the smegma itself acts as a local irritant which can cause inflammation.
- It is common for stone to form among those with neurologic impairment and paraparesis or paraplegia [9]; this may be due to urinary incontinence and improper preputial cleaning.

In the reported female cases; the prepuce was usually long, and bulging, with an excessive smegma production, and retraction showed the presence of a smegmolith, lying on the one side of the clitoris.

Complications

- Balanoposthitis is common with both smegmoliths and smegma pearls accumulations [10].
- Preputial ulceration and perforations
- Neglected cases may leads to an upper urinary tract obstructive uropathy, such as hydronephrosis and renal failure [2].

Treatment

Treatment involves removal of the calculi, as well as the treatment of the urinary obstruction and stasis which are the primary causes. Opening of the preputial sac through either circumcision or a dorsal slit procedure generally reveals multiple smooth, rounded calculi, which are brittle on examination (Fig. 26.4).

According to patient's wishes either a dorsal slit with preputioplasty or a formal circumcision should be firstly done, and through which the calculi are extracted and any other causative pathology is removed. The recurrence is unlikely specially in cases of properly performed circumcision, which usually suffices to relieve the obstructive uropathy as well.

If there are any other associated causes such as calculi higher up in the urinary tract, it should be managed either in the same setting or shortly latter on. Treatment should be directed to the metabolic abnormality when such abnormality is found on evaluation [11].

References

1. Cut Through Smegma. Horse J;2007, pp. 19–20.
2. Tuğlu D, Yuvanç E, Yılmaz E, Batislam E, Gürer YK. Unknown complication of preputial calculi: preputial skin fistula. Int Urol Nephrol. 2013;45(5):1253–5. https://doi.org/10.1007/s11255-013-0496-x.

3. Mohapatra TP, Kumar S. Concurrent preputial calculi and penile carcinoma—a rare association. Postgrad Med J. 1989;65(762):256–7. https://doi.org/10.1136/pgmj.65.762.256.
4. Kaan GW. Bull. Free Hosp. Women;1903, i, 17.
5. Central Union Bank Building, Evansville, Indiana REFERENCES CABOT, HUGH: Modern Urology;1918, p. 225.
6. Bhat GS. Preputial calculi: a case report and review of literature. Indian J Surg. 2017;79(1):70–2. https://doi.org/10.1007/s12262-016-1452-7.
7. Ellis DJ, Siegel AL, Elder JS, Duckett JW. Preputial calculus: a case report. J Urol. 1986;136(2):464–5.
8. Kekre GA, Kothari PR, Gupta AR, Patil PS, Kamble RS, Dikshit KV, et al. A rare case of preputial calculi in a child with balanitis xerotica obliterans: a short communication. Afr J Urol. 2016;22:227–9. https://doi.org/10.1016/j.afju.2015.05.002.
9. Chong TH, Asyraf MZ, Hayati F, et al. Giant preputial calculus: the first reported case in Malaysia. Case Rep Surg. 2018;2018:4606259. https://doi.org/10.1155/2018/4606259, 3 pages.
10. Sonnex C, Croucher PE, Dockerty WG. Balanoposthitis associated with the presence of subpreputial "smegma stones". Genitourin Med. 1997;73:567.
11. Kim SO, Juag GD, Jang CS, Paick JS, Lee MS. Preputial calculi associated with urethral calculi, bladder calculi and bladder transitional cell carcinoma: a case report. Korean J Urol. 1983;24(3):487–90.

Part IV

Preputial Neoplasm

27 Preputial Angiokeratomas

Definition and Synonym

Angiokeratoma is a vascular expansion with a hyperkeratotic surface, it may be multiple lesions and affect the scrotum and hence called Angiokeratoma Scroti or the vulva; Angiokeratoma Vulvae, prepuce may be involved along the scrotal skin, or very rarely angiokeratoma may be an isolated pathology of the prepuce and usually poses a diagnostic challenge (Fig. 27.1).

Multiple angiokeratomas of the scrotal skin are common in older men, such cases are presented with a bright red or more blue-red hemangiectases, 1–5 mm in size, of slowly increasing numbers, with varying verrucous components.

In females angiokeratomas are small vascular papules found on the labia majora, and rarely may be extended to involve the clitoris or preputial hood. They vary in colour from red to blue-black and are normally asymptomatic, but can become quite large and bleed if traumatised, particularly during pregnancy.

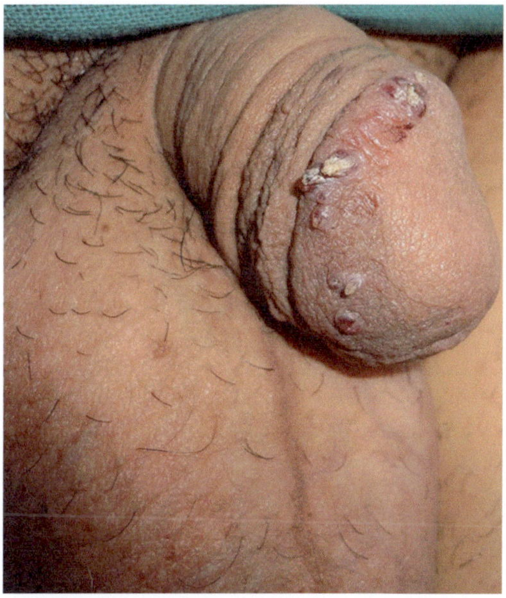

Fig. 27.1 Angiokeratomas appear as a multiple, bluish purple hyperkeratotic papules at the coronal sulcus

Epidemiology

Genital angiokeratomas are frequent in adult patients, appearing at about 30–40 years of age.

Etiology

It is the result of the dilatation of dermal papillae vessels. Possible pathogenetic mechanisms include venous hypertension, vascular malformations and vascular fragility.

M. A. B. Fahmy, *Normal and Abnormal Prepuce*, https://doi.org/10.1007/978-3-030-37621-5_27

Clinical Findings and Course

This nevoid malformation usually exists at birth. A telangiectatic nevus of a red-blue- blackish color is found, usually on the leg, as a result of the multiplication and dilatation of the papillary capillaries, and is covered by a wart-like hyperkeratosis. Occasionally it also shows a linear or zosteriform arrangement. They consist of one or more vascular papular lesions with a hyperkeratotic surface and a maximum diameter of 1–5 mm. They are mainly localized on the scrotum, less often on the penis and prepuce.

Clinical Course

Although angiokeratomas are generally benign, in rare cases they can reveal systemic disorders, such as Fabry's disease (Fabry disease is an X-linked lysosomal storage disorder caused by pathogenic variants in GLA gene encoding the lysosomal enzyme α-galactosidase) [1]. Cases diagnosed at childhood will shows growth parallels the growth of the affected area, occasionally lesions reveal a spontaneous growth in adolescence or later. There is no tendency for spontaneous regression.

Diagnosis

It is generally clinical, in dermatoscopy, angiokeratoma is characterized by the presence of a whitish veil and red or dark lacunae. A histopathological examination can be helpful in certain cases to distinguish angiokeratomas from other vascular tumors.

Histopathology

Ectatic capillaries in the subepidermal space with hyperkeratotic epidermis.

Differential Diagnosis

This solitary verrucous, can be confused with a verrucous malignant melanoma and angiokeratoma corporis diffusum [2].

Treatment

Excision is only indicated for aesthetic reasons. It can be achieved by electric coagulation or laser therapy.

References

1. Saha M, Barlow R, Bunker CB. Angiokeratoma circumscriptum of the penis. Br J Dermatol. 2006;154:775–6.
2. Kelly B, Kelly E. Angiokeratoma corporis diffusum in a patient with no recognizable enzyme abnormalities. Arch Dermatol. 2006;142:615–8.

28 Preputial Warts

Abbreviations

AGW	Anogenital warts
DM	Diabetes mellitus
MMR	Measles, mumps, and rubella
HPV	Human papilloma virus
STI	Sexually transmitted infection
VEGAS	Verruciform genital-associated xanthoma

Definition

Apart from a few exceptions, warts are benign infectious epithelial proliferations. Underlying them is a virus-induced reactive epithelial hyperplasia (acanthosis, hyperkeratosis), capable of regression, with associated expansion of the connective tissue papillary body (papillomatosis), warts occur on skin and mucous membranes, as a rule they heal without scarring and generally confer immunity. Penile warts are the most common sexually transmitted disease in males. HPV is the most common STI worldwide and genital warts are a manifestation of infection by this virus. More than 90% of cases of AGW are caused by HPV types 6 and 11 [1].

Penile warts are either:

- Viral warts
- Seborrheic warts

Seborrheic keratosis of the penis is a rare entity, it has been mistaken as genital warts and differentiation is only made on histopathology. It is typically presents as an asymptomatic, well-demarcated, round or oval, brown plaque with a 'stuck on' warty appearance (Fig. 28.1). Oftenly, lesions may appear shiny and oily and, hence, the misnomer 'seborrheic' (greasy) keratosis. Sites of predilection include the face and chest. Occurrence on the penis is rare but has been reported. HPV is found in approximately 70% of cases of seborrheic keratosis in the genital area versus 5% in nongenital areas [2].

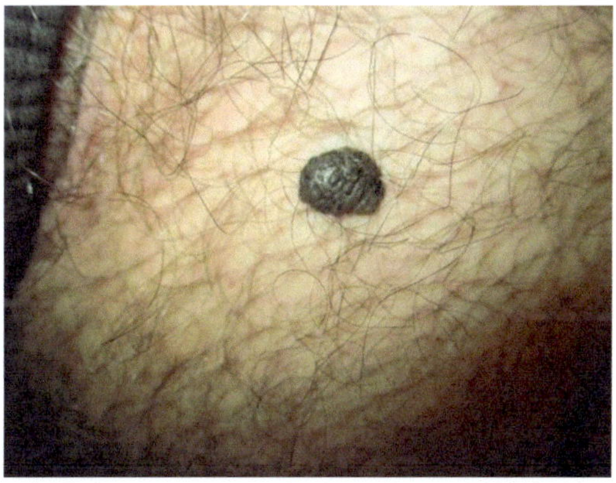

Fig. 28.1 Pedunculated seborrheic genital wart [3]

M. A. B. Fahmy, *Normal and Abnormal Prepuce*, https://doi.org/10.1007/978-3-030-37621-5_28

Rarely seborrheic keratosis may be presented with a multiple pedunculated warts, this condition should be considered in the differential diagnosis for the warty lesions of the penis and histopathology after shave excision will help in the diagnosis [3].

Nomenclatures

Anogenital warts (AGWs), also known as condyloma acuminata, however, AGW and condyloma acuminata are often used as synonyms, other names which are not commonly in use are; Verrugas anogenitais, Condiloma acuminado, Common warts (verruca vulgaris)

Incidence

The incidence of AGW in children has increased in recent decades, it is greatly associated with sexual abuse, and represent a possible long-term complications of this condition. A concomitant increase in adults is also reported [4].

Prenatal transmission of HPV to the fetus, and perinatal transmission may occur during childbirth by the direct contact with the infected genital tract of the mother, which is known as vertical transmission, while horizontal transmission is particularly a contamination by the parents or caregivers of the child, by direct contact [5].

AGW represent a failure of immune recognition, although they only rarely have oncogenic potential. Although the transmission of HPV does not necessitate clinical lesions to be present, the viral burden of AGW is usually high and can therefore facilitate transmission.

The warts grow via a virally induced increase in cell number, leading to the thickening of the basal, spinous, and granular layers of the epidermis. Utilizing the keratinization process, the virus crosses the skin layers and is released with dead cells from the upper layer [5].

Clinically

The warts usually appear as skin-colored verrucous papules approximately 1–5 mm in diameter (Fig. 28.2). They can be pedicled, and, if extremely exophytic, they may have a cauliflower-like appearance. Giant tumor masses that occupy the anogenital area are known as Buschke-Lowenstein tumors [4]. Warts are usually asymptomatic; however, they may bleed, become painful, or pruritic.

Diagnosis

The diagnosis of AGW is primarily clinical, but it may be aided by magnification instruments, together with the application of acetic acid or dyes such as lugol dye [6].

Biopsy and histological examination should be conducted in case of doubt. Molecular biology methods, such as polymerase chain reaction (PCR) and hybrid capture, can detect genomic HPV sequences in different lesions produced by the virus, thus enabling the screening of genetic material in epithelial cells and genotyping.

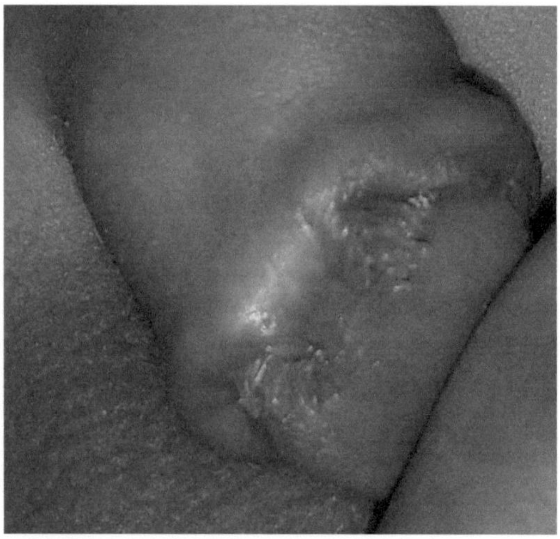

Fig. 28.2 Fine genital worts affecting the prepuce and the coronal sulcus, with a skin bridge between the warts

Predisposing Factors

Although it is well known that DM is a predisposing factor for infection in general, and for AGW in particular, the mechanisms for this predisposition are not completely understood, but it could be related to depressed immunity.

Many cases diagnoses at childhood are secondary to child abuse, and homosexuality at adulthood [6].

Clinically

The warts presented as exophytic growths, with rooster comb appearance and completely circled the preputial ring in most cases. Maceration, fissures and bleeding could often be observed on the prepuce.

The condition may cause physical problems such as pain, itching, burning, irritation. In addition, AGW can impact the sexual activity of patients, either through fear of transmission or embarrassment of lesions. Furthermore, AGW are associated with substantial direct and indirect costs. Overall genital warts represent a frustrating challenge for both patients and physicians. Apart from the psychological aspects, extensive genital warts on prepuce can cause discomfort during sexual intercourse, bleeding, ulceration, or even phimosis in severe cases. The treatment itself can cause scarring and phimosis if used incorrectly or aggressively.

Phimosis and/or paraphimosis were often present (Fig. 28.3). The frenulum could also be covered with warts. The coronal sulcus and glans were seldom involved.

Balanitis was commonly seen, especially as candidal balanitis, balanitis was found in (71.4%) patients, and of these (83.3%) cases were candidal balanitis as confirmed by fungal culture [7].

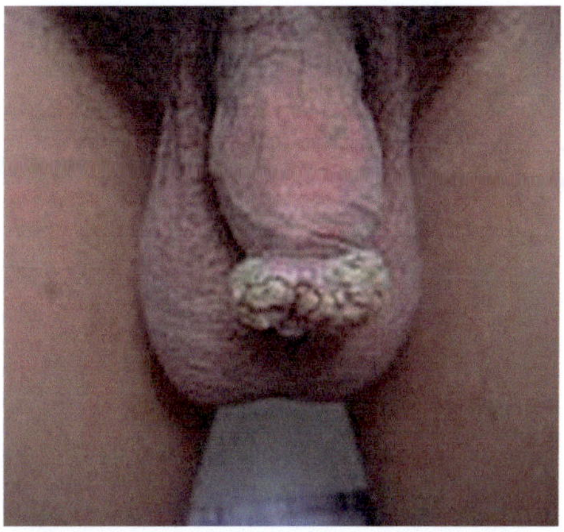

Fig. 28.3 Condylomata acuminata of the prepuce. The warts presented as exophytic growths circling the preputial ring. Phimosis and candidal balanitis was also present

Management

Most AWs disappear spontaneously within a few months or years in children with healthy immune systems. Therefore, active non-intervention is an option in children with asymptomatic lesions. However, studies suggest that lesions should be actively treated in cases in which they persist for more than 2 years or are symptomatic [6].

Treatment is important to avoid malignant transformation and to decrease the risk of further transmission. Treatments can be divided into surgical and non-surgical methods. Surgical methods involve the non-specific elimination of infected tissue, including cryotherapy, CO_2 laser therapy, pulsed- light therapy, electrocoagulation, and surgical excision. These procedures often require local or general anesthesia [7].

Local application of cytotoxic agents, such as podophyllotoxin, is recommended as initial treatment. Remaining warts are usually removed surgically by cautery, diathermy, laser, or excision. Genital condylomata, as well as warts located in the vagina or on the cervix, are preferably removed surgically without pretreatment with podophyllotoxin [8].

There are multiple treatment options available depending on the number and location of lesions, response to previous treatments, local availability of the medications, cost, and patient's wishes. For fewer lesions, and in compliant patients, topical therapy such as podofilox solution or imiquimod works well. But these have a long response time and if applied incorrectly can cause damage.

Destructive modalities such as cryotherapy and electrofulguration have the advantage of rapid response, but in cases of extensive lesions, these may have to be done in a phased manner to avoid patient trauma and mutilation [9].

Twice daily applications of 1% 5-fluorouracil (5-FU) in 70% ethanol on penile condylomas, with complete cures were obtained in 37% and marked regression in 42% of the patients. The most pronounced effect was seen on warts in the preputial cavity and on the adjacent foreskin [10].

In the cases of condylomata acuminata associated with DM, management of DM was carried out during the same therapy session [11].

Intralesional immunotherapy has shown promising efficacy in the treatment of warts including the following: Bacille Calmette–Guerin vaccine, candida antigen, and measles, mumps, and rubella (MMR) vaccine. Meena D et al. reported two cases of genital warts, with an excellent response after intralesional MMR vaccine [12].

References

1. O'Mahony C, Gomberg M, Skerlev M, Alraddadi A, Heras-Alonso M, Majewski S, Nicolaidou E, Serdaroğlu S, Kutlubay Z, Tawara M, Stary A, Al Hammadi A, Cusini M. Position statement for the diagnosis and management of anogenital warts. J Eur Acad Dermatol Venereol. 2019;33:1006–19. https://doi.org/10.1111/jdv.15570.
2. Leung AK, Barankin B, Leong KF, Hon KL. Penile warts: an update on their evaluation and management. Drugs Context. 2018;7:212563. https://doi.org/10.7573/dic.212563.
3. Thakur JS, Thakur A, Chauhan CGS, Diwana VK, Chauhan DC, Giant pedunculated seborrheic keratosis of penis. Indian J Dermatol. 2008;53(1):37–8. https://doi.org/10.4103/0019-5154.39743.
4. Costa-Silva M, Rodrigues AG. Anogenital warts in pediatric population. An Bras Dermatol. 2017;92(5):675–81. https://doi.org/10.1590/abd1806-4841.201756411.
5. Steinberg JL, Cibley LJ, Rice PA. Genital warts: diagnosis, treatment, and counselling for the patient. Curr Clin Top Infect Dis. 1993;13:99–122.
6. Drezett J, Vasconcellos RM, Pedroso D, Blake MT, Oliveira AG, Abreu LZ. Transmission of anogenital warts in children and association with sexual abuse. Rev Bras Crescimento Desenvolv Hum. 2012;22:34–40.
7. Lopaschuk CC. New approach to managing genital warts. Can Fam Physician. 2013;59:731–6.
8. Hallén A, Ljunghall K, Wallin J. Topical anaesthesia with local anaesthetic (lidocaine and prilocaine, EMLA) cream for cautery of genital warts. Genitourin Med. 1987;63(5):316–9.
9. Summary of the 2012 CDC Sexually Transmitted Diseases (STD). Treatment guidelines new Hampshire infectious disease prevention, investigation and care services section. Accessed 20 Sep 2014. http://www.dermakuwait.com/Summary_STDs_tt_Guidelines_2010.
10. von Krogh G. The beneficial effect of 1% 5-fluorouracil in 70% ethanol on therapeutically refractory condylomas in the preputial cavity. Sex Transm Dis. 1978;5(4):137–40.
11. Wang XL, Wang HW, Hillemanns P, Hamblin MR. Distinctive features of foreskin condylomata acuminata associated with diabetes mellitus. Acta Derm Venereol. 2008;88(6):578–83. https://doi.org/10.2340/00015555-0537.
12. Meena D, Sharma S, Chauhan P. Measles, mumps, and rubella vaccine in genital warts: a case report of two patients. Indian J Sex Transm Dis AIDS. 2018;39(2):133–5. https://doi.org/10.4103/ijstd.IJSTD_44_16.

29 Preputial Xanthoma and Rare Preputial Tumors

Xanthomas in general are reactive yellowish tumors caused by the extravasation of serum lipoproteins through the vascular walls and through local ingestion by scavenger receptor-mediated endocytosis and macrophages.

The conditions causing xanthomas are:

- In most cases, pathological concentrations of lipoproteins in the plasma
- Abnormal permeability of the vascular walls.
- Penetration of serum lipoproteins through the vascular walls and their deposition in perivascular connective tissue.
- Ingestion and processing by pericytes and accumulating macrophages.

Genital xanthoma could be:

- Papular Xanthoma: This is a syndrome of normolipemic papular xanthomatosis of skin and mucous membrane with a benign, self-healing course in which no early histocyte phase has been recognized.
- Verruciform Xanthoma

Definition

This is a very rare neoplasia, occurring in both sexes and in all age groups, the lesions are located preferentially on the oral or genital skin.

Clinical Findings

It becomes manifest as a wart-like lesion which is diagnosed only after histopathological examination, with characteristic acanthokeratotic lesion and a dense accumulation of foam cells in the dermis [1].

Verruciform xanthoma mainly affects the mouth, and the genitalia are the next most frequently involved area, where it presents as a painless, yellow-brown or red, verrucous, sessile or papillary plaque. Fewer than 20 cases have been reported. The histological findings are hyperkeratosis, focal parakeratosis, acanthosis and fat-filled foam cells in the papillary dermis. Verruciform xanthoma is thought to represent epidermal degeneration, with keratinocyte lipid then taken up by dermal macrophages or fibroblasts to form the foam cells. HPV type 6 has been implicated in one case but excluded in another. Treatment is by surgical excision [2].

Clinically, they present as solitary plaques or warty lesions and vary in colour from yellow to grey or pink. There is acanthosis, papillomatosis and parakeratosis, and the presence of foamy macrophages in the papillary dermis and tips of the elongated rete ridges distinguishes this entity from a viral wart. Nodular fasciitis presents as a painless mass and has rarely been reported on the vulva.

M. A. B. Fahmy, *Normal and Abnormal Prepuce*, https://doi.org/10.1007/978-3-030-37621-5_29

Other conditions affecting mucous membranes (e.g., verruciform xanthoma) may rarely also affect the foreskin and glans penis. Verruciform genital-associated xanthoma (VEGAS) is an asymptomatic wart-like benign lesion of unknown pathogenesis. The classic histologic appearance consists of foamy histiocytes within elongated dermal papillae and epithelial acanthosis. A biopsy is required and complete excision by surgery, fractionated CO_2 laser or treatment with imiquimod cream have all been described as a curative modality if the lesion is completely excised otherwise recurrent cases have also been reported [3].

Rare Preputial Neoplastic Lesions

Apocrine Hidrocystoma

Apocrine hidrocystoma is a benign adenomatous cystic proliferation of apocrine glands, which rarely occurs on the genitalia and is most prevalent in adults between 30 and 70 years of age. It is subdivided into proliferative or non-proliferative. In the proliferative type, true complex papillae with a fibrous core are seen and usually associated with atypia and mitotic activity, whereas, in the non proliferative type, there may be some structures that resemble papillary projections but lack the fibrous core. Excision of apocrine hidrocystoma is generally curative with recurrence as a remote possibility. Other treatments described are electrodesiccation, anticholinergic creams, and CO_2 laser treatment [4].

Preputial Neurofibroma

Primary neurofibroma of the prepuce is a rare benign lesion, detected in some children. It arises from Schwann cell proliferation, which is positive for SI00 marker, Clinically, it has been described as an asymptomatic penile mass along with multiple cafe-au-lait spots and complete resection is curative and a key is to avoid recurrence [5]. Preputial hood neurofibroma will be described with the female prepuce (Chap. 34).

Penile Traumatic Neuroma

Clinically, the differential diagnosis for single or multiple penile papules is broad and includes condyloma acuminatum, pearly penile papules, Bowenoid papulosis and sebaceous gland hyperplasia. Rarely, a traumatic neuroma may also present as a papular penile lesion.

Traumatic neuromas are benign and develop as a consequence of trauma to a nerve, commonly detected after circumcision. The normal reparative process of the damaged nerve is disrupted leading to a disorganised exuberant proliferation of axons and nerve sheath cells [6].

Benign spindle cell tumors is a very rare neoplasm, which may affect the penis and the prepuce, we encountered only one case of such tumor developed in the edges of preputial remnants, one year after circumcision and histopathology proved the benign nature of the swelling (Fig. 29.1).

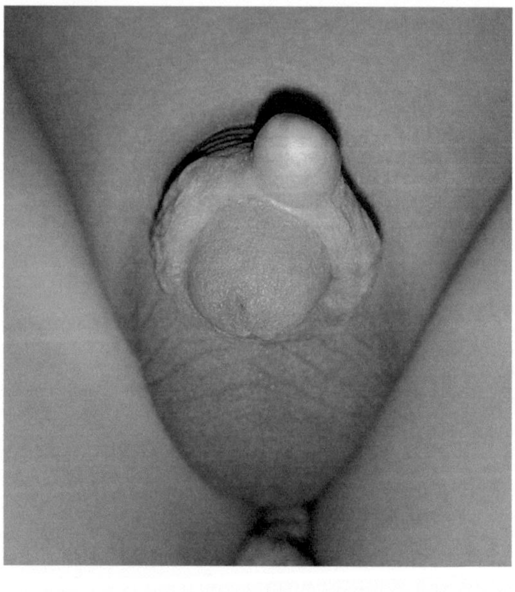

Fig. 29.1 Benign spindle cell tumor at the preputial edge in a 5 years circumcised boy (with a kind permission from Dr. Ahmed Al Shamy, AlAzhar University, Cairo)

References

1. Caputo R, Passoni E, Cavicchini S. Papular xanthoma associated with angiokeratoma of Fordyce: considerations on the nosography of this rare non-Langerhans cell histiocytoxanthomatosis. Dermatology. 2003;206:165–8.
2. Ers ̦ahin C, Szpaderska AM, Foreman K, Yong S. Verucciform xanthoma of the penis not associated with human papillomavirus infection. Arch Pathol Lab Med. 2005;129:e62–4.
3. Stiff KM, Cohen PR. Vegas (verruciform genital-associated) xanthoma: a comprehensive literature review. Dermatol Ther. 2017;7:65–79.
4. Sarabi K, Khachemoune A. Hidrocystomas—a brief review. MedGenMed. 2006;8:57.
5. Littlejohn JO, Belman AB, Selby D. Plexiform neurofibroma of the penis in a child. Urology. 2000;56:669.
6. Cardoso TA, dos Santos KR, Franzotti AM, Avelar JC, Tebcherani AJ, Pegas JR. Traumatic neuroma of the penis after circumcision - case report. Bras Dermatol. 2015;90:397–9.

30 Preputial Hyperpigmentation

Abbreviation

MSH Melanocyte stimulating hormone

Hyperpigmented Prepuce

It is more common in black persons, it is present in 20% of Mongolian and in 5% of Caucasian infants, hyperpigmentation of the linea nigra can coexist [1] (Fig. 30.1).

The hyperpigmentation is believed to be due to a MSH stimulation in the uterus, but the precise pathogenetic mechanism is not clear. The physiological hyperpigmentation of the prepuce is usually identical to the scrotal pigmentation and corrugation. Physiological cases must be differentiated from the rare hyperpigmentation due to a congenital adrenal hyperplasia (Fig. 30.2).

A unique hyperpigmentation of the penis in the form of a transverse circular bands alternated with bands of normal or hypopigmented color which gives the penis a tiger tail look is very rare [2] (Fig. 30.3).

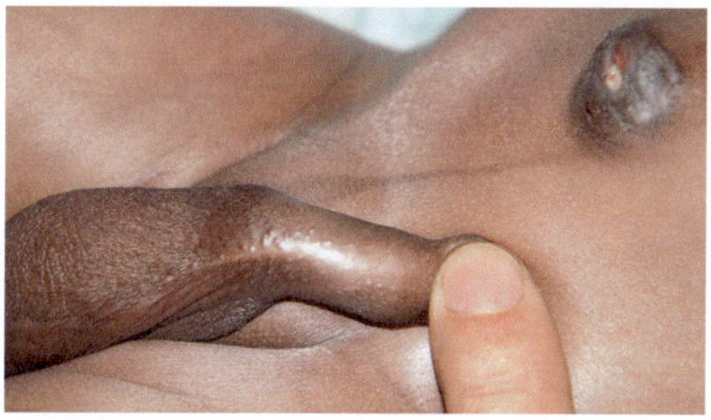

Fig. 30.1 Preputial hyperpigmentation usually associated with a wide pigmented linea nigra

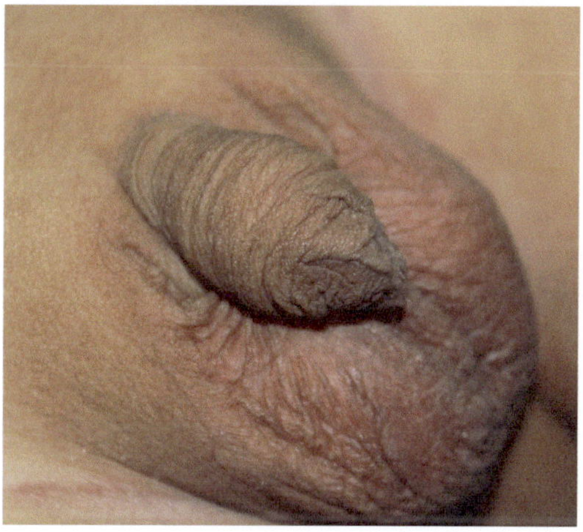

Fig. 30.2 Normal preputial hyperpigmentation of the redundant prepuce, with corrugation looks like the scrotum

M. A. B. Fahmy, *Normal and Abnormal Prepuce*, https://doi.org/10.1007/978-3-030-37621-5_30

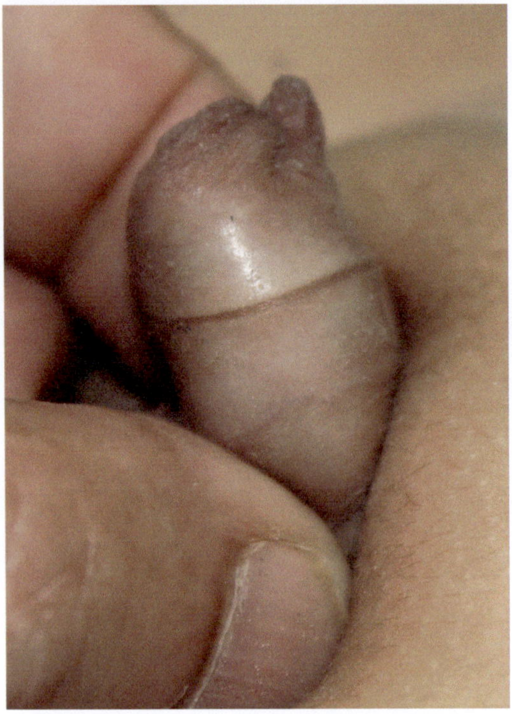

Fig. 30.3 Circular liner hyperpigmentation of the prepuce

Preputial Melanosis

Definition

Melanosis is a benign pigmented lesion of mucosa and skin characterized by pigmentation of basal keratinocytes with normal, or a slightly increased number of melanocytes.

Congenital and acquired melanocytic nevi are respectively benign neoplasms or hamartomas, composed of melanocytes. In acquired lesions, nevus cells may form some peculiar clusters at the dermal junction (junctional nevi), in the dermis (dermal and blue nevi), or in both (compound nevi).

Etiology

It remains unknown, both genetic and environmental (sun exposure) factors seem to be involved in the development of melanocytic nevi. It is considered idiopathic, but some cases have been described in the literature related to trauma, irritation or PUVA therapy [3].

It is possible that naevi on the penis occur more frequently in patients with the atypical naevus syndrome, but this has not been formally documented.

Epidemiology

There is no data available about the exact incidence of preputial melanosis, but it is not a rare lesions, in a series of 372 consecutive circumcisions for phimosis performed during the period of 2 years; Val-Bernal et al. [4] detected preputial melanocytic nevi in (1.1%) of the patients.

Cullen [5] states that 9% of males have at least one acquired melanocytic nevus in the area of genitalia during lifetime.

Classifications

Melanocytic nevi localized in the genital area may be congenital and acquired. Acquired melanocytic nevi usually appear firstly in early childhood and reach a maximum in adolescence (Fig. 30.4). Nevi decline in numbers after the age of 50 years, and by the age of 90 years, they are usually none to be detected, as they have faded [6].

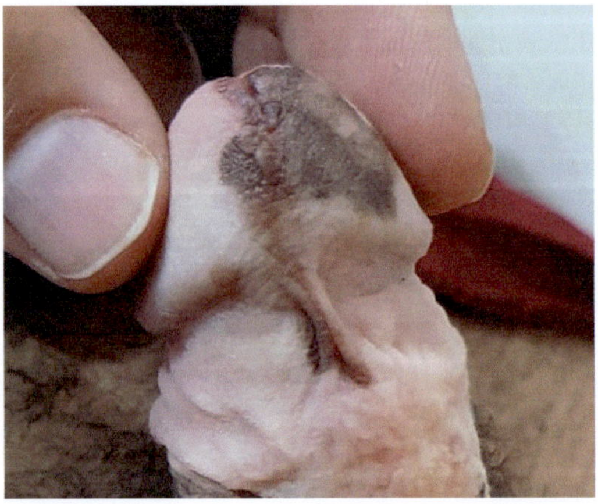

Fig. 30.4 Large nevus at the under surface of the glans with frenular affection with a vitiligo affecting the rest of the penis

Congenital nevi have been classified into 3 groups according to size:

- Small nevi are less than 1.5 cm in greatest diameter.
- Medium nevi are 1.5–19.9 cm in greatest diameter.
- Large or giant nevi are greater than 20 cm in greatest diameter.

Junctional nevi are sharply marginated, tan to dark brown macules, only a few millimetres in diameter. Compound and dermal nevi are soft, sharply marginated, and brown to skin coloured. Blue nevi are bluish to gray-brown papules (Fig. 30.5).

Congenital nevi, depending on size and location, may have a significant impact on cosmoses. There is no racial predilection recognized for congenital nevi, it occurs equally in both sexes.

Giant congenital melanocytic nevi (CMN) also known as “bathing trunk nevi” or “garment nevi” are large macular lesions with diameters over 20 cm that are present since birth and develop coarse terminal hair over a period of years. The surface was rugose, leathery, and with fine hairs [7].

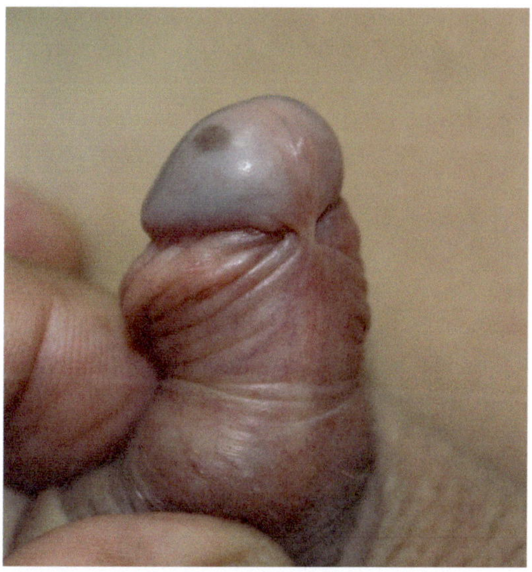

Fig. 30.5 Small congenital nevus of the glans penis, frenulum brave is also noticeable

Genital melanosis may be a part of systemic hyperpigmentation, or the genitalia may be involved along the course of giant melanoma of the abdominal wall or buttock (Fig. 30.6).

Post circumcision hyperpigmentation, is an acquired melanosis, which may be secondary to the irritation or surgical trauma, it is not rare, but not frequently reported. It may be presented as a localised pigmentations or freckles at the inner mucosal remnant of the prepuce (Fig. 30.7).

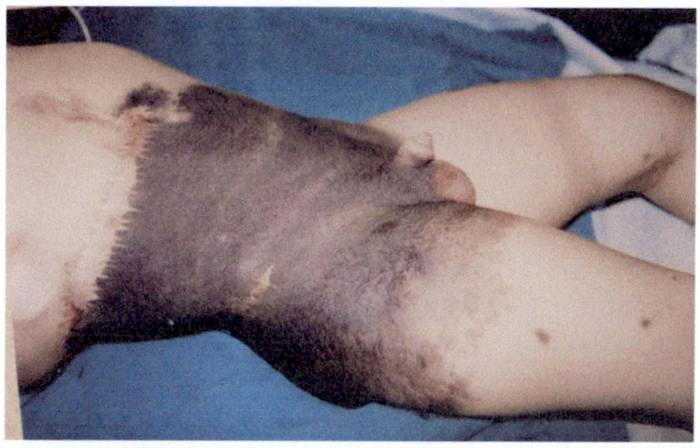

Fig. 30.6 Penile involvement along a giant abdominal wall melanocytic nevus

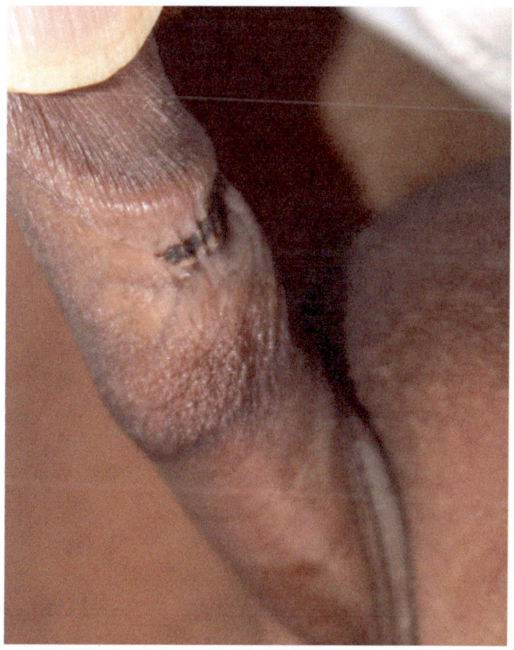

Fig. 30.7 A raised hyperpigmented freckle at the mucosal remnant detected 1 year after circumcision

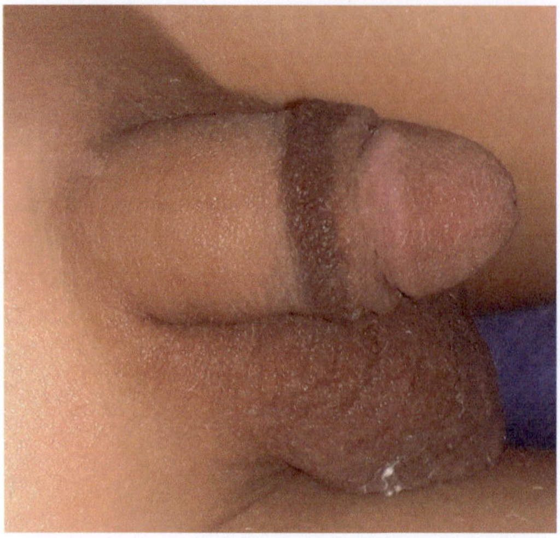

Fig. 30.8 Post circumcision circular hyperpigmentation

Also post circumcision preputial hyperpigmentation may attributes a ring formed around the scar line; such cases may end at adulthood with the picture of Two-Toned penis, where the post circumcision scar looks hyperpigmented in comparison to the rest of penile skin [8] (Fig. 30.8).

This over-toned penis may be considered an ugly or non aesthetic for some men. In a survey completed by National Organization of Restoring Men, in UK, 74% of the respondents were dissatisfied with the appearance of their circumcised penises, and particularly, 26% complained about the variation in skin colour [9].

General Features

Penile melanosis are nonneoplastic hyperpigmented lesions that can clinically be confused with benign and malignant melanocytic proliferations. They are usually found in the glans, the prepuce, or both. Penile melanosis usually manifests as a large, single, pigmented macule with irregular borders. Rarely the lesions are multiple, asymptomatic, dyschromic, and with irregular borders [10]. Melanosis, particularly when occurring on the genitalia, can clinically mimic mucosal melanoma, creating concern in both the patient and the physician.

It is very rarely to detect a large melanoma in the prepuce and/or the penis, also prepuce is very rarely affected by hypopigmentation or vitiligo (Fig. 30.4).

Clinical Course

Little is known about the natural history or the risk of developing melanoma. Most of the lesions remain stable over decades, and evolution into genital melanoma is rare and occurs in the elderly.

Microscopic

The histological picture is similar in all entities. Melanocytic hyperplasia with more or less prominent hyperpigmentation of basal layers in an otherwise normal epidermis is the typical finding [11].

Diagnosis

It is generally made on the basis of clinical findings, dermatoscopy is often important for the differential diagnosis with other pigmented skin lesions and for the individuation of atypical lesions. Sometimes, multiple biopsies may be necessary to avoid misdiagnosis and to confirm the benign nature of the condition by the lack of atypical features on histopathological examination.

Differential Diagnosis

These hyperpigmented lesions should be distinguished from acral malignant melanoma. The diagnosis is made by histological examination of the lesion.

Special Forms of Genital Melanosis

Spitz naevus has been rarely described in genitalia. It is often suspected clinically by its characteristic small size, raised, pink, red or brown nodule, dome-shaped appearance and rapid growth over a few weeks to months. It may resemble hemangioma or pyogenic granuloma. Several new data indicate that these tumors are genetically more diverse than was previously thought [12].

Divided or kissing naevus (analogous to the entity recognized naevus on the eyelids) has been reported, with one component located on the dorsal or dorsolateral side of the glans and the other on the distal penile shaft or inner face of the prepuce, and separated by uninvolved skin across the coronal sulcus. It has been hypothesized that melanoblasts migrate to the lesion before the embryological separation of epithelial preputial placode, just following the completion of the preputial epithelial placode invagination at the twelfth gestation week [13] (Fig. 30.9).

Therapy

Treatment depends on the type of the nevi, its location and abnormal features detected in the dermatoscopic examination [14]. For small lesions, which can easily be removed, surgery is the best option. Large or multiple lesions should be monitored with videodermatoscopy before planning treatment, to evaluate clinical changes such as enlargement or discolouration [15]. Definitely all atypical lesions require surgical excision.

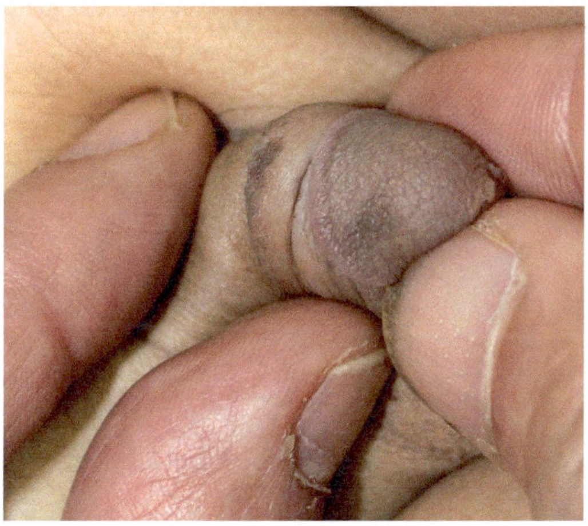

Fig. 30.9 Small divided neavi (kissing naevus) affecting both the glans and the prepuce

Preputial Freckles

Freckles are clusters of concentrated melaninized cells which are most easily visible on people with a fair complexion. Freckles do not have an increased number of melanocytes, but instead have melanocytes that overproduce melanin granules (melanosomes) results in changing the coloration of the outer skin cells (keratinocytes). As such, freckles are different from lentigines and moles, which are caused by accumulation of melanocytes in a small area. Freckles can appear on all types of skin tones, and in all races and rarely it may affect the genitalia or the prepuce.

Preputial Lentigo

A lentigo (/lɛnˈtaɪgoʊ/) (plural lentigines, /lɛnˈtɪdʒɪniːz/) is a small pigmented spot on the skin with a clearly defined edge, surrounded by normal-appearing skin. It is a harmless (benign) hyperplasia of melanocytes which is linear in its spread. This means the hyperplasia of melanocytes is restricted to the cell layer directly above the basement membrane of the epidermis where melanocytes normally reside. This is in contrast to the "nests" of multi-layer melanocytes found in moles (melanocytic nevi). Stromal melanophages can occasionally be seen, especially in penile lentiginosis [16].

Lentigoes are distinguished from freckles based on the proliferation of melanocytes. Freckles have a relatively normal number of melanocytes but an increased amount of melanin. A lentigo has an increased number of melanocytes. Freckles will increase in number and darkness with sunlight exposure, whereas lentigines will stay stable in their color regardless of sunlight exposure.

Penile lentiginosis is characterized by the presence of multiple hyperpigmented small-to medium-size lesions with uniform or variegated pigmentation [17] (Fig. 30.10).

Histopathology

Elongation of rete ridges with basal layer hyperpigmentation, slight melanocytic hyperplasia, epithelial hyperplasia and stromal melanophages, no atypia. Lymphocytes, which are found in close apposition, destroy melanocytes and surrounding keratinocytes lack pigmentation.

Management

Generally, there is no treatment required for Lentiginosis of penis, since it is a benign and harmless condition with no significant signs and symptoms or complications. Individuals, in whom it causes significant cosmetic issues, or psychic concern may undergo a surgical excision or laser therapy to have them removed [4]. Surgical excision may be problematic in terms of scarring and subsequent functional restriction.

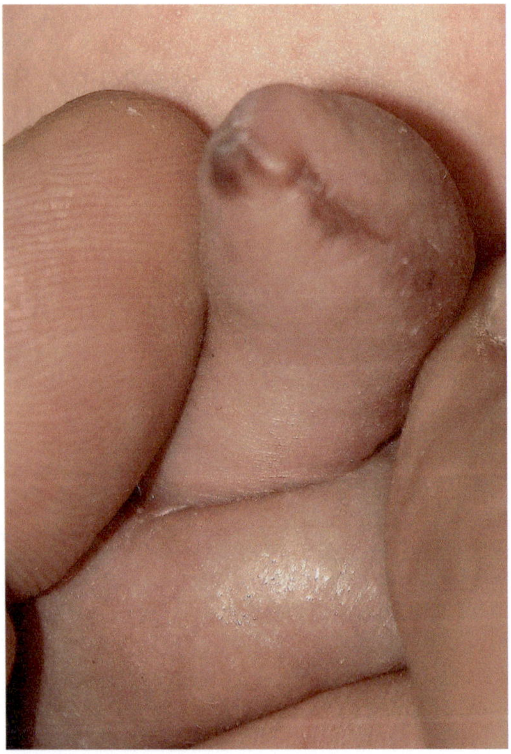

Fig. 30.10 Liner lentigo affecting the ventral surface and meatus of the prepuce

References

1. Rivers JK, Frederiksen PC, Dibdin C. A prevalence survey of dermatoses in the Australian neonate. J Am Acad Dermatol. 1990;23:77–81.
2. Cutrone M, Milano A, Rovatti G, Bonifazi E. Genital and anal anatomical variants. Eur J Pediatr Dermatol. 2013;23:29–45.
3. Fitzpatrick TB, et al. Chapter 75. Hypomelanoses and hypermelanoses. In: Fitzpatrick's dermatology in general medicine. New York: McGraw Hill Companies; 2012. ISBN 978-0-07-166904-7.
4. Val-Bernal F, Val D, Garijo MF. Clinically unapparent melanocytic nevi on the prepuce. J Cutan Pathol. 2009;36:444–7. https://doi.org/10.1111/j.1600-0560.2008.01070.x.
5. Cullen SI. Incidence of nevi. Report of survey of the palms, soles, and genitalia of 10,000 young men. Arch Dermatol. 1962;86:40–3.
6. McGovern VJ, Lane Brown MM. The nature of melanoma, vol. 69. Springfield, IL: Charles C. Thomas; 1969.
7. Reyes-Múgica M, Beckwith M, Etchevers HC. Etiology of congenital melanocytic nevi and related conditions. In: Marghoob AA, editor. Nevogenesis (practical clinical medicine series). Berlin: Springer; 2012. p. 73–97.
8. Allan JA. Chapter 11: Circumcision scars and aesthetic concerns. In: Fahmy M, editor. Complications in male circumcision. St. Louis: Elsevier; 2019. https://doi.org/10.1016/B978-0-323-68127-8.00011-9.
9. Warren JP. NORM UK and the medical case against circumcision. In: Denniston GC, Milos MF, editors. Sexual mutilations: a human tragedy, vol. 95. New York: Plenum Press; 1997.
10. Sopena Barona J, Gamo Villegas R, Guerra Tapia A, Iglesias Díez L. Acromelanosis. An Pediatr. 2003;58:277–80.
11. Cervigón I, Palomo A, Torres LM. Melanotic macules of the penis. Actas Dermosifiliogr. 2007;98:722–3.
12. Aoyagi S, Sato-Matsumura KS, Akiyama M, et al. Spitz naevus of the glans penis: an unusual location. Acta Derm Venereol. 2004;84:324–5.
13. Kono T, Nozaki M, Kikuchi Y, et al. Divided naevus of the penis: a hypothesis on the embryological mechanism of its development. Acta Derm Venereol. 2003;83:155–6.
14. Hengge UR, Meurer M. Pigmented lesions of the genital mucosa. Hautarzt. 2005;56:540–9.
15. Laguna C, Pitarch G, Roche E, Fortea JM. Atypical pigmented penile macules. Actas Dermosifiliogr. 2006;97:470–2.
16. El Shabrawi-Caelen L, Soyer HP, Schaeppi H, et al. Genital lentigines and melanocytic nevi with superimposed lichen sclerosus: a diagnostic challenge. J Am Acad Dermatol. 2004;50:690–4.
17. Mahto M, Woolley PD, Ashworth J. Pigmented penile macules. Int J STD AIDS. 2004;15:717–9.

31 Preputial Malignancy

Abbreviatisons

AABP	Adult acquired buried penis
HPV	Human Papilloma virus
MALToma	Mucosal-associated lymphoid tissue lymphoma
PCB	Plasma cell balanitis
PeIN	Penile intraepithelial neoplasia
SCC	Penile squamous cell carcinoma
WHO	The World Health Organisation
ZB	Zoon's balanitis

Incidence

In general penile cancer is an uncommon genitourinary malignancy with an incidence rate that increases with age, in England the age standardised incidence rate for penile cancer is 1.3 per 100,000 males [1]. Geographical disparities in incidence of penile cancer are evident with high rates concentrated in the developing world (2.8–6.8 per 100,000) where neonatal circumcision is low and the socioeconomic conditions may predispose patients to multiple risk factors [2].

Risk Factors

Risk factors for penile SCC have been heavily scrutinised. Of mention in particular is the affects attributed to neonatal circumcision, the risk associated with pathological phimosis, the rather debated carcinogenic effects of smegma and the close association with lichen sclerosis (LS).

Human Papilloma Virus

The association of human papilloma virus (HPV) with certain penile neoplastic diseases is well known. A systemic review estimates that HPV is found in 48% of penile cancer specimens. Specifically high risk serotypes 16 and 18 were found in 36.7% of the samples examined [3]. In a recent study the human papilloma virus (HPV) has been linked to nearly 40% of cases and molecular mediators continue to be investigated [2].

Phimosis

Phimosis is frequently present in patients with invasive penile cancer. Neoplastic changes of the prepuce may result from chronic balanitis, lichen sclerosis, or other systemic conditions. There is a huge debate about the protective effect of circumcision at birth, which may be related to the prevention of phimosis (Chap. 18) (Fig. 31.1).

The presence of lichen sclerosis is significantly associated with some special subtypes of HPV-unrelated penile carcinomas such as usual, pseudohyperplastic, verrucous, and papillary

M. A. B. Fahmy, *Normal and Abnormal Prepuce*, https://doi.org/10.1007/978-3-030-37621-5_31

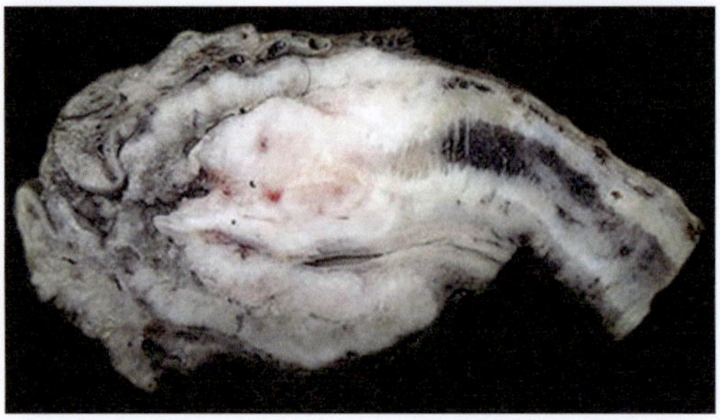

Fig. 31.1 Phimosis. Cut surface of a partial penectomy specimen showing complete obliteration of the preputial orifice due to severe phimosis. The glans and the tumor are concealed [24]

SCCs, especially when located exclusively in the foreskin. Almost 10% of patients with long-standing lichen sclerosus will develop a penile carcinoma [2].

Other risk factors are antecedents of penile tears, abrasions, injuries, chronic balanitis, genital warts, immunosuppression, and human immunodeficiency virus (HIV) infection [4].

To compare the foreskin in the general population and patients with penile cancer, Velazquez et al. examined the foreskin of 215 uncircumcised males without cancer (age range 15–93 years) and the foreskin of 23 patients with cancer (age range 31–90 years), and they found that cancer patients showed a long foreskin in 78% of the cases, and phimosis was significantly frequent in this group (52%) as compared with the other ($p < 0.001$) [5].

In some geographic regions a coexistence of a long foreskin and phimosis with a high incidence of penile cancer is evident, however, the presence of long foreskin may be a necessary but not a sufficient condition for cancer development. So authors supporting preventive circumcision in patients with long and phimotic foreskins living in high-risk areas [5]. Cancers not related to long foreskins, and phimosis may be causally different.

UVA Phototherapy

Treatment with Psoralen UV-A phototherapy (PUVA) for psoriasis and other dermatological conditions poses an increased risk of squamous cell carcinoma on non-sun-exposed skin, few studies have examined its specific association with penile cancer. A recent systematic review reiterated that the risk is dose dependent and can persist even after cessation of treatment [6].

Penile Hygiene

A number of studies have attributed an increase in penile cancer to poor penile hygiene [7].
There is a definite link between long phimotic prepuce, buried penis, accumulation of smegma, retention of urinary excreted smoking carcinogens and poor penile hygiene.

Smoking

Cigarette smoking has been linked to penile cancer, and several epidemiological studies have established a dose–response relation, with heavy smokers at higher risk.
Smoking has been implicated as a risk factor for multiple malignancy sites and penile cancer is no exception. Hellberg et al. [8] showed that smoking could be an independent risk factor after adjusting for confounding factors. In addition, a dose-response effect was also observed with a relative risk (RR) of 1.88 for heavy smokers when compared to light smokers and RR of 2.22 compared to non-smokers.

Buried Penis

The prevalence of penile cancer appears to be higher in patients with adult acquired buried penis (AABP), Because the penile shaft is hidden under overhanging adipose tissue, it oftentimes cannot be exhumed for urination or hygiene. Patients with AABP have urinary dribbling and pooling within the adipose layers of lower abdominal wall, that bury the glans leading to an environment of chronic inflammation, recurrent infections, and ultimately poor quality of life. Patients with AABP may inherently possess multiple risk factors for penile cancer including functional phimosis, poor genital hygiene, morbid obesity and chronic inflammation of the penile skin and glans [9].

Akroposthia

Cancer patients showed a long foreskin in 78% of the cases, and phimosis was significantly frequent in this group (52%) as compared with the other ($p < 0.001$) [5].

Elderly males with redundant prepuce, usually have a hyperplasia and hypertrophy, which may be a precancerous lesions (Chap. 11).

Benign and Pre-Neoplastic Lesions of the Foreskin

- **Penile Lichen Sclerosis**
  Penile lichen sclerosis is a chronic progressive inflammatory condition characterised by a lymphocytic response with a bimodal distribution affecting young boys and middle-aged men. However, more recent literature indicates that 28–50% of penile cancer patients had a history of BXO and estimates a risk of 2–15% for developing a penile squamous cell carcinoma [10] (Chap. 21).
- **Plasma Cell Balanitis**
  Plasma cell balanitis (PCB), also known as balanitis circumscripta plasmacellularis, was first described by Zoon, a Dutch dermatologist in 1952, and is now commonly referred to as Zoon's balanitis. This uncommon dermatosis typically affects uncircumcised middle-aged to elderly men. It presents as a well defined, erythematous plaque with purpuric spots creating a "cayenne pepper" appearance on the glans and inner foreskin [11] (Chap. 22).

  The disease is generally considered benign although, at least three cases of Erythroplasia of Queyrat and one of carcinoma of the penis arising on lesions of ZB have been reported [12].
- **Condyloma Acuminatum**
  Condylomas are warty, exophytic, squamoproliferative sexually transmitted lesions. They may affect any part of the anogenital region and are commonly found on the foreskin and shaft of the penis. They present as single or multiple soft and friable papules. Condylomas are considered as a benign lesion and in 90% of cases are associated with HPV subtypes 6 and 11. However, co infection with high risk oncogenic subtypes, particularly HPV 16 can lead to an increasing the risk of invasive SCC [13].

Pathology and Pathogenesis

Primary Malignancies

Penile intraepithelial neoplasia (PeIN) is the precursor lesion of penile squamous cell carcinoma (SCC). The World Health Organisation (WHO) classifies PeIN into two subtypes based on the association with HPV; these include differentiated and undifferentiated PeIN. These subtypes of PeIN can be differentiated by specific cytological and architectural characteristics [14].

PeIN is also classified into differentiated ("simplex") and undifferentiated, the latter subclassified to warty, basaloid, and warty–basaloid types. There are cases of mixed differentiated–undifferentiated PeIN in the same specimen. Less frequent patterns are clear cell, pagetoid, and pleomorphic, among others. Differentiated PeIN are usually negative for HPV whereas undifferentiated PeIN are frequently associated with the virus. PeIN is frequently found in association with penile carcinomas, either merging with the invasive component or adjacent to it. However, PeIN can also be detected as a single lesion during clinical examination for other conditions or during peniscopy.

Early disease (stage I–II) is curable in most patients, who can be treated by conventional penile amputation or, in selected cases, by organ preserving techniques. For more advanced primary tumours, penile amputation is required [15].

Differentiated PeIN preferentially occurs in the foreskin of older individuals, but the glans is also affected. Undifferentiated PeIN involves preferentially the glans of patients younger than those with differentiated PeIN.

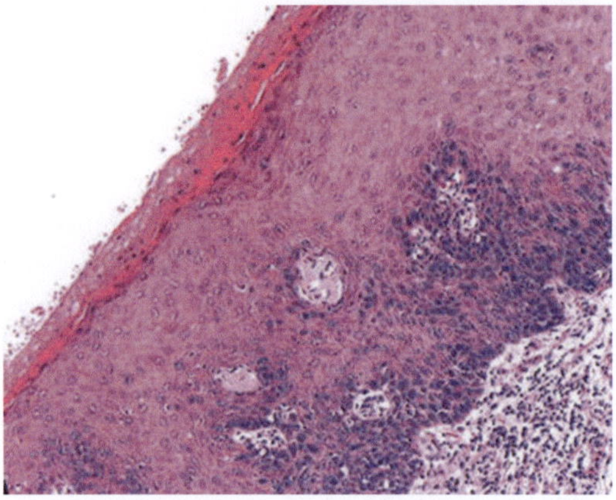

Fig. 31.2 Differentiated PeIN, with hyper and parakeratosis and epithelial thickening, squamous maturation is noted, with mild atypical cells in the basal layers

The vast majority of invasive neoplasms of the penis are squamous cell carcinoma (SCC). Other primary malignancies include but are not limited to basal cell carcinoma, extra-mammary Paget's disease, melanoma, lymphoma and various rare mesenchymal tumours (Fig. 31.2).

Basal Cell Carcinoma of Foreskin

Genital basal cell carcinoma (BCC) is very rare with only 22 reported cases. BCC involves the penile shaft with scrotum and pubic area, and it spreads occasionally. Proposed risk factors include trauma, HPV infection, and ageing. The treatment is surgical excision with complete recovery [16].

Malignant Lymphoma

Penile malignant lymphomas are very rare and can originate in the penis (primary lymphoma) or be secondary to systemic dissemination (secondary lymphoma). All penile compartments can be affected. Priapism and Peyronie disease have been reported in association. Clinically, a flesh-white or ulcerated lesion is the commonest presentation. Most of the cases correspond to diffuse large cell lymphomas, although other types, such as MALT, T-cell, anaplastic and large cell lymphomas, have been reported. Morphological and immunohistochemical criteria for differential diagnosis are similar to those applied for lymphoma elsewhere [17].

Mucosal-Associated Lymphoid Tissue Lymphoma (MALToma)

Extranodal marginal zone B cell (MALT) lymphoma of the foreskin is extremely unusual. In general, Maltoma is the third most common non-Hodgkin lymphoma accounting for up to 8% of cases. Clinically, it has been reported to present as a painless lobulated lesion without lymphadenopathy. The histopathologic characteristics are a neoplastic expansion of marginal zone B cells. The most effective treatment is surgical excision, local radiotherapy, or chemotherapy [17].

Rare Malignant Lesions

Mesenchymal tumors are rare in the male external genitalia. Eisner BH et al. [18] reported two cases with mesenchymal penile malignancy; one of them had a combined dermatofibrosarcoma protuberans, giant cell fibroblastoma, and fibrosarcoma, which is a malignant tumor, the second case was myofibroma, a benign fibroblastic tumor with a prominent myofibroblastic component that is congenital and tends to occur within the first few months after birth [18].

Myeloid Sarcoma

Foreskin myeloid sarcoma is a very rare presentation of myeloid sarcoma. In acute or chronic leukaemia, myeloid cells can proliferate outside the bone marrow, giving rise to cutaneous lesions including erythematous to violaceous papules, nodules, plaques, or persistent non-healing ulcer. The condition is subdivided into well or poorly differentiated types based on the presence of numerous maturing myeloid elements or blasts, respectively. In neonates, the lesion is associated with TORCH (Toxoplasma, Rubella, and Herpesvirus) infection. In adults, myelofibrosis often coexists with rare association with chronic myeloid leukemia. In the setting of an unknown hematological malignancy, the diagnosis of myeloid sarcoma is often challenging. Local therapy may improve symptoms but does not influence survival [19].

Kaposi's Sarcoma

Is a human immune-deficiency virus-related malignant neoplasm that is extremely rare in the foreskin, therefore poses a diagnostic and management challenge. It has been reported to present as paraphimosis and painless purple papule or macule on the foreskin without urethral discharge or lymphadenopathy. Biopsy showing groups of spindle cells, extravascular erythrocytes, and macrophages filled with hemosiderin and immunohistochemistry for human herpesvirus-8 provides a diagnosis. Besides treating the patient with highly active antiretroviral therapy, for small and single lesions, surgical excision is recommended, while for multiple skin lesions or large-size radiation therapy has been recommended [20].

Also few cases of leiomyosarcoma and fibrosarcoma of the penis had been reported, with only 6 cases reported for preputial involvement [21].

Metastasis

The foreskin has rich vascularization and an extensive lymphatic network with the adjacent organs, yet penile metastasis is extremely rare, and the main source is primary pelvic tumors, including 70% with primary tumor in the genitourinary tract, 21% in the gastrointestinal tract; 5% in the respiratory system, and the remaining 4% as metastases from primary bone tumors and malignant melanoma. Metastasis to the foreskin should be differentiated from superficial spread of malignant melanoma, penile koilocytosis, pagetoid dyskeratosis, clear-cell papulosis, and mucinous metaplasia. Therefore, positive immunostaining can help distinguish a metastasis from primary penile lesions [22].

Clinical

Preputial cancer is a rare neoplasm most commonly detected in men aged 50–70 years old. The most common site for penile cancer is the glans, which accounts for 48% of diagnoses, followed by prepuce (21%), glans and prepuce (9%), coronal sulcus (6%) and uncommonly the shaft (<2%) [15].

Patients note changes of the glans or foreskin, but experience no pain. In many cases, the diagnosis of exophytic penile cancer is established by inspection. Superficial stages of penile cancer are often limited to surface changes.

Some patients may present with malignant priapism, penile masses or nodules, ulceration, obstructive or irritative urinary symptoms, and hematuria. Early suspicion and biopsy are necessary to prevent delays in treatment initiation.

Management

Maximally organ-preserving surgery with safety margins of no more than a few millimetres is the current therapeutic standard, because a local recurrence, if it arises, can still be treated locally with curative intent. Local radiotherapy can be performed in early stages. Lymphogenic metastasis must be treated with radical lymphadenectomy and adjuvant chemotherapy. Penile cancer is curable in all early stages with the appropriate treatment, but its prognosis depends crucially on the proper management of the regional (i.e., inguinal) lymph nodes. In many countries, the treatment of this rare disease entity has been centralized [23].

Conclusion

There is a definite link between long phimotic prepuce, buried penis, accumulation of smegma, retention of urinary excreted smoking carcinogens and poor penile hygiene; which is associated with high incidence of penile and preputial malignancy. Many studies indicated that circumcision lowers the risk of penile cancer (hazard ratio: 0.33).

References

1. Montes Cardona CE, Garcia-Perdomo HA. Incidence of penile cancer worldwide: systematic review and meta-analysis. Rev Panam Salud Publica. 2017;41:e117.
2. Douglawi A, Masterson TA. Penile cancer epidemiology and risk factors: a contemporary review. Curr Opin Urol. 2019;29(2):145–9. https://doi.org/10.1097/MOU.0000000000000581.
3. Flaherty A, Kim T, Giuliano A, Magliocco A, Hakky TS, Pagliaro LC, Spiess PE. Implications for human papillomavirus in penile cancer. Urol Oncol. 2014;32(1):53.e1–8.
4. Madsen BS, van den Brule AJC, Jensen HL, Wohlfahrt J, Frisch M. Risk factors for squamous cell carcinoma of the penis—population-based case-control study in Denmark. Cancer Epidemiol Biomark Prev. 2008;17(10):2683.
5. Velazquez EF, Bock A, Soskin A, Codas R, Arbo M, Cubilla AL. Preputial variability and preferential association of long phimotic foreskins with penile cancer: an anatomic comparative study of types of foreskin in a general population and cancer patients. Am J Surg Pathol. 2003;27(7):994–8.
6. Archier E, Devaux S, Castela E, Gallini A, Aubin F, Le Maître M, Aractingi S, Bachelez H, Cribier B, Joly P, Jullien D, Misery L, Paul C, Ortonne JP, Richard MA. Carcinogenic risks of psoralen UV-A therapy and narrowband UV-B therapy in chronic plaque psoriasis: a systematic literature review. J Eur Acad Dermatol Venereol. 2012;26(Suppl 3):22–31.
7. Frisch M, Friis S, Kjaer SK, Melbye M. Falling incidence of penis cancer in an uncircumcised population (Denmark 1943-90). BMJ. 1995;311(7018):1471.
8. Hellberg D, Valentin J, Eklund T, Nilsson S. Penile cancer: is there an epidemiological role for smoking and sexual behaviour? Br Med J. 1987;295(6609):1306–8.
9. Pekala KR, et al. The prevalence of penile cancer in patients with adult acquired buried penis. Urology. 2019;133:229–33. https://doi.org/10.1016/j.urology.2019.07.019.
10. Bunker CB, Shim TN. Male genital lichen sclerosus. Indian J Dermatol. 2015;60(2):111–7.
11. Buechner S. Common skin disorders of the penis. BJU Int. 2002;90:498–506. https://doi.org/10.1046/j.1464-410X.2002.02962.x.
12. Starritt E, Lee S. Erythroplasia of Queyrat of the glans penis on a background of Zoon's plasma cell balanitis. Australas J Dermatol. 2008;49:103–5.
13. Anic GM, Giuliano AR. Genital HPV infection and related lesions in men. Prev Med. 2011;53(Suppl 1):S36–41.
14. Sewell A, Oxley J. An overview of benign and premalignant lesions of the foreskin. Diagn Histopathol. 2019;25:390. https://doi.org/10.1016/j.mpdhp.2019.07.002.
15. Mosconi AM, Roila F, Gatta G, Theodore C, et al. Crit Rev Oncol Hematol. 2005;53(2):165–77.
16. Manavi K, Kemmett D. A case of penile superficial basal cell carcinoma involving the inner surface of foreskin. Int J STD AIDS. 2005;16:766–7.
17. Haque S, Noble J, Wotherspoon A, Woodhouse C, Cunningham D. MALT lymphoma of the foreskin. Leuk Lymphoma. 2004;45:1699–701.
18. Eisner BH, McAleer SJ, Gargollo PC, Perez-Atayde A, Diamond DA, Elder JS. Pediatric penile tumors of mesenchymal origin. Urology. 2006;68(6):1327–30.
19. Lan TY, Lin DT, Tien HF, Yang RS, Chen CY, Wu K. Prognostic factors of treatment outcomes in patients with granulocytic sarcoma. Acta Haematol. 2009;122:238–46.
20. Schwartz RA, Micali G, Nasca MR, Scuderi L. Kaposi sarcoma: a continuing conundrum. J Am Acad Dermatol. 2008;59:179–206; quiz 7-8.
21. Kathuria S, Jablokow VR, Molnar Z. Leiomyosarcoma of penile prepuce with ultrastructural study. Urology. 1986;27(6):556–7.
22. Zhang K, Da J, Yao HJ, Zheng DC, Cai ZK, Jiang YQ, Xu MX, Wang Z. Metastatic tumors of the penis: a report of 8 cases and review of the literature. Medicine (Baltimore). 2015;94:e132.
23. Hakenberg OW, Dräger DL, Erbersdobler A, Naumann CM, Jünemann KP, Protzel C. The diagnosis and treatment of penile cancer. Dtsch Arztebl Int. 2018;115(39):646–52. https://doi.org/10.3238/arztebl.2018.0646.
24. Cheng L, Bostwick DG, editors. Essentials of anatomic pathology. Cham: Springer; 2016. https://doi.org/10.1007/978-3-319-23380-2_40.

Part V

Frenulum

32 Frenulum Anomalies and Diseases

Abbreviations

FB Frenulum breve
PE Premature ejaculation

Nomenclatures

Frenulum preputii penis. The word "frenulum" is a diminutive of the Latin word "frenum" which means bridle, pl. frenula. In female it is called the frenulum of clitoridis.

Definition

Frenulum is an elastic band of tissue under the glans penis that connects to the prepuce and helps to retract the prepuce over the glans, it is formed by ruffle of inner mucosa of the prepuce (Fig. 32.1). It is a bridge-like structure that joins the ventral prepuce to the glans, the point of attachment of the prepuce is advanced towards the meatus; which usually assumes a longitudinal direction on the same line with the frenulum, frenulum is continuous with the ridged band proximally.

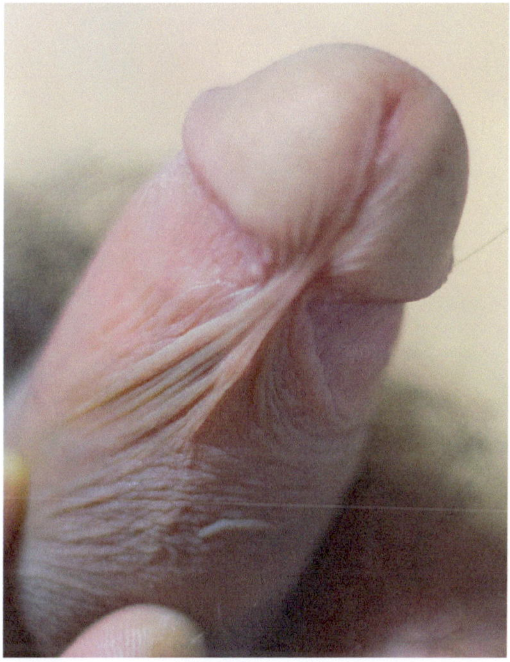

Fig. 32.1 Normal anatomy of the frenulum in intact prepuce

Anatomy of the Frenulum

The ridged band is continuous with the frenulum, being a radial band over about 60% of the penile diameter—the dorsal and lateral aspects—then turning distally to form a 'V' shape in the ventral aspect whilst smoothly reducing its width to merge with the frenulum. This continuity is the

M. A. B. Fahmy, *Normal and Abnormal Prepuce*, https://doi.org/10.1007/978-3-030-37621-5_32

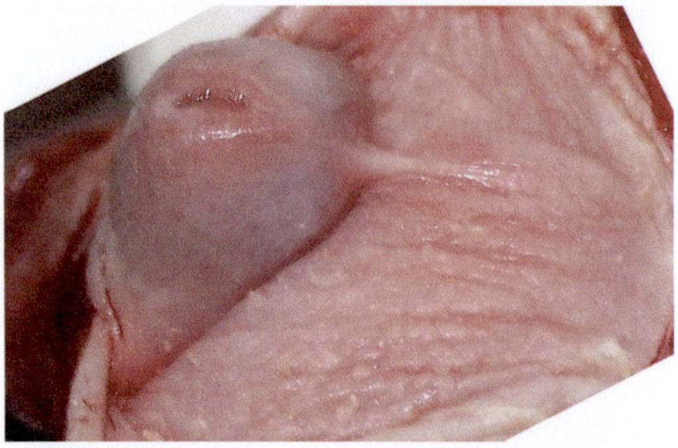

Fig. 32.2 The frenulum looks as a midline folding of the ridged band of inner preputial mucosa

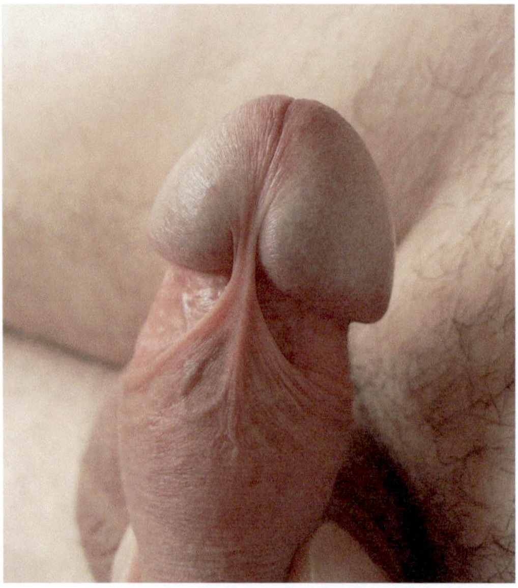

Fig. 32.3 Frenular delta

reason why the ridged band is also known as the frenular band (Fig. 32.2).

The preputial mucosa of triangular shape distal to the ridged band in the ventral aspect having the frenulum at its point, and its sides defined by the ridged band is called *Frenular Delta*. The frenular delta is noted by some men as the most sensitive area of their penis (Fig. 32.3) (Chap. 5).

Regardless of the pattern and numbers of superficial vessels in the ventral aspect of the prepuce, there are two medium-sized branches curve from each side of the outer prepuce to course through the frenulum closer to the median raphe, eventually to lie on either side of the frenulum before disappearing into its depths. In this way, they appear eventually to flank the frenular artery

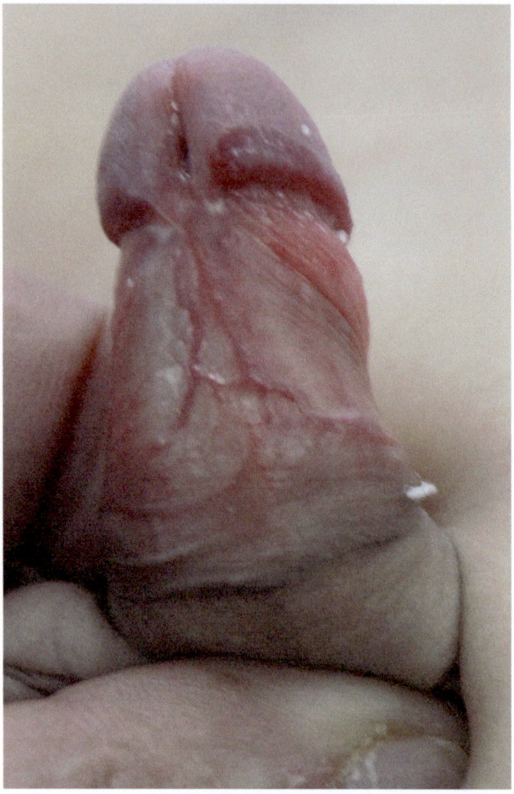

Fig. 32.4 A visible branched frenular artery

to form a triplet analogous to the two dorsal arteries and deep dorsal vein of the penile shaft [1] (Fig. 32.4).

The anatomical configuration of the female frenulum is different; it will never fused, and forming a two leaflets attached to the labia minora (Chap. 33).

MRI study has confirmed that the glans wings do not fuse at the ventral midline and they are separated by a fibrous tissue (septum glandis). This fibrous tissue is connected to the frenulum, traversing the wings of the glans penis [2].

The frenulum is in a confrontation to the preputial raphe outside, so the median raphe of the prepuce lies at the same sagittal plane of the frenulum.

Embryology

In the 65 mm fetus (fourth month of intra-uterine life) the urogenital ostium is confined to the under surface of the glans and the preputial fold has rolled over the base of the glans except in the region of the urogenital ostium, with the further distal development of the glandular urethra and closure of its edges, the perpetual fold close ventrally to form the frenulum which is attached to the undersurface of the glans at the inner mucosal aspect and preputial raphe at the outer surface. The distal migration of the glanulo-preputial lamella, which forms the prepuce, causes the fusion of the edges of the glanular groove as well, forming the floor of the glanular urethra under the frenulum.

Function of the Frenulum

Generally the frenula of the body is a small fold of tissue that secures or restricts the motion of other mobile organs, the most common example is lingual frenulum. Genital frenulum helps along with the dartos muscle, to tether the prepuce and help its return to the anatomically correct position after deployment during erection or after manual retraction.

In female the frenulum of the clitoridis, helps to stabilize the clitoris in its position.

The frenulum preputi and the associated tissue delta on the underside of the penis below the corona has been described in sexuality textbooks as "very reactive" and "particularly responsive to touch that is light and soft, meaning the distal surface of the glans below the corona" is a "source of distinct pleasure". Crooks and Baur [3] observe that two extremely sensitive specific locations that many men find particularly responsive to stimulation are the corona, and the frenulum. Repeated stimulation of this structure will cause orgasm and ejaculation in some men. In men with spinal cord injury, preventing sensations from reaching the brain, the frenulum just below the glans can be stimulated to produce orgasm and peri-ejaculatory response [4].

According to Van Howe [5], meatal stenosis requiring surgical correction (meatotomy) may be a common complication of circumcision in children, and frenular artery damage resulting in meatal ischemia which has been suggested as a possible cause of this problem [6]. Therefore, frenular artery preservation during circumcision, or the use of alternative procedures to conventional circumcision might be recommended in young patients (Fig. 32.5).

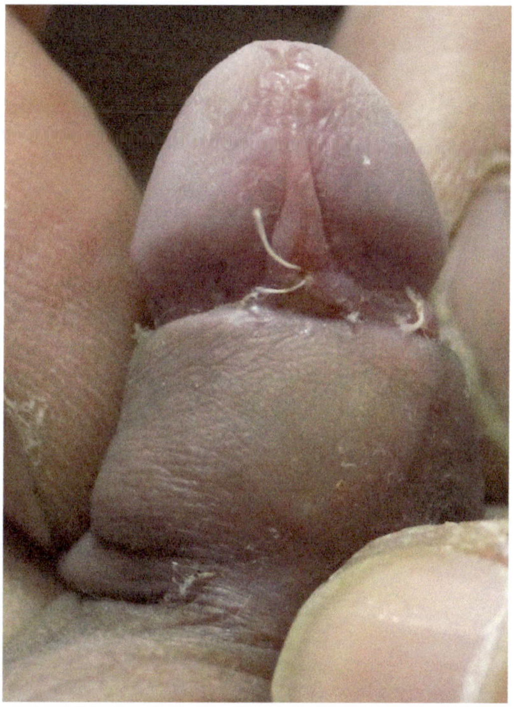

Fig. 32.5 Preserved frenulum in dissection method of circumcision

Congenital Anomalies: Absent Frenulum

Almost always most cases of acquired absent or partially deficient frenulum are secondary to circumcision, as the frenulum usually sacrificed during guillotine circumcision, and also it may be torn during plastibell applications.

Recently with recognition of its importance, many surgeons are trying to preserve frenulum during circumcision and trying to create a frenulum like structure from the mucosal collar during distal hypospadias repair (Fig. 32.5).

Frenulum is congenitally absent or deficient in almost all cases of hypospadias, along the ventrally deficient prepuce (Fig. 32.6).

In cases of megameatus intact prepuce (MIP), there is a normal development of the preputial-glanular lamella, but it fails to fuse with the deep glanular groove and the floor of the glanular ure-

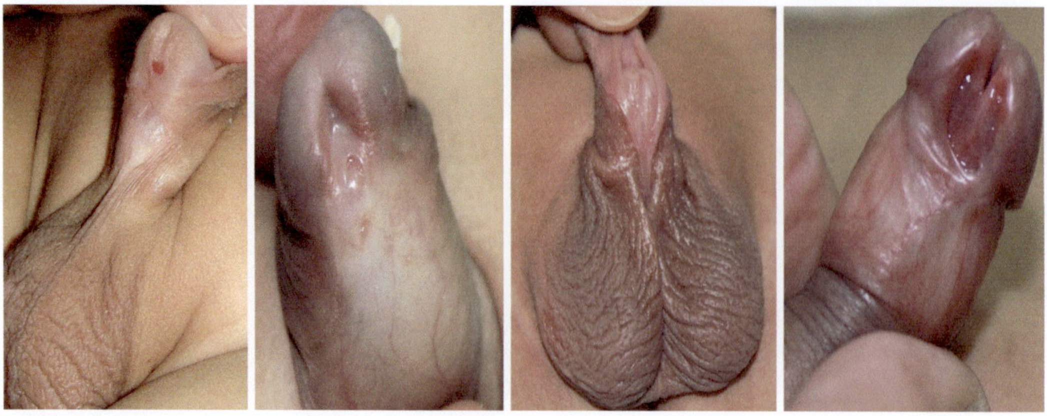

Fig. 32.6 Congenitally deficient frenulum in all forms of hypospadias and cases of megameatus intact prepuce

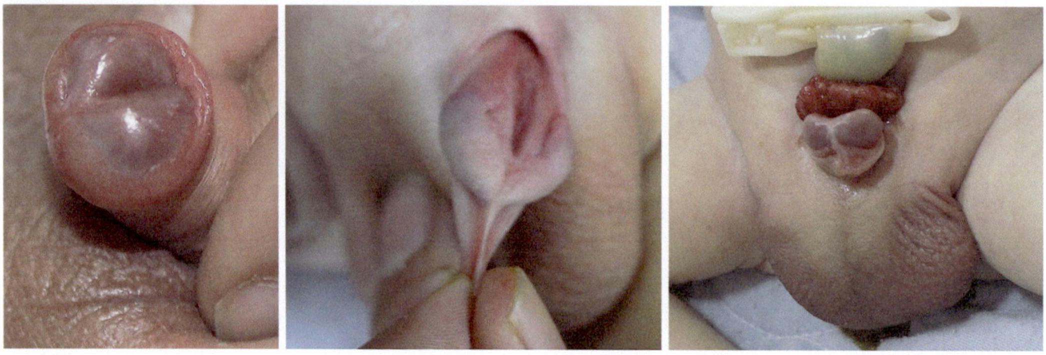

Fig. 32.7 A preserved frenulum in different grades of isolated epispadias and cases of bladder exstrophy epispadias complex

thra as well the frenulum is not developed. In contrary almost all cases of either an isolated epispadias or epispadias associated with bladder exstrophy; the glans penis had no urethra or meatus, but had a well preserved frenulum (Fig. 32.7).

We encountered few cases of deficient or nearly absent frenulum in cases of ventrally deficient prepuce without hypospadias (microposthia), in such anomaly the incomplete prepuce is attached directly to the glanular epithelium (Fig. 32.8). In Fig. 32.9 another rare case of triangular megameatus with ventrally deficient prepuce; the frenulum is absent with a direct insertion of the preputial edges to the glanular surface. It seems that ventrally deficient prepuce usually associated with deficient frenulum.

Frenulum Breve (Fig. 32.10)

Nomenclature

"Breve" is Spanish term means "short", this condition also known as a frenular chordee.

Frenulum breve is a condition in which the frenulum is short and restricts the backward movement of the foreskin, which may or may not interfere with normal sexual activity (Fig. 32.10). Having a short frenulum is commonly associated with having a short ridged band.

Frenulum breve may contribute to frenular chordee, where the glans is pulled toward the vernal body of the penis.

The diagnosis of frenulum breve is almost always confused with that of phimosis and a generally tight

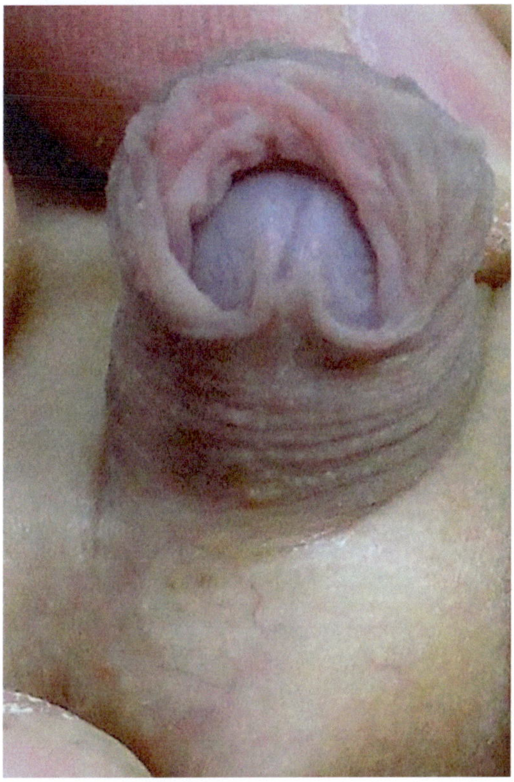

Fig. 32.8 Absent frenulum in a case of hooded prepuce without hypospadias and a normally positioned meatus

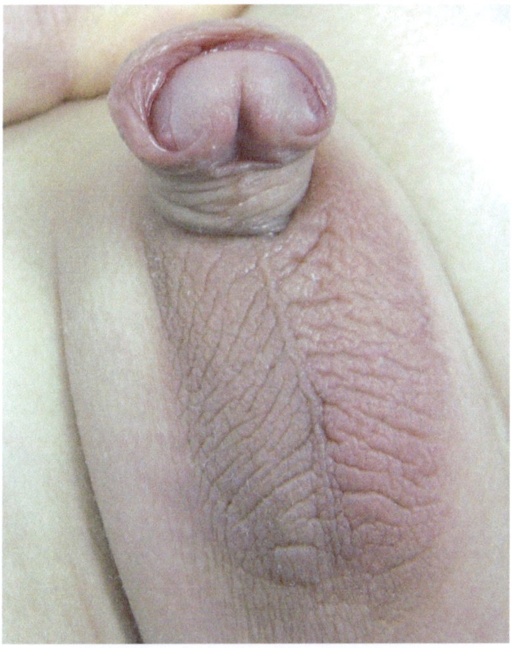

Fig. 32.9 A rare case of triangular megameatus with a direct insertion of the prepuce in to the glans penis without frenulum

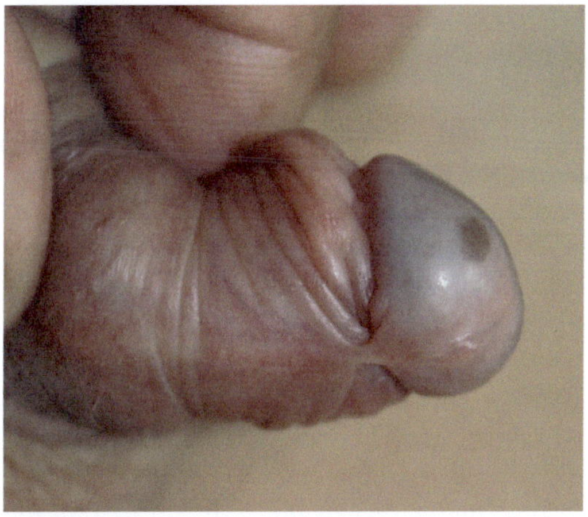

Fig. 32.10 A case of frenulum breve, the limitedly retracted prepuce revealed a melanoma in the glans

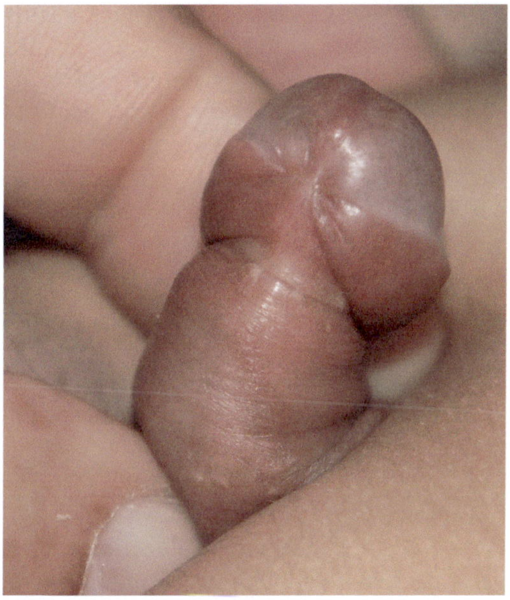

Fig. 32.11 Frenulum breve with a limited preputial retraction

foreskin, since the symptom is common: difficulty in retracting the foreskin. Most men with phimosis also have frenulum breve to a certain extent (Fig. 32.11).

Frenulum breve may be complicated by tearing of the frenulum during sexual or other activity and is a cause of man dyspareunia. The torn frenulum may result in healing with scar tissue that is less flexible after the incident causing further difficulties. However, this tearing can also solve the problem, healing such that the frenulum is longer and therefore no longer problematic.

Frenulum breve may be treated by manually expanding the shaft skin by stretching. But most cases have to be treated with surgery. There are several different techniques to treat this condition. Threading a suture through the lower membrane, and then tying a tight knot around the frenulum itself is a procedure that minimizes invasive action, after a few days the frenulum will weaken and eventually break apart to allow the prepuce to fully retract. Other procedures involve the cutting of the skin and require the use of sutures to help in the healing process. Stretching exercises and steroid creams may also be helpful. Alternatively, it may be treated by a reparative surgical procedure called a frenuloplasty.

Old trend is to treat such case by complete circumcision including resection of the frenulum (frenectomy), but this is not acceptable recently with the trend of most surgeons to preserve frenulum; emphasising its significant importance.

Frenuloplasty

The goal of treatment is to allow normal retraction of the foreskin.

The procedure usually involves the removal of the frenulum or the creation of an incision in the frenulum that is then stretched to lengthen it and stitched closed. The incision can be z-shaped, y-shaped or a single horizontal cut. Once healed, the procedure effectively elongates the frenulum, allowing normal function. Under normal circumstances the incision heals completely in around 4 weeks, after which time normal sexual activity can be resumed. Other methods of treatment include horizontal stitches in the frenulum which over the course of a week cut through the tight skin, elongating it. This is generally more painful than the standard procedure, but heals faster [7].

The Frenuloplasty can be conducted under both general or local anesthesia. It is possible that frenuloplasty may avoid the need for circumcision even when a clinician felt circumcision to be indicated at presentation.

Laser frenuloplasty, consisting of frenulum vaporization by laser CO2, is an alternative simple, safe and efficacious procedure [8].

Fleshy Frenulum

In a very few cases the frenulum may acquires an abnormal thickness, and it may looks fleshy, such cases may give the same picture of FB, with restriction of the normal preputial retractability. (Fig. 32.12).

Frenular Deviation

During our survey for cases of megameatus among children before retail circumcision, we came across this rare case of frenular deviation from the normal midline position, which is also associated with a minimal degree of urinary meatus widening [9] (Fig. 32.13).

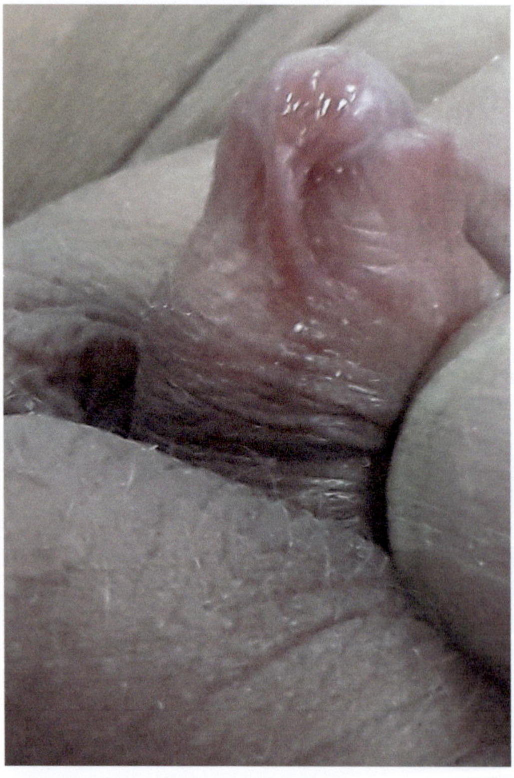

Fig. 32.12 Thickened flashy frenulum

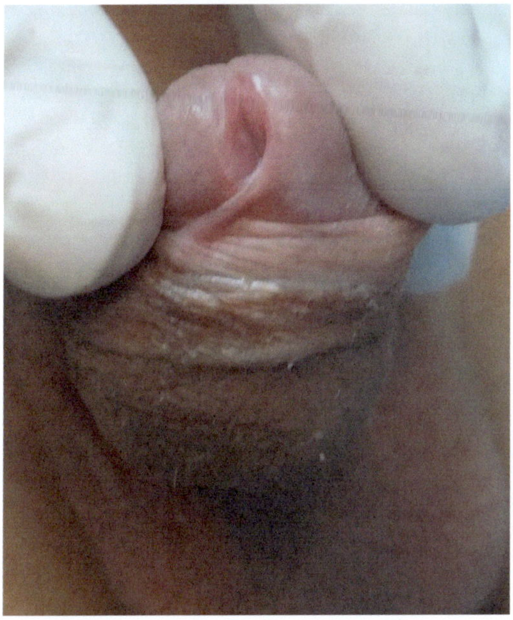

Fig. 32.13 Deviated frenulum with relatively wide meatus

Infectious Diseases

Frenulum is the favourable site for settlement of many genital infectious and sexually transmitted diseases; it is affected fairly often with condyloma acuminata, syphilis and gonorrhoea [10].

Frenular Piercing

Frenulum piercing is a type of body piercing located on the underside of the shaft of the penis. A series of parallel piercings is known as a frenum ladder. A frenum ladder also known as a Jacob's Ladder, which may be extended to include transscrotal piercings or any underside of the shaft of the penis.

Frenulum piercings rarely reject if pierced properly, although they may migrate, or get infected. It is common for a frenulum piercing to start to close soon after the jewellery has been removed (Fig. 32.14).

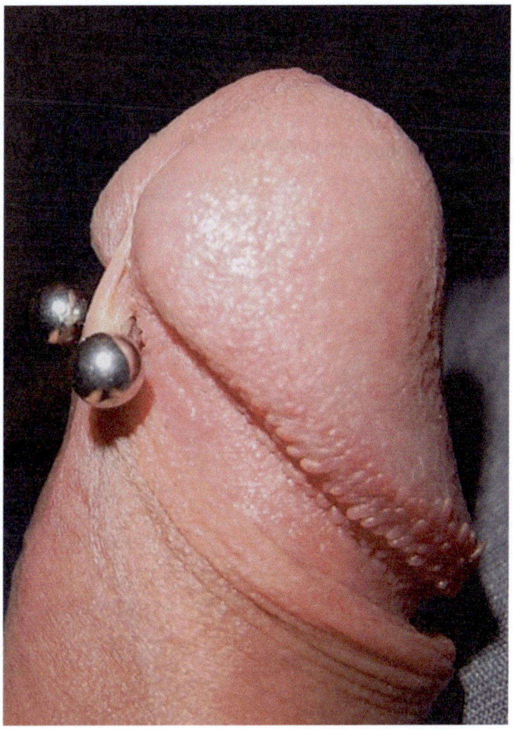

Fig. 32.14 Frenular piercing. Wikipedia file: This file is licensed under the Creative Commons Attribution-Share Alike 3.0 Unprotected license

References

1. McGrath K. The frenular delta. In: Denniston GC, Hodges FM, Milos MF, editors. Understanding circumcision. Boston: Springer; 2001. https://doi.org/10.1007/978-1-4757-3351-8_11.
2. Özbey H, Kumbasar A. Glans wings are separated ventrally by the septum glandis and frenulum penis: MRI documentation and surgical implications. Turk J Urol. 2017;43(4):525–9. www.turkishjournalofurology.com.
3. Crooks R, Baur K. Our sexuality. 5th ed. Benjamin/Cummings: Redwood City; 1993. p. 129. ISBN 0-534-59567-7.
4. Pryor JL, Leroy SC, Nagel TC, Hensleigh HC. Vibratory stimulation for treatment of anejaculation in quadriplegic men. Arch Phys Med Rehabil. 1995;76(1):59–64. https://doi.org/10.1016/S0003-9993(95)80044-1.
5. Van Howe RS. Incidence of meatal stenosis following neonatal circumcision in a primary care setting. Clin Pediatr (Phila). 2006;45:49–54.

6. Persad R, Sharma S, McTavish J, Imber C, Mouriquand PD. Clinical presentation and pathophysiology of meatal stenosis following circumcision. Br J Urol. 1995;75:91–3.
7. Rajan P, Alan McNeill S, Turner KJ. Is frenuloplasty worthwhile? A 12-year experience. Ann R Coll Surg Engl. 2006;88(6):583–4. https://doi.org/10.1308/003588406X130633.
8. Duarte AF, Correia O. Laser CO_2 frenuloplasty: a safe alternative treatment for a short frenulum. J Cosmet Laser Ther. 2009;11:151. https://doi.org/10.1080/14764170902777356.
9. Fahmy MAB. Spectrum of megameatus anomaly, a new classification. Eur Urol Suppl. 2018;17(9):e2467. https://doi.org/10.1016/S1569-9056(18)32838-0.
10. Braun-Falco O, Plewig G, Wolff HH. Dermatologie und Venerologie. 3rd (revised) ed. Berlin: Springer; 1984.

Part VI

Female Prepuce

33 Normal Female Prepuce

Abbreviations

CAH	Congenital adrenal hyperplasia
DSD	Disorders of sex development
FGM	Female genital mutilation

Nomenclature The clitoral hood also called preputium clitoridis, preputial sheath and clitoral prepuce.

Definition Female prepuce is a fold of skin that surrounds and protects the external shaft of the clitoris completely and the clitorial hood is the distal part of this prepuce which partially cover the glans, it develops as an external lamella around the genital tubercle, it is composed of mucocutaneous tissues; these tissues are between the mucosa and the skin, and it has an immunological importance. The clitoral hood is also important not only in protection of the clitoral glans, but also in sexual pleasure, as it is an erogenous tissue.

Embryology of Female Prepuce (Fig. 33.1)

The clitoral hood is formed during the fetal life as a cellular lamella, which grows down on the dorsal side of the clitoris and is eventually covering both sides while fused with the clitoris. It is formed from the same tissues that form the foreskin in human males.

It starts to appear at the eighth week of development, as a slight lamellar proliferation, referred to as the ectoblastic preputial plate, penetrating more or less deeply, from the surface epithelium, develops at the ectoblastic epithelial layer which covers the genital tubercle. Vacuoles appear in this lamina following apoptosis phenomena. The convergence of these vacuoles creates a space around the glans, which ends up separating, on the periphery, the glans and the portion of the prepuce which envelopes it, the preputial chamber of the glans clitoridis is thus created. It is bordered by the same epithelium corresponding to the internal layer of the hood and, on the other side, to the surface covering of the glans.

The clitoris will also undergoes an intrauterine reduction, thus modelling its shape and reducing its size, it was longer and more voluminous than the penis at same stage. Thus, in a 4-month-old female foetus, and in relation to a normal development, the clitoris will have already acquired its final aspect: minuscule formation covered by the prepuce and whose end, the glans, is hidden under the hood. Its embryological origin is separate from the labial structures; as the urogenital fold becomes the labia minora and the labioscrotal fold becomes the labia majora, whereas the clitoral hood originates from a cellular lamella that grows on the dorsum of the clitoris (Fig. 33.2) [1].

M. A. B. Fahmy, *Normal and Abnormal Prepuce*, https://doi.org/10.1007/978-3-030-37621-5_33

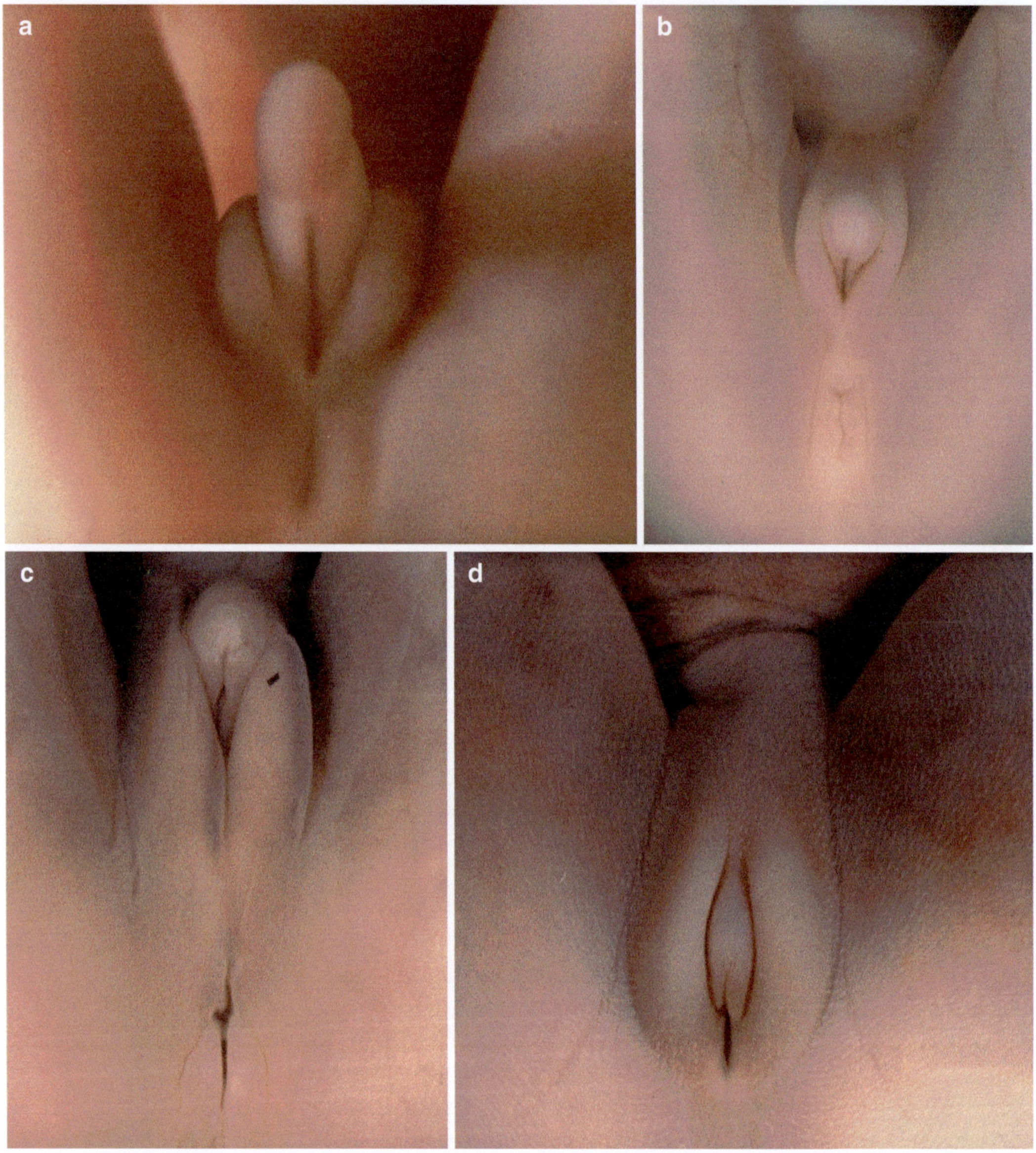

Fig. 33.1 Development of the external genitalia in females between 8 and 20 weeks. (**a**) Ambisexual stage at 8–9 weeks. (**b**) The genital tubercle grows slower than the foetus at 9 weeks, making it looks progressively smaller. The genital folds remain unfused to show the developing vestibule. (**c**) By week 17 the folding of genital tubercle shows that it is now has the appearance of a clitoris. (**d**) By week 20 the external anatomy is fully formed as female (reproduced with permission: https://s100.copyright.com/AppDispatchServlet)

Like male prepuce; the female prepuce also continue to develops, evolves and maturates after delivery, the neonatal prepuce is completely different from that we see at adulthood, due to neonatal hyperestrogenemia, the prepuce and clitorial hood are markedly oedematous and it is extremely difficult in many occasions to recognise the clitoris, from the oedematous prepuce (Fig. 33.3).

Clitorial prepuce and hood is an analogue to the penile skin and the prepuce, where the clitoris is a homologue to the penis. The labioscrotal swellings, which are separate early and will become the labia majora. The pelvic portion of the female urogenital sinus becomes the vestibule, into which emerges, at its cranial part, the external orifice of the urethra and directly below

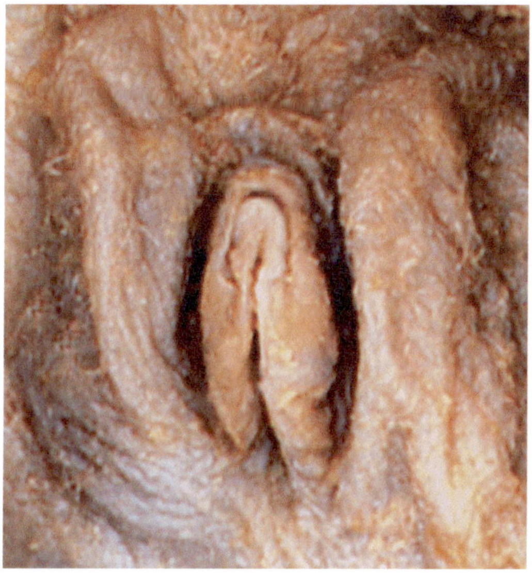

Fig. 33.2 Female human foetus at the end of the fourth month (18 weeks of amenorrhea). Macrophotography of the external genitalia Biometry of the foetus; length vertex-coccyx: 14 cm. All structures (greater and lesser lips, clitoris, frenula, commissures) are in place, normally developed. The genital tubercle declined, turned into clitoral glans [16]

it, is the external orifice of the vagina. The genital tubercle protrudes below the ventral commissure of the labia. Inside of the labia majora, the labia minora, which are connected to the bottom surface of the genital tubercle. The epithelium which covers the medial surface of labia minora comes from the phallic portion of the urogenital sinus. It is thus of endodermal in origin [2].

Sexual dimorphism of external genitalia in humans is particularly profound in humans; as size and morphology of the penis and clitoris are strikingly different even though both structures develop from the remarkably similar ambisexual genital tubercle.

Anatomy

The prepuce, clitoral hood, clitoris and labia minora were observed to be distinctly separate structures. An anatomically accurate description of any structure is of paramount significance for reconstructive surgeons, and this rationale the

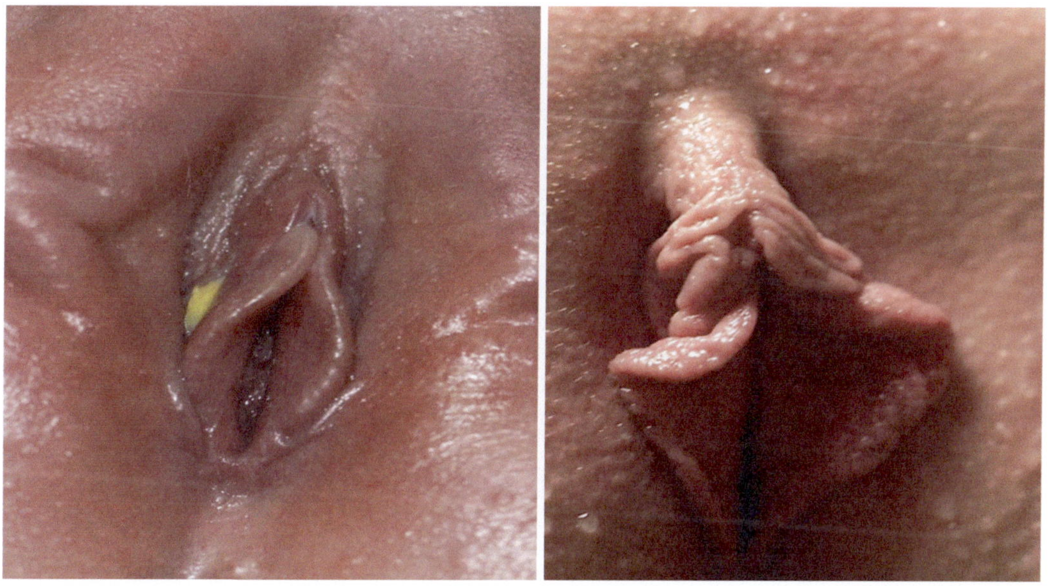

Fig. 33.3 Difference between neonatal and adult prepuce; neonatal one is smaller, dip with the clitoris, which is completely hidden by the prepuce dorsally and the labia ventrally, adult prepuce overhangs and more prominent, directed forward and caudally

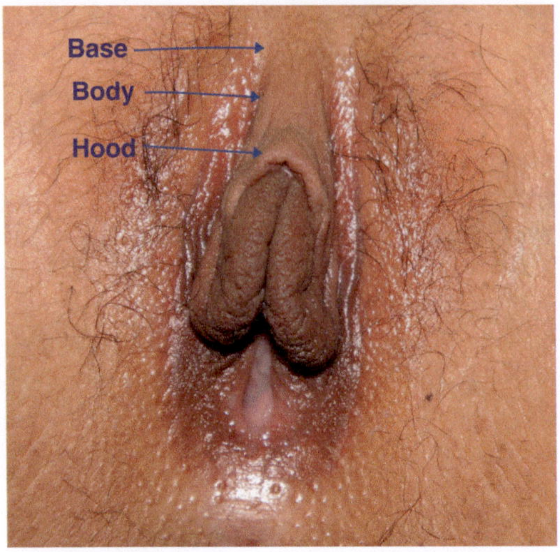

Fig. 33.4 Female prepuce; formed of three parts, the base in continuity with mons pubis, the body and the free edge known as clitorial hood

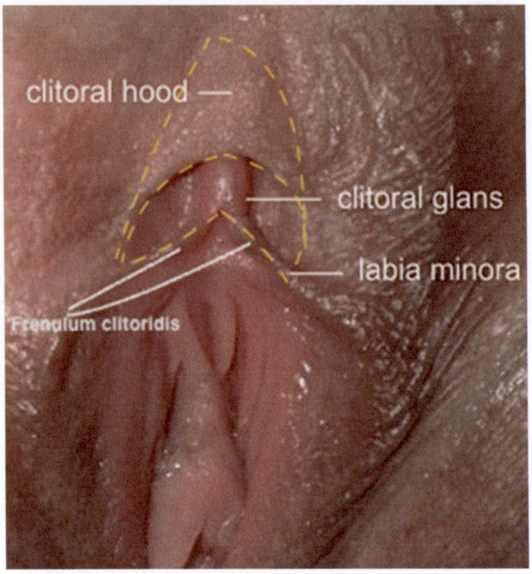

Fig. 33.5 Two lateral triangular spaces are formed by the clitorial hood in relation to the glans clitoris

continuous anatomical investigation on the female prepuce.

Almost all descriptions of the female prepuce are confined only to the distal portion, the clitorial hood, but actually the prepuce in female is formed of three distinct parts: the base (sometimes called the apex), which is in continuity proximally with mons pubis and cover the most proximal part of the clitoris and suspensory ligament, preputial body covering the shaft of the clitoris, this part is sometimes called the clitoral prepuce and the term clitorial hood is reserved for the only cutaneous and nearly circular fold at the loose end of this prepuce (Fig. 33.4).

Labium minus splits cranially into the superior (the preputium of the clitoridis) and the inferior frenulum of the clitoridis (the clitoral frenulum). The inferior branch of the labium minus (nymphea), called the frenulum clitoridis, is attached to the ventral surface of the clitoral glans.

The two leaflets of the clitoral hood were observed to intersect the labia minora at an angle, forming a bilateral depressions at sides of the clitoris. Normally the prepuce forming three depressions around the clitoris, two are more or less triangular, and one semicircular just above the clitorial glans (Fig. 33.5). The hood can slide along the surface of the glans, so that the latter can be retracted (such as with the male prepuce). A cavity is therefore formed between the glans and the internal surface of the hood, the preputial chamber. The bottom of this chamber is an arc-shaped groove, which stops, such as the hood, at the level of its inferior surface (due to the presence of the frenula): it is the neck of the glans clitoridis (equivalent to the balano-preputial groove of the male penis). It is at the level of this neck that the external epithelium of the glans is reflected on the internal coating of the hood (Fig. 33.6).

The lateral parts of the hood extend beneath the glans and are gradually incorporated into the lateral surface of the labia minora. The fusion with the labia minora can be precocious (high fusion). It can also occur at a lower level, at the top-third to mid-third junction of the labia minora (low fusion). This case corresponds to a lateral extension of the hood, sliding on the lateral surface of the labium minus, before merging with the latter. Low preputial insertion is usually associated with a large clitoris (Fig. 33.7).

Generally, there is no symmetry between the right and left levels of the junctions between the lateral extension of the hood and the homolateral labium minus [2].

The clitorial frenulum (frenulum clitoridis, crus glandis clitoridis) is completely different from the male one; as its two leaflets are widely separated and incorporated laterally with labia minora bilaterally (in male the two edges of the frenulum are adherent and only separated proximally form the frenular delta "Chap. 32").

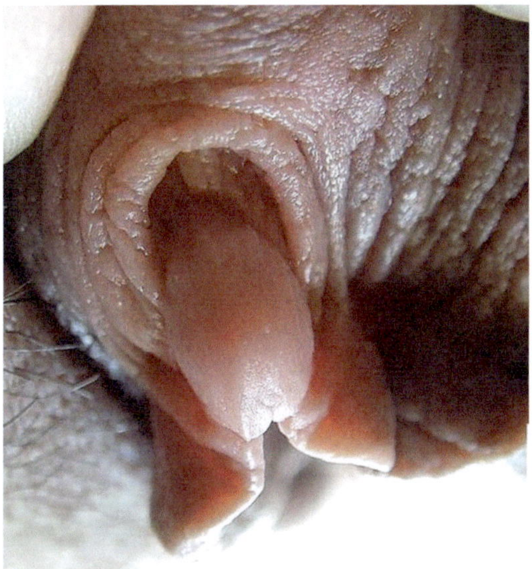

Fig. 33.6 Semicircular space between the free edge of the clitorial hood and the dorsum of the glans of the clitoris, the separated two leaflets of the clitorial frenulum are also obvious

The clitoral frenulum surrounding the clitoris, it varies greatly in size between women, it maintaining the clitoral glans in its natural position and preventing it from aquiring mobility (Fig. 33.6).

The proximal part of the superficial clitoral frenulum stratum inserts into the posterior clitoral glans and the distal part fuses with the labium minus bifurcation. The inferior edge of the clitoral frenulum is firmly fused to the infrafrenulum structure, in some women the frenula are very short, in others it is almost non-existent.

In a recent study of 85 girls aged from one to thirteen years, Brodie et al. [3] found that clitoral hood became more retractile and had more layers of rugae, as the age increase. The clitoral hood skin color was noted to be the same color as the skin of the labia minora in 55% of girls, and a lighter color in 43%. The clitoral hood was observed to have the same level of keratinization in 60% of patients, and was more keratinized in 34% of patients (Fig. 33.8).

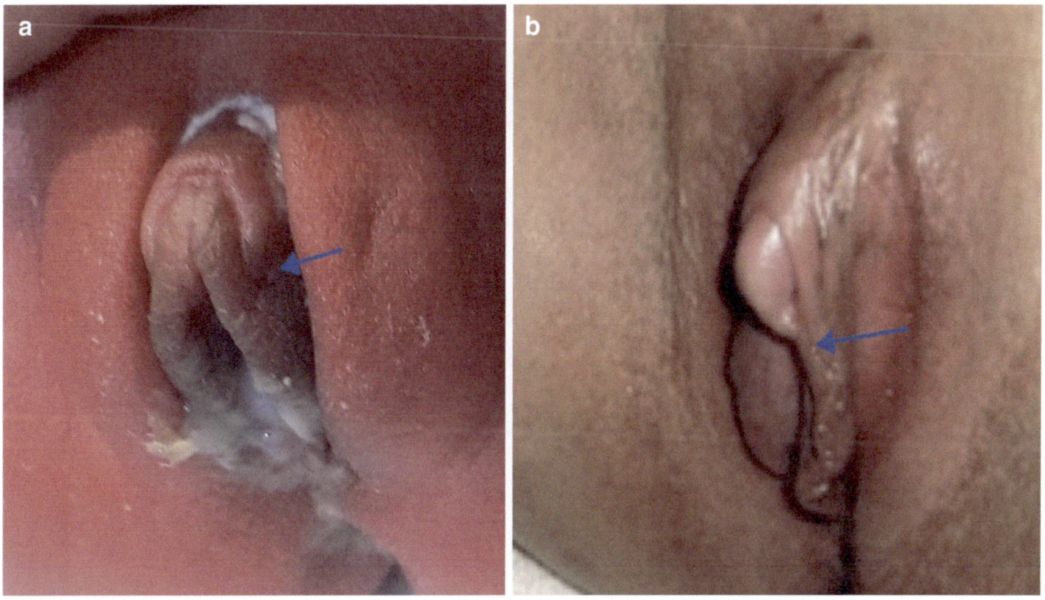

Fig. 33.7 Different levels of the insertion of the lateral edge of the clitorial hood in the labia minora (arrows); (**a**) high insertion in neonate, (**b**) low insertion associated with large protruded clitoris

There were four observed shapes of the clitoral hood: horseshoe, trumpet, coffee bean, and tent (Fig. 33.9).

The most commonly observed shape of the clitoral hood was the tent shape, which occurred in 50% of patients (the clitoral hood forms a peak then divides into right and left leaflets, with a linear opening between the two sides where the clitoral glans is situated) (Fig. 33.10). In infants, the most commonly observed shape (61%) was a coffee bean (right and left sides of the clitoral hood were fused over the clitoral glans) [4]. That means the shape of the hood is changeable with maturity, the horseshoe and trumpet shapes of clitoral hood were seen across all age categories.

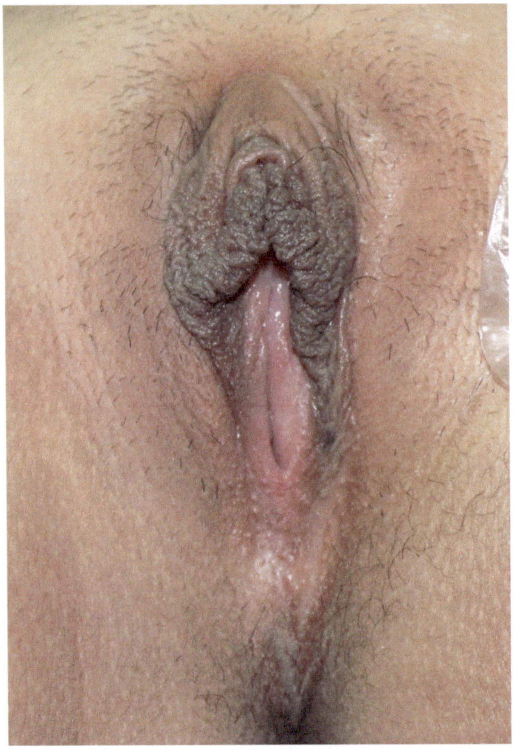

Fig. 33.8 Long redundant prepuce, with a corrugated and dark brown labia similar to the scrotal skin

Clitoris

Anatomy of the female prepuce cannot be launched without highlighting the anatomy of the clitoris, which is a short, cylindrical, erectile structure, 2–3 cm in length, at the superior portion of the vestibule. It is situated beneath the anterior labial commissure, partially hidden between the anterior segments of the labia minora. The clitoris consists of a base of two crura that attach to the periosteum of the symphysis pubis. Like the penis, the clitoris has a suspensory ligament and two small muscles, the ischiocavernosi, which are inserted into the crura of the clitoris. The body of the clitoris consists of two cylindrical corpora cavernosa composed of thin-walled, vascular channels that function as erectile tissue. The distal one-third of the clitoris is a small rounded tubercle (glans clitoridis) that consists of spongy erectile tissue with many nerve endings. The junction between the clitorial glans and the body of the clitoris is demarcated by the presence of the glans corona, similar to the coronal sulcus in male, this corona is mainly visible in women with a well formed clitoris immediately under the preputial hood. Usually, only the glans is visible, with the body of the clitoris

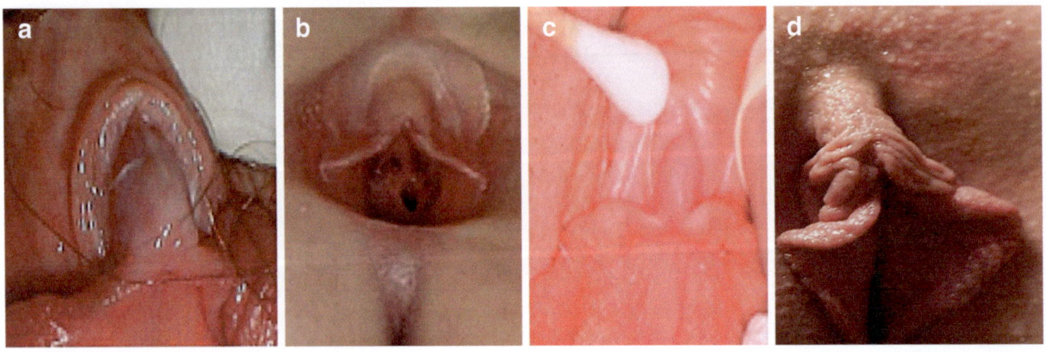

Fig. 33.9 Different shapes of the female prepuces, (**a**) horseshoe, (**b**) trumpet shape, (**c**) coffee bean, and (**d**) tent shape

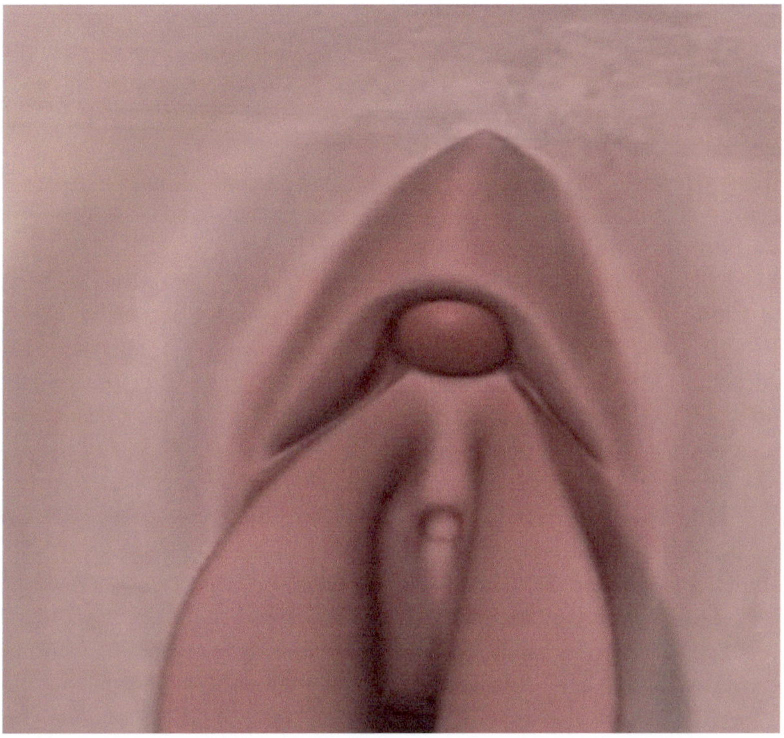

Fig. 33.10 Tent shaped clitoral hood, which forms a peak then divides into right and left leaflets, with a linear opening between the two sides where the clitoral glans is situated

positioned beneath the skin of the preputial body and hood. The normal glans clitoridis in adult women has a width less than 1 cm, with an average length of 2–3 cm. Age, weight, and oral contraceptive usage do not change its anatomic dimensions [5]. Childbearing may influence the size of the clitoris, among women of reproductive age, there is significant variation in the size of the clitoris, its glans and the labia minora, which are relatively more prominent in children and postmenopausal women (Fig. 33.3).

Also with age, the prepuce tissues tend to undergo a ptosis and distension. This causes the formation of a sort of withered sheath, inside which the glans is often completely hidden. The clitoris is the most elaborate sensory organ of the female body. It is provided with highly specialised tactile sensitivity receptors, in connection with the sexual function. With its invaluable sensors, the clitoris has only one function: the reception of pleasure stimuli for a single purpose: to generate sexual excitation in women in all types of contexts (masturbation, foreplay and sexual intercourse).

Histologically, the labia minora are composed of dense connective tissue, erectile tissue, and elastic fibers. Unlike the labia majora, they do not contain adipose tissue. The skin of the opposed surfaces of labia minora has numerous sebaceous glands but few hair follicles and sweat glands.

The clitoral prepuce consists of the same skin forming the labia, the hood often has several folds, and in most cases it is not very thick, but sometimes it may thicken and adopt a dysmorphic aspect, even in young women. The external surface of the prepuce is covered by a keratinised squamous epithelium. In young girls, a mucous layer is generally present on the internal surface of the hood. In a women of an age to procreate, this layer is gradually replaced by a non-keratinised squamous epithelium.

The cutaneous epithelium of the female prepuce is consists of four layers:

1. A basal germinative layer (stratum basale), which rests on the basal lamina between the epidermis and the dermis.
2. A spinous or prickle cell layer, forming the bulk of the epidermal thickness (stratum spinosum).
3. A granular layer (stratum granulosum).
4. A surface layer of flattened, keratinized cells embedded in hydrophobic intercellular lipid (stratum corneum).

Histologically, the clitoral frenulum comprises two layers, the superficial stratum consists of the dermis, subdermis, and cutis appendages (sebaceous and apocrine glands). There is squamous mucosa with erectile tissue between the skin folds. The deep stratum of the clitoral frenulum (the infrafrenulum fascia bundle) consists of fibroconnective adipose tissue with intermittent layers of adipose cells and fibrous bands [6].

Three specialized cells; melanocytes, Langerhans cells, and Merkel cells are also reside in the epidermis of the prepuce. Melanocytes represent one-tenth to one-fifth of the cells in the cutaneous basal layer. They convert tyrosine to melanin pigment, which protects the basal cells from ultraviolet damage. Melanocytes respond regionally to hormones: at puberty, pigmentation of the mons pubis and labia majora increases; also during pregnancy steroid hormones stimulate melanogenesis [7].

Langerhans cells (LCs) are a dendritic cells found in the epidermis, in thymic and mucosal tissues, and in lymph nodes. Their chief function is to sample antigen at the epithelial surface, process it, and present it to circulating T lymphocytes, the activation of which initiates the cell-mediated immune response, it have a highly protective and necessary function for survival. Immune inactivation of the LCs render the mammal in a perilous and vulnerable state. Specialized immunological properties should be noted by the presence of Langerhans cells and other lytic materials, which defend against common microbes, and there is robust evidence supporting HIV protection [8].

Merkel cells are found in the basal epidermal layer. Their cell bodies form synapse-like contacts with the terminal endings of myelinated nerve fibers. They release neurotransmitters in response to sensory excitation. Merkel cells serve as skin mechanoreceptors that shape sensitivity to soft touch.

In the female, there is no mesenchymal proliferation in the prepuce to form a dartos muscle layer.

The presence of sebaceous glands (preputial glands) is observed at the neck of the clitorial glans, which explains the accumulation of smegma, especially if the hood is fully covering the clitoris or if the level of hygiene is not satisfactory.

Hormonal Receptors of the Prepuce

Generally vulvar skin has a higher concentration of epidermal androgen receptors than skin at nongenital sites. At puberty, androgens direct the maturation of preputial sebaceous glands and hair follicles. Progesterone receptors are restricted to the transitional epithelium of the inner aspect of the labia minora and to the nonkeratinized epithelia of the vagina and vulvar vestibule [9].

There is an extensive circumstantial evidences that estradiol and also progesterone influence the postnatal physiology of extra genital and, especially, genital skin in the human female. Studies have demonstrated effects of oestrogen treatment on human skin thickness, collagen content and blood flow [10].

Innervation

The clitoral glans is a particularly sensitive receptor and transmitter of sexual stimuli. There was a study published at 1999, which claimed that the clitoris had more nerve endings than the penis [11]; however, this has been disproven with more recent studies. The difference is that the glans clitoridis packs nerve endings into a volume only about one-tenth the size of the glans penis. In addition, the glans clitoridis has greater variability in cutaneous corpuscular receptor density (1–14 per 100× high-powered field) compared with the glans penis (1–3 per 100× high-powered field). This concentration of nerves makes the glans clitoridis more sensitive than the glans penis. As a result, many women can feel discomfort—even pain—with anything more than a gentle touch. In fact, most women do not enjoy direct stimulation of the glans and prefer stimulation through the clitorial hood [12].

Female prepuce have a considerable number of free nervous endings and sensory receptors. The genital corpuscles are most important for the perception of erogenous sensibility, but Pacinian and Meissner corpuscles are also present.

Function of Female Prepuce

Normally, the clitoral glans itself is an erogenous tissue, it is too sensitive to be stimulated directly, such as in cases where the hood is retracted. Women with hoods covering most of the clitoral glans can often masturbate by stimulating the hood over the clitoral glans; those with smaller, or more compact, structures tend to rub the clitoral glans and hood together as one item. The clitoral hood additionally provides protection to the clitoral glans, like foreskin on the penile glans, it internalizing the glans, thus preventing irritation or oversensitization.

During sexual stimulation, the hood may also prevent the penis from coming into direct contact with the glans clitoris, which is usually stimulated by the pressure of the partners pubis. Most mammals and primates approach copulation from the rear instead of the common frontal position that humans often assume, so the clitoral stimulation is directly created by glans contact with the scrotum at the base of the penis and the different contractions of its corrugated dartos muscles [13].

The preputial hood lubricated the clitoral glans by the naturally provided sebum, if a woman's clitoris is not lubricated the hood may not caress it during sexual stimulation, or the female may experience pain rather than pleasure [13].

During sexual arousal, the female prepuce does not retract as it does in males, because it is continuous with the labia minora. So with erection of the body of the clitoris, there is the apparent disappearance of the glans within the prepuce.

Self-assessment reports on genital anatomy and sexual function have underlined the importance of the clitoris and the skin above/beside the clitoris for sexual sensitivity. This is consistent with the results of neuroanatomical studies of the fetal clitoris showing that the highest nerve density is located within the tunica of the dorsal aspect of the clitoris. Thus, in feminizing procedures, preservation of the clitoris, including its nerve supply, is recommended for maintenance of this sexually sensitive area [14].

During sexual stimulation, the clitoral hood has a stimulating effect on the engorged clitoris, but also covers the clitoris from direct contact. These observations are suggestive of a delicate balance between pleasure and pain. Nonphysiological conditions, like the absence of a clitoral hood, can disrupt this equilibrium, resulting in both discomfort and diminished sexual sensitivity [15].

As stated before, the prepuce had a supportive role in stabilising the clitoris and limiting its excessive mobility. Also the prepuce protect the clitoris and the uppermost part of the introits mechanically and immunologically; as the genital area is in a direct contact with the other partner and vulnerable to a uncountable different pathogens, so this can explain the immunological importance of the different structure of the genital tract and the prepuce in particular.

Normal Variation of Clitoral Hood

Variations between women in the development of the clitoral hood are very wide not only in the anatomical orientation, but also in the function and perception, some women may had a clitoral hood covered by the labia when standing upright, but others may had a protruding clitoral hood.

The clitoral hood varies in the size, shape, thickness, and other aesthetic areas. Clitorial hood size usually coincides with the size of the clitoris, but in few occasions this is not the case; a redundant prepuce with a rudimentary clitoris or a small retracted prepuce partially encircling a

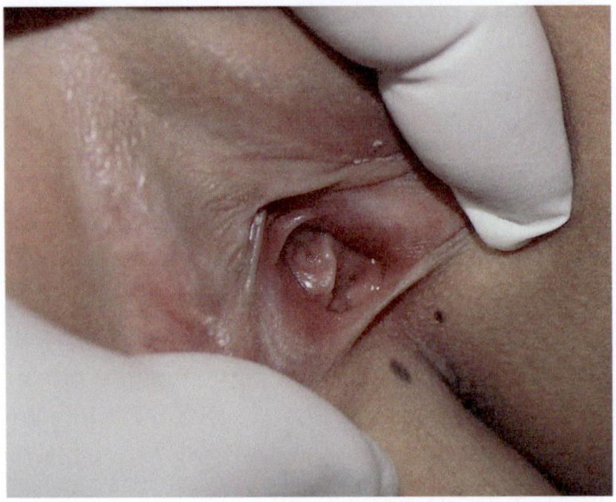

Fig. 33.11 Infant with a completely hidden clitoris under the prepuce

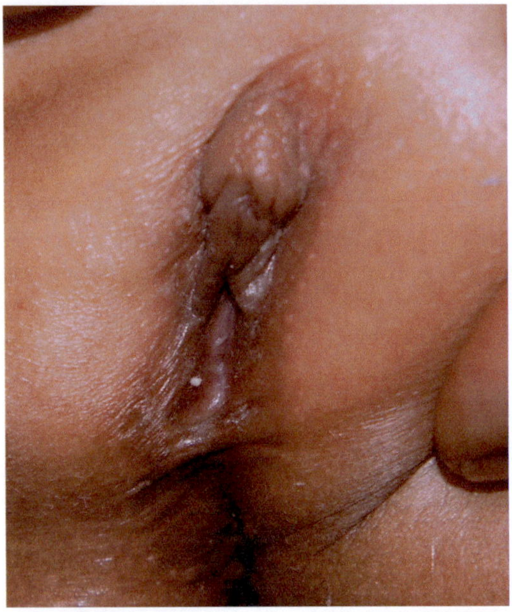

Fig. 33.12 Long prepuce covering the clitoris completely in a 5 years old girl

prominent clitoris are not rare. Females may have a large clitoral hoods that completely cover the clitoral glans, some of these can be retracted to expose the clitoral glans, such as for hygiene purposes or for pleasure; others do not retract (Figs. 33.11 and 33.12). Other women have smaller hoods that do not cover the full length of the clitoral glans, leaving it exposed all the time. As in the male, sticky bands of tissue adhesions can form between the hood and the glans; these stick the hood onto the glans so the hood cannot be pulled back to expose the glans, and strongly scented smegma can accumulate.

Caudal or cephalic displacement of the clitorial hood either with or without labial displacement is a rare positional anomalies, which may not had any clinical impaction. These anomaly may be due to disproportionate growth of one side, or due to failure of the symmetrical migration of the labioscrotal fold during early fetal development.

References

1. Robboy SJ, Bernhardt PF, Parmley T. Embryology of the female genital tract and disorders of abnormal sexual development. In: Blaustein's pathology of the female genital tract. New York: Springer; 1994. p. 10e2.
2. Di Marino V, Lepidi H. Anatomic study of the clitoris and the bulbo-clitoral organ. Cham: Springer; 2014. https://doi.org/10.1007/978-3-319-04894-9_4.
3. Brodie KE, Grantham EC, Huguelet PS, Caldwell BT, Westfall NJ, Wilcox DT. Study of clitoral hood anatomy in the pediatric population. J Pediatr Urol. 2016;12:177.e1–5.
4. Chalmers DJ, O'Donnell CI, Casperson KJ, Bernard SC, Hou AH, Nuss GR, et al. Normal anatomic relationships in prepubescent female external genitalia. J Pediatr Urol. 2014;10(6):1117–21.
5. Ashton-Miller JA, De Lancey JOL. Functional anatomy of the female pelvic floor. Ann N Y Acad Sci. 2007;1101:266–96. https://www.scopus.com/inward/record.uri?eid=2-s2.0-
6. Ostrzenski A. The clitoral infrafrenulum fascial bundle. The anatomy and histology. Clin Anat. 2018;31:907–12. https://doi.org/10.1002/ca.23215.
7. Williams GL. The significance and function of preputial Langerhans cells. In: Oenniston GC, Hodges FM, Milos MF, editors. Male and female circumcision: medical, legal and ethical considerations in pediatric practice. 5th ed. New York: Kluwer Academic/Plenum Publishers; 1998. p. 43.
8. Patton DL, et al. Epithelial cell layer thickness and immune cell populations in the normal human vagina at different stages of the menstrual cycle. Am J Obstet Gynecol. 2000;183:967.
9. Harper WF, McNicol EM. A histological study of normal vulval skin from infancy to old age. Br J Dermatol. 1977;96:249.
10. Hodgins MB, Spike RC, Mackie RM, MacLean AB. An immunohistochemical study of androgen, oestrogen and progesterone receptors in the vulva and vagina. BJOG Int J Obstet Gynaecol. 1998;105:216–22. https://doi.org/10.1111/j.1471-0528.1998.tb10056.x.

11. Angier N. Woman: an intimate geography. New York: Houghton Mifflin Company; 1999. ISBN 0395691303
12. Puppo V. Anatomy and physiology of the clitoris, vestibular bulbs, and labia minora with a review of the female orgasm and the prevention of female sexual dysfunction. Clin Anat. 2013;26:134–52.
13. Schober JM, Meyer-Bahlburg HF, Ransley PG. Self-assessment of genital anatomy, sexual sensitivity and function in women: implications for genitoplasty. BJU Int. 2004;94:589–94.
14. Bronselaer G, Callens N, De Sutter P, De Cuypere G, T'Sjoen G, Cools M, et al. Self-assessment of genital anatomy and sexual function within a Belgian, Dutch-speaking female population: a validation study. J Sex Med. 2013;10:3006–18.
15. Di Marino V, Lepidi H. Anatomic study of the clitoris and the bulbo-clitoral organ. Cham: Springer International; 2014. p. 13. https://doi.org/10.1007/978-3-319-04894-9_2.
16. Shih C, Cold CJ, Yang CC. Cutaneous corpuscular receptors of the human glans clitoris: descriptive characteristics and comparison with the glans penis. J Sex Med. 2013;10:1783.

34 Preputial Hood Anomalies

Abbreviations

CAH	Congenital Adrenal Hyperplasia
CP	Clitorial Phimosis
DSD	disorders of sex development
FGM	Female Genital mutation
LS	Lichen sclerosis
PGAD	Persistent Genital arousal Disorder
TS	Turner syndrome

Phimosis of the Female Prepuce: (Clitorial Phimosis CP)

The fetal development of the prepuce and the glans in male and females are similar; they are fused together and a space under prepuce is formed during the first year after birth and if they do not separate, it is possible, as in the male, for adhesions and resultant phimosis or synechia of the clitoris to result. As the preputial hood is not completely encircling the clitoris, normally the ventral surface of the later is exposed, so entire phimosis of the female prepuce has seldom been reported, except few cases has been reported in the post-pubertal female with diabetes [1].

In the past there were a limited data in the gynecologic literature concerning the prevalence, pathophysiology, or management of clitoral phimosis, only during the last 10 years few studies oriented with this issue start to emerge.

Clitoral phimosis is generally undiagnosed and unrecognized; as most cases are usually not complaining of sexual dysfunction or urinary manifestations. On rare occasions, however, clitoral phimosis may be associated with a clitoral pain disorder. It is unclear whether clitoral phimosis of any degree would blunt the sensory perception and lead to orgasmic dysfunction.

On the other hand clitorial synechiae; in which an adhesion is appreciated between the shaft of the clitoris and prepuce, with focal adhesion between the clitorial glans and the preputial hood, at different levels, distal to the balanopreputial sulcus is more common than the reported cases. Theses adhesions will prevent full exposure of the clitoris and result in bad preputial hygiene, with accumulation of smegma and dirts which results in different forms of dermatitis, not only at adulthood, but also at younger ages.

Clitoral adhesions documented during physical examination by failure to visualize the entire glans corona. There is a spectrum of clitoral adhesions, ranging from mild to severe, but in all cases, there is a closed compartment covering some portion of the glans corona. Evaluation of 614 individual patients demonstrated clitoral adhesions detected in 140 women (23%) of whom 44%, 34%, and 22% demonstrated mild, moderate, and severe clitoral adhesions, respectively [2].

M. A. B. Fahmy, *Normal and Abnormal Prepuce*, https://doi.org/10.1007/978-3-030-37621-5_34

Incidence Female preputial phimosis is a common presentation of lichen sclerosis (LS) at different age groups, studies had a wide variations about prevalence of phimosis without LS in normal population; the average rate was identified in one study as 22% of the women had different grades of phimosis [3].

Various forms of CP were found in 46 of 3650 patients (1.3%), and severe forms were found in only 9 cases [4]. Another study looked at a group of 589 college-age students seen in a student health clinic, found the rate of clitoral adhesions to be 33% of those with adhesions, 58% were considered mild [5].

Clinically Clitoral phimosis may be associated with clitoral pain syndromes and dyspareunia [6].

The closed compartment space under the clitoral adhesions can prevent adequate drainage of keratinaceous desquamation. Smegma and squamous cells can accumulate underneath the prepuce resulting in smegmatic pseudocysts and/or keratin pearls, in which squamous cells actually form concentric layers and result in several millimetre sized masses. Thus, the closed compartment between the prepuce and the clitoris can become irritated, erythematous, or infected. Any of these changes can be associated with a persistent foreign body sensation (described as similar to grains of sand in the eye), balanitis, discomfort, hypersensitivity, clitorodynia sexual pain disorder, and even persistent genital arousal disorder (PGAD) [6].

CP associating lichen sclerosis is usually present with itching and pain. Clitoral pain on arousal was ascribed to an entrapped clitoral erection. Other than its link to sexual pain, the clinical significance of this finding, in particular the relation to diminished sensitivity and impaired orgasm, is enough for diagnosis of CP. Sometimes itching or discharge is the dominant complaint.

Phimosis may be suspected in adults female who experienced to retract her prepuce smoothy by inability to retract it, or retract the hood only with difficulty or painfully.

CP classified to three grades; mild, moderate and severe according to the degree of retractability of the prepuce and its adhesions with the glans (Fig. 34.1).

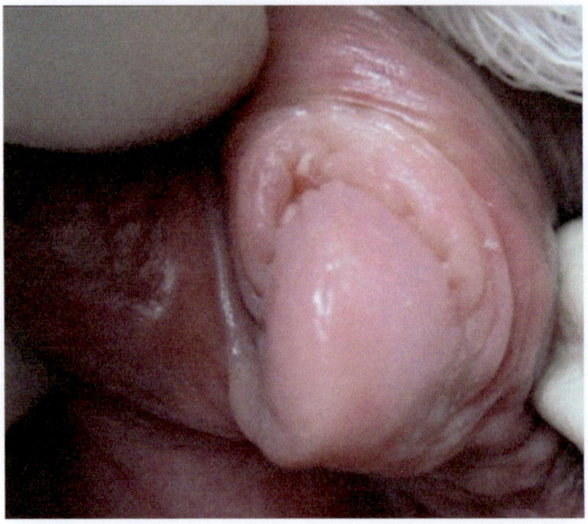

Fig. 34.1 Mild Degree of CP, with partially retracted preputial hood and inability to expose the clitorial corona

Predisposing Factors The most likely pathophysiology of clitoral phimosis is scarring and relative inelastic mechanical property of the prepuce. The most common cause of CP is lichen sclerosis, phimosis in such cases is associated with narrowing of the introitus, thinning, fusion of labia, and vulvar fissures surrounded by purple or red borders. A biopsy is recommended to confirm the diagnosis and to rule out other pathologies [7].

Blunt perineal or genital trauma changing prepucial elasticity, recurrent genital fungal or bacterial infections, specially in diabetic women, genital dermatologic conditions such as lichen sclerosis, and insufficient sex steroid hormones are a possible factors which may predispose to CP. Future research will need to determine whether these risk factors are causally related.

Smegma in infants and preadolescent girls may develop under the prepuce, and the irritation caused by its accumulation may result in forming adhesions between the glans and prepuce, in smegmatic pseudocyst, and in phimosis of the clitoris, therefore, it is important to maintain proper hygiene of the vulva (Smegma discussed in details in Chap. 17).

Labial adhesions which is a common acquired condition secondary to hypoestrogenism, vulvovaginitis, and exposure to exogenous androgens usually affecting girls at or before adolescent [8], and manifested by labia minora agglutination,

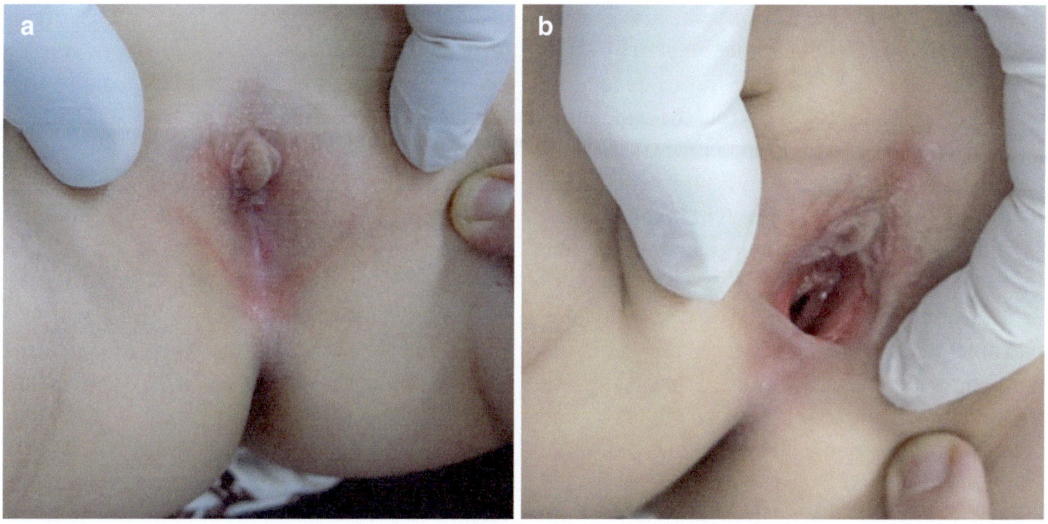

Fig. 34.2 (**a**) Extensive labial adhesion in a 6 years old girl, extended to the prepuce and results in preputial phimosis, (**b**) adhesiolysis revealed an inflamed labial mucosa extended to the prepuce

but sometimes the pathology extended cranially to involve the preputial hood and results in a form of preputial phimosis (Fig. 34.2).

In communities still practising FGM, and among some migrants in European countries scaring after this infibulation usually entrapping the leftover clitoris between the scared labial remnants, with a permanent concealment of the clitoris, and results in a cicatricial form of CP (Fig. 34.3).

Treatment Any predisposing or associated dermatitis should be treated first, proper hygienic and genital cleaning should be followed. Mild and moderated cases may respond to topical steroids. Severe or recurrent cases of CP are treated by hoodectomy or dorsal slit. An alternative and easy surgical treatment is hoodplasty. The hood of the clitoris is approached via dorsal incision resulting in two preputial flaps, which are de-epithelialized, reflected laterally and sutured. The outcomes of this procedure were assessed objectively based on symptomatology regression, recurrence, and subjectively by assessing the surgical success and patient satisfaction, with a favourable results. The two preputial flaps avoid retracting scars, recurrence or adhesions, or re-submerged clitoris [9].

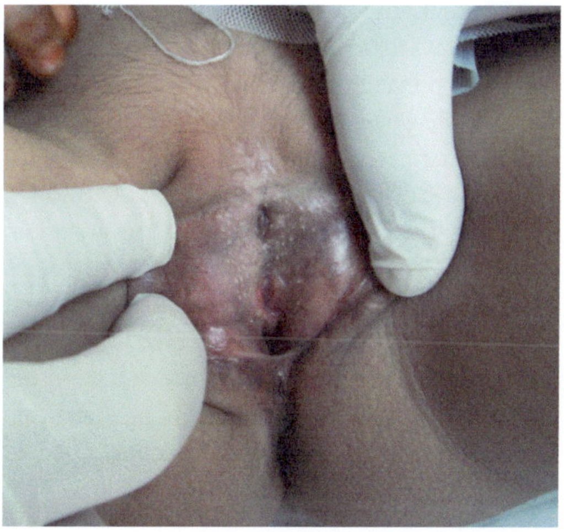

Fig. 34.3 Post circumcision extensive scaring affecting the labia, partially closing the introits, and entrapping the clitorial remnants in a scar tissue

Lichen Sclerosis (LS)

Lichen sclerosis is a cutaneous disease that has an affinity for the anogenital region. The exact etiology is unknown but there is evidence that it is autoimmune in nature. There might also be a genetic component, as it can be found in mother-daughter pairs. LS can occur at anytime through the lifespan, it is an intensely pruritic disease, and sleep disturbance is a common complaint [7].

Vulvar appearance with LS varies depending on the severity and length of time the patient has had this condition. The disease process disrupts the normal vulvar anatomy; typical changes include phimosis of the clitoral hood, involution of the labia minora, and scarring of the introitus.

The affected skin can have a thin, white, parchment paper-like appearance, it can be thin and red, or it could be thickened and white. All these skin variations can appear on the vulvar and anogenital region together. There may be an "hourglass" pattern seen over the anogenital region, which can extend into the genitocrural folds. These architectural changes can lead to recurrent tearing during intercourse (vulvar granuloma fissuratum) and decreased clitoral sensation [10]. A vulvar biopsy may be useful in diagnosing LS.

Treatment for LS is aimed at alleviating symptoms and preventing disease progression. Low-to-moderate-potency steroid ointments are useful. There is evidence that 0.1% tacrolimus ointment (Protopicw, Astellas Pharma U.S., Inc., Deerfield, IL, U.S.A.) is useful in the treatment of LS [11]. Symptom management strategies include following strict vulvar skin care and hygiene guidelines, using lukewarm water baking soda or colloidal oatmeal soaks, and applying an occlusive skin protectant daily to prevent urine and vaginal discharge from contacting affected skin [12].

Hypertrophy of Clitoral Hood: (Preputomegaly, Megaloprepuce)

Most of literature are mainly discussing clitoromegaly and few attention were given to preputomegaly, also the subsequent therapeutic measures are directed to reduce the size of the clitoris and few aesthetic surgeons give a concern to remould the large prepuce. Abnormally large prepuce, is not a well known disease, this is in contrary to male with megaloprepuce; which is a recognised entity with different names (Akroposthia, megaloprepuce and macroposthia) (Chap. 10). Most cases of clitoromegaly in menarchal women are due to excess androgen stimulation either from steroid producing ovarian tumors or late presentation of congenital defects in the cortisol synthesis pathway.

We can classify preputomegaly from etiological point of view to:

- Primary cases
- Secondary cases; in which the primary cause could be either systemic or local.

Differentiating potential aetiologies of clitoromegaly and preputomegaly requires a careful history, physical examination, select hormone levels determination, imaging, and pathological studies, which allows for appropriate management.

Although clitoromegaly is usually associated with preputomegaly, but it is not rare to have a pathologically enlarged prepuce without a corresponded clitoromegaly, on the other hand many cases of isolated preputomegaly may mimic a clitoromegaly.

Enlarged prepuce without a compatible clitoromegaly may results in phimosis and entrapment of the normal clitoris between the edges of adherent hood (Fig. 34.4).

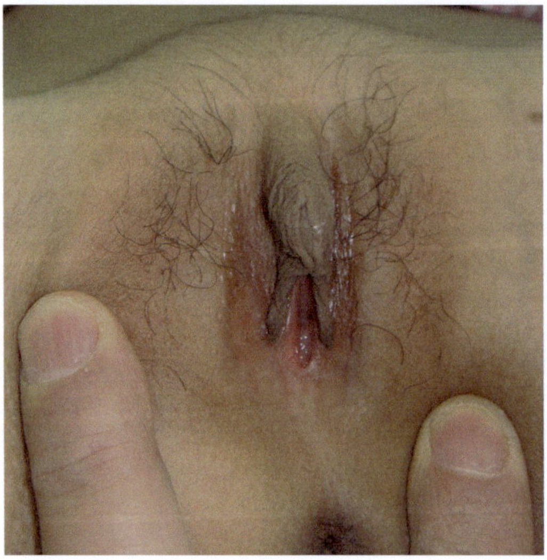

Fig. 34.4 An enlarged prepuce covering completely the tip of the normal sized clitorial glans with a consequent phimosis

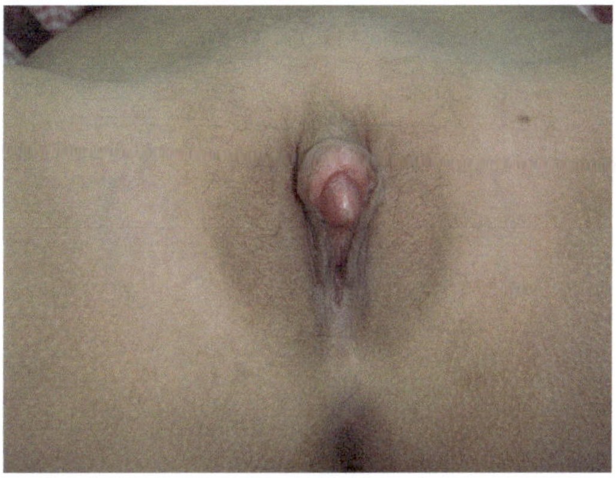

Fig. 34.5 Clitorial enlargement without an equivalent preputomegaly with an exposed clitorial glans

On the other hand an enlarged clitoris without a corresponding preputomegaly may results in an exposed clitorial glans without any preputial coverage (Fig. 34.5).

As the term preputomegaly is not a commonly used expression, many reports are confused between this anomaly and clitoromegaly, which is defined as the measurement of the clitoral index (width length, in millimetres) larger than 15 mm^2 in the newborn or over 21 mm^2 in adults [13]. The definition of clitoromegaly is indefinite in literature, there may be racial differences between clitoral length values. In neonates a clitoris length above 1 cm has traditionally been defined as clitoromegaly [14].

Neonatal benign enlargement of the clitoris, with or without preputial enlargement is associated with antenatal exposure to exogenous or endogenous androgens, it is a well recognized condition, and its self resolution is the usual fate [15].

Preputomegaly could be a transient condition, or a long standing chronic disease. There are local and systemic disorders which may be associated with preputomegaly, but in few cases no primary factor could be detected and the enlargement is considered idiopathic.

Some congenital anomalies like anorectal malformations may be associated with an idiopathic clitorial and preputial engagement (Fig. 34.6).

Following a brief preoperative investigation, early surgical correction provides an adequate aesthetic aspect of the vulva and lessens the family's and the patient's anxiety. In adults preputomegaly have to be differentiated from clitoral priapism.

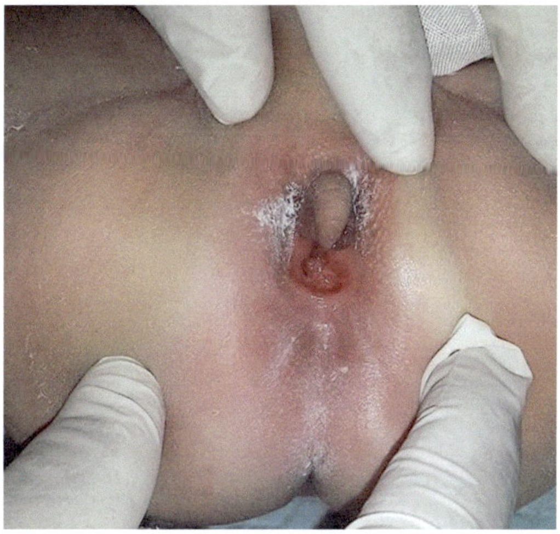

Fig. 34.6 Idiopathic preputomegaly and clitoromegaly associating a case of imperforate anus

Female preputial hypertrophy can be either congenital or acquired, and it is commonly associated with clitoromegaly, but rare focal lesions may result in selective preputial engagement. The congenital forms are caused by hormonal disturbances or intersex states with gonadal or chromosomal alteration, present mainly in disorders of sex development (DSD). Such case are usually obvious at birth. When the hypertrophy develops later on, the underlying aetiology should be explored and an acquired causes should also be considered. These acquired forms are either hormonal or non-hormonal, in the hormonal cases, an androgen excess is the main contributing factor, and the most common congenital disease associated with both preputial and clitorial engagement is Congenital Adrenal Hyperplasia (CAH), which results from an increase in size and metabolic activity of the adrenal cortex or medulla due to inherited enzymatic disorders. The enzymes implicated in this disorder are steroid 21-hydroxylase (21-OH), 11b-Hydroxylase and 3b-hydroxysteroid dehydrogenase. This rare condition is present in 1 of 15,000–16,000 live births worldwide, and 11% of all the patients develops clitoromegaly [16]. The main management is either surgical or medical treatment with

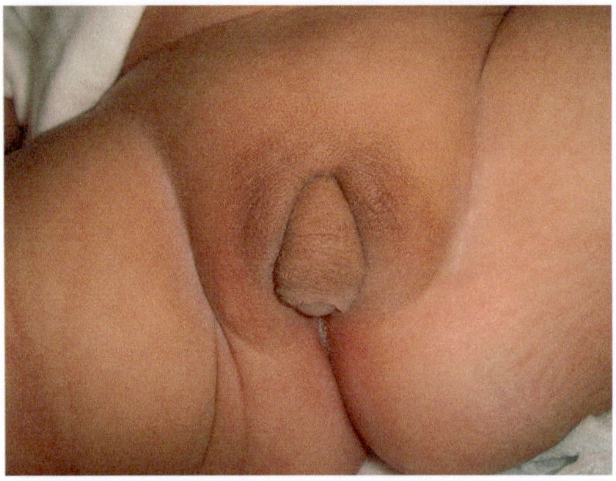

Fig. 34.7 An obvious preputomegaly covering an enlarged clitoris in a female child with CAH

the normalization of the genitalia as the objective. The surgical approaching is based on many techniques aimed to create normal looking female external genitalia, and focused on fixing the volume and size of clitoris and prepuce with preservation of the clitorial sensitivity. Many outcomes for clitroplasty and hoodplasty reported good results following different procedures [17] (Fig. 34.7).

Cases of Persistent urogenital sinus (a rare urogenital abnormality in which the urethral and vaginal tracts open into a common channel and share a single opening) either with or without CAH usually associated with a significant preputomegaly, we found in such cases that the preputial enlargement usually exceed the clitorial hypertrophy (this just an observational finding without an objective explanation) (Fig. 34.8).

Turner syndrome (TS), also known as congenital ovarian hypoplasia syndrome, occurs when the X chromosome is partially or completely missing in females. Its main clinical manifestations include growth disorders, reproductive system abnormalities, cardiovascular abnormalities, and autoimmune diseases [18].

In cases of TS which may be presented with either clitoromegaly, preputomegaly or both the defect in such cases is mainly a chromosomal anomaly; due to presence of Y chromosome or its fragments in a female child [19] (Fig. 34.9).

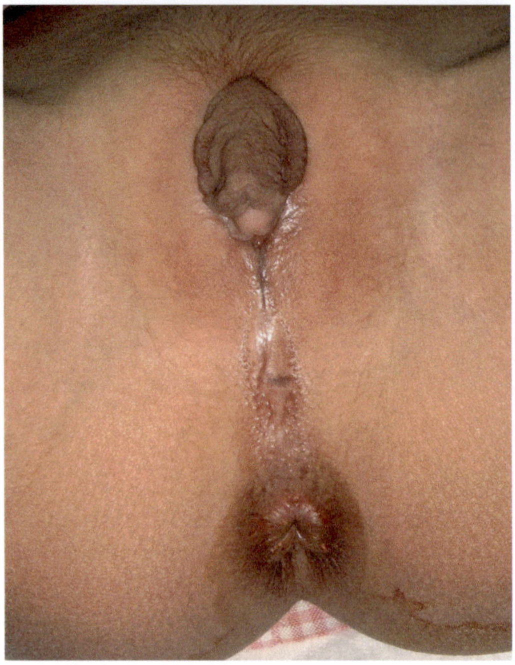

Fig. 34.8 A case of persistent urogenital sinus with a significant preputomegaly exceeding the clitoromegaly, an excess suprapubic hair is visible

Hormonal Preputomegaly In adults the most important endocrinopathies associated with preputomegaly are non-polycystic ovarian hypertestosteronism and polycystic ovarian syndrome. Four groups of post hormonal preputomegaly should be distinguished:

- Endocrinopathies; Leydig-cell tumors, virilizing cortical adenocarcinoma or adenoma.
- Masculizing tumours.
- Polycystic ovary syndrome.
- Self-injection of long acting synthetic androgens, and Gonadotropic pituitary extract and testosterone injection [20].

Use of anabolic steroids by bodybuilders and other athletes can result in significant enlargement of the prepuce and/or clitoris in concert with other masculinizing effects on their bodies.

Those taking hormones or other medications as part of female-to-male transition usually experience dramatic preputial and clitoral growth.

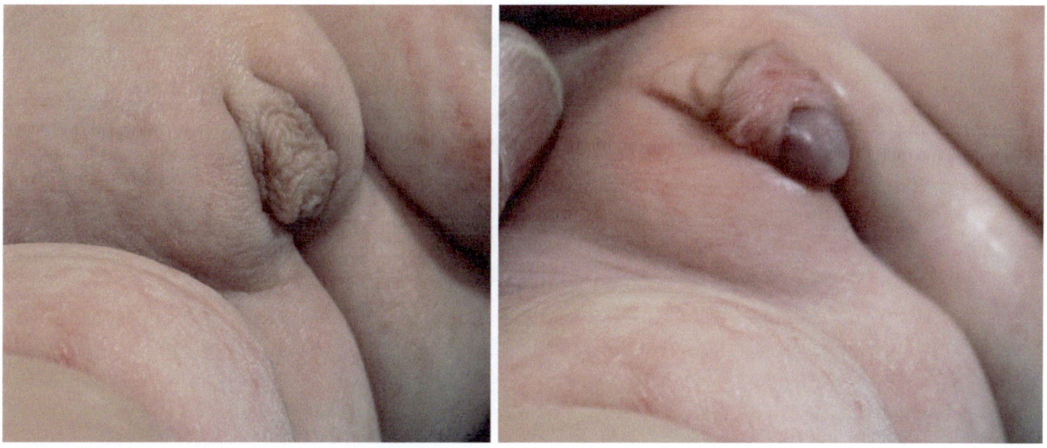

Fig. 34.9 A 5 month girl with Turner's syndrome with a redundant preputomegaly and prominent clitoris

Local Lesions Associated with Preputomegaly Clitoromegaly due to tumor infiltration is exceptionally rare. Literature review up to 2015 for cases of clitoromegaly secondary to other benign clitoral lesions in the pediatric population revealed one case of angiokeratoma, 1 hemangiopericytoma, 1 granular cell tumor, 6 hemangiomas, and approximately 30 neurofibromas. Clitoral malignancies in the pediatric population are even more rare with only 3 cases of clitoral schwannomas, 2 rhabdomyosarcomas, 1 lymphoma, and 1 endodermal sinus tumor documented in the literature [21].

Other clitoral anomalies or tumors are rarely reported, they are present within an ample spectrum, include fibroma, leiomyoma, pseudolymphoma, myiasis. Whereas malignancies include carcinoma, sarcoma, epitheloid hemangioendothelioma and lymphoma.

There is a paucity of literature on cancer of clitoris, among 360 patients diagnosed with vulvar cancer, 40 cases were found to have clitoral cancer. The histologic features of a carcinoma of clitoris were found to be different from squamous cell carcinoma of vulva, with large areas showing a transitional cell carcinoma pattern and foci of spindle and anaplastic cells. Some authors blaming any abnormality of clitoris, whether it is inclusion cysts, FGM or other causes of clitoromegaly as a predisposing factors for clitoral malignancy [22].

Clitoral cysts must be considered as a possible cause of clitoral enlargement in the prepubertal population. Clitoral tumors are distinguished clinically from hormonal abnormalities and intersex disorders by their hormonal profile, and the presence of an underlying mass. Ultrasound and magnetic resonance imaging might be useful imaging modalities to further characterize the clitoral and preputial enlargement.

Epidermoid Cyst of the Prepuce Most of literature reporting epidermoid cyst as it affect the clitoris, but I think—and after dealing with 15 cases—that the main scene of this inclusion cyst is the preputial remnants and not the clitorial one.

Epidermoid cyst of the prepuce is not common in European countries, as most reported cases are commonly reported after female genital mutilation, and clitorial or preputial piercing [23]. There are some case reports secondary to aesthetic procedures and traumas. Yannis et al. [24] reported the first case of preputial epidermoid cyst in a postmenopausal woman with no previous history of female genital cutting or infection.

The development of epidermal clitoral inclusion cyst after type III FGM is one of the most common long-term complications. The formation of the cyst results from the epidermal embedding, invagination and proliferation of keratinized epithelial cells and sebaceous glands in the line of scar. They grow slowly and usually do not cause symptoms, but they may become infected, causing pain and discomfort. In addition to the physical complications, inclusion cysts may cause psychological problems, including disfigurement, shame, and fear of cancer, and they may affect the personal and family life of the patient [25].

Many families may interpret preputial cyst as an enlarged phallus and even physicians unaware about these uncommon pathologies of clitorial and preputial enlargement may thought that the affected girl had a sort of DSD; as some cyst, may gives an impression of intersex problems (Fig. 34.10).

Cases of post FGM epidermoid cyst may acquire a large size and usually associated with other scars in the vulva, mainly in the labia minora (Fig. 34.11).

Embryonic Cyst Most embryonic cysts of the vulva are located in the hymen, vestibule, labia minora, and periclitorial tissues; they are usually solitary, superficial, and thin walled. As a rule, embryonic cysts are smaller than 3 cm in diameter; although, a few may reach 10 cm [26].

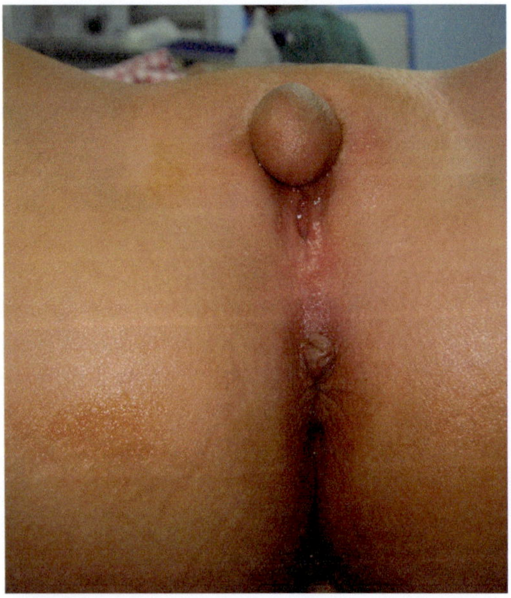

Fig. 34.10 A large inclusion epidermoid cyst involving the preputial remnants after type II FGM

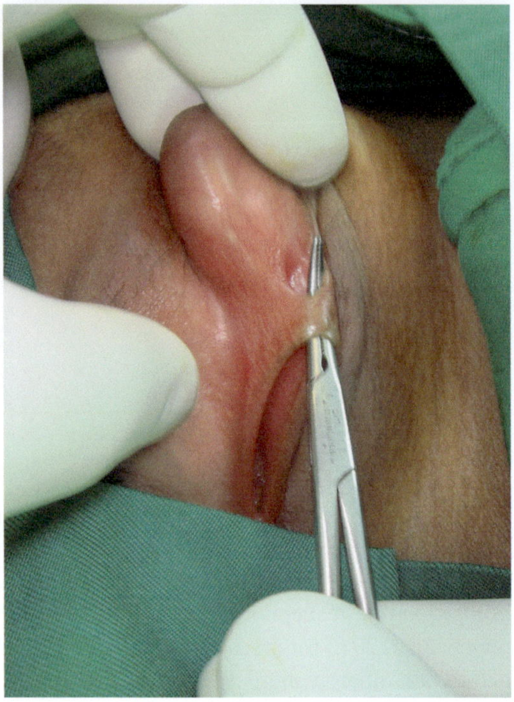

Fig. 34.11 Scar bridge between labia minora in association with an epidermoid inclusion cyst of the prepuce

Dermoid and pilonidal cysts of the clitoris and prepuce are a very rare entity and only few cases had been reported [27, 28].

Cysts affecting the prepuce should be excised precisely with great caution to preserve the blood and nerve supply of the clitorial remnant as well as the prepuce and to maintain a near normal architecture of the preputial hood, usually the long standing of such cysts is fortunately expanding the preputial skin, and giving a chance for possible hoodplasty (Fig. 34.12).

Neurofibromatosis Clitoral neurofibroma was first reported in 1960 by Haddad and Jones [29], Labardini et al. [30] reviewed six cases of female genital involvement, and many cases had an associated urinary bladder involvement, and some cases may had a renovascular hypertension. In neurofibromatosis, a nodules of various sizes occur along small nerve branches, which generally make appearance on skin, in some cases it involves the clitoris and/or the prepuce.

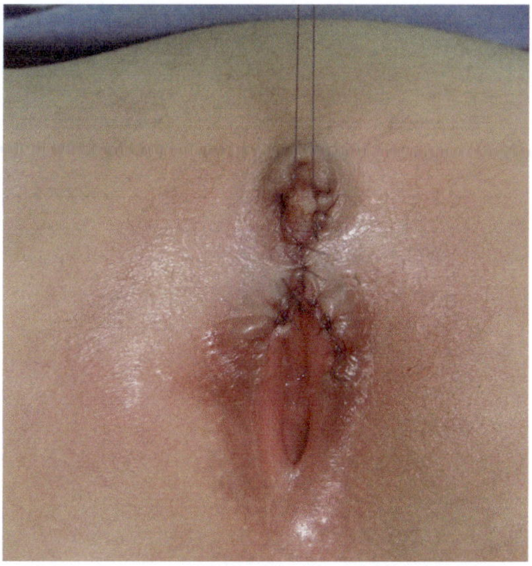

Fig. 34.12 Excised preputial cyst with preservation of the clitoris and prepuce

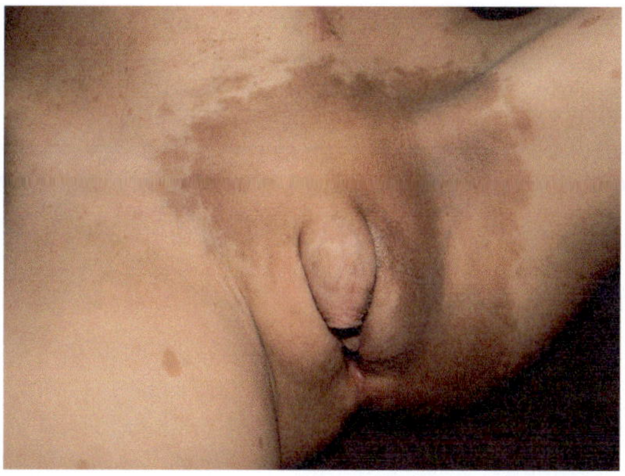

Fig. 34.13 11 years girl had a von Recklinghausen's, with a characteristic cafe-eu-lait skin colouration in the suprapubic region and a large neurofibromas of the genitals ended with a significant preputomegaly

Till 2008 literature reports documented 26 patients with neurofibromas with clitoral involvement [22].

Either systemic or only localised neurofibromatosis of the preputial hood may be manifested as hypertrophy of the prepuce, such cases usually associated with clitorial involvement.

Von Recklinghausen's disease is an autosomal dominant inherited disorder, with neurofibromatosis well described in the cutaneous, osseous, and central nervous systems, and urogenital involvement have been reported as rare manifestations [31]. Such cases usually mistaken for congenital adrenal hyperplasia (Fig. 34.13).

Plexiform schwannoma is a painless tumor of clitoris. Although it is rare, it should be included in the differential diagnosis of a clitoral enlargement or mass. Chuang et al. [32] found plexiform schwannoma in a 41 year old woman, without any other neurofibromatosis.

Haemangioma and Vascular Malformations (Fig. 34.14) Hemangiomas are still one of the most common skin lesions in infancy and early childhood.

Hemangiomas in the sensitive genital area of the female body are a constant major cosmetic concern. In the majority of cases they are even complicated by ulceration and/or haemorrhage as well. In addition, their delicate location make genital hemangiomas like their facial counterparts prone to psychosocial disorders, too.

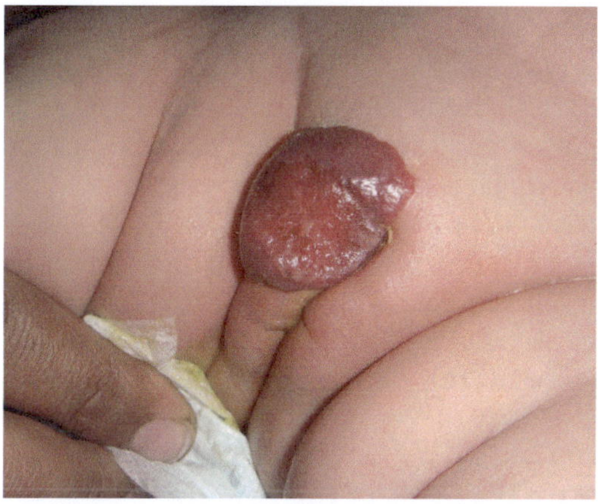

Fig. 34.14 Neonate with a large haemangioma affecting the prepuce and uppermost uppermost part of the labia, mainly to the right side

Cavernous hemangioma of clitoris is an extremely rare cause of clitoromegaly and, only few cases have been reported, all cases have been observed in young and adolescent patients, and none of them have been diagnosed before pathologic examination of the mass [33].

Epithelioid hemangiomas was first described in 1969, as a rare, slowly growing, benign vascular lesions that typically occur during early and mid-adult life. The lesions are well-circumscribed with abundant, well-formed vascular spaces with open lumina and a distinctive eosinophilic inflammatory infiltrate. The characteristic feature of epithelioid hemangioma is the epithelioid endothelial cells with large oval nuclei and abundant eosinophilic cytoplasm [34]. Surgical management with close clinical follow-up for local recurrence is essential.

Traditional wait and see approach is not applicable for genital haemangiomas as final involution and residuum might be considered as absolutely unacceptable. The risk of a small physical scar, resulting out of a well-planned early active treatment, should always be weighted up against the sequelae a lifelong emotional scar will have. Especially, when nowadays we are able to treat genital hemangiomas more safe and easily with injection or by laser application [35].

In Germany indeed, in order to prevent maceration and infection of hemangiomas in the anogenital area, and by supporting the philosophy of considering such hemangiomas as a "cosmetic emergency", the use of cryosurgery is recommended as early as possible, and not found to be associated with an increased scarring potential [36].

Rare Diseases of the Female Prepuce

Clitoral priapism, also known as clitorism, is a rare, potentially painful medical condition and is sometimes described as an aspect of PGAD (Persistent genital arousal disorder), in which the erect clitoris does not return to its relaxed state for an unusually extended period of time (ranging from minutes to days), despite the absence of both physical and psychological stimulation; PGAD can also be associated with morphometric and vascular modifications of the clitoris. Drugs may cause or affect clitoral priapism. The drug trazodone is known to cause male priapism as a side effect, but there is only one documented report that it may have caused clitoral priapism, in which case discontinuing the medication may be a remedy [37].

Because PGAD is relatively rare and, as its own concept apart from clitoral priapism, has only been researched since 2001, there is little research into what may cure or remedy the disorder.

As in male patients, clitoral priapism can be treated by alpha adrenergic agonists to promote vasoconstriction either by direct injection into the corpus or oral treatment with imipramine hydrochloride.

Bifid Prepuce Bifid clitoris (Fig. 34.15) is usually seen in association with exstrophy of the bladder. Exstrophy of the bladder occurs rarely (1 per 30,000 births) and has a male predominance (3,1). However, when it occurs in females, it is often associated with bifid clitoris. It is noted that 43% of 70 female patients with bladder exstrophy had associated reproductive tract anomalies, these included vaginal anomalies and Mullerian duct fusion problems [38]. Such cases, of bifid clitoris and prepuce may be overlooked during exstrophy reconstruction, specially in a tiny girl, but female survivors should receive a special attention before adulthood to reconstruct her clitoris and prepuce

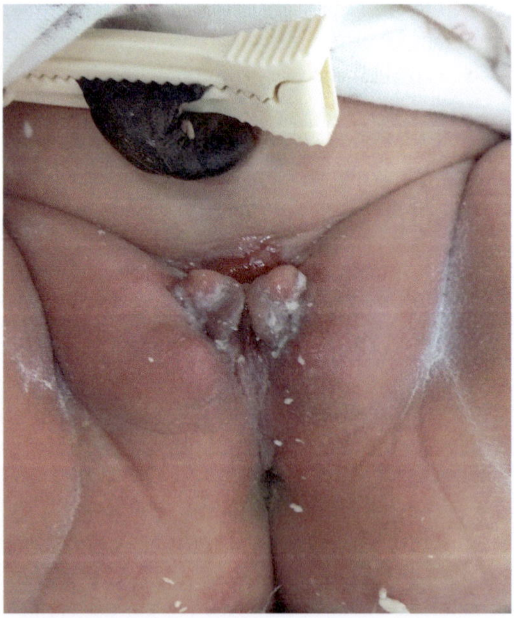

Fig. 34.15 Case of bifid both clitoris and prepuce in a neonate girl with bladder exstrophy

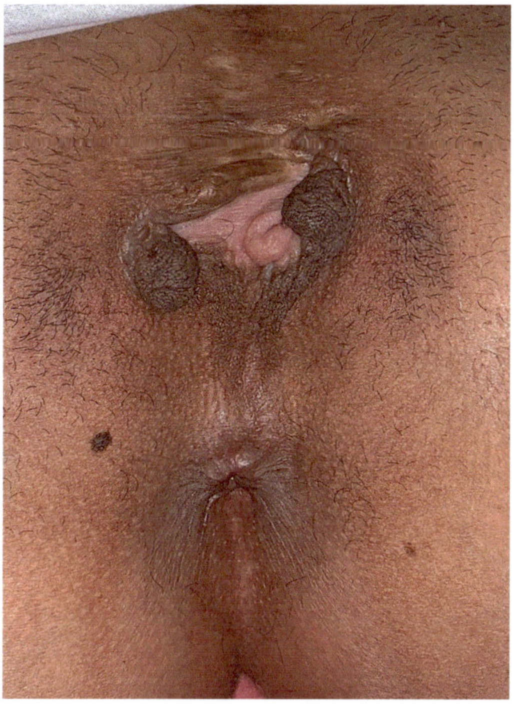

Fig. 34.16 A persistent non repaired bifid prepuce in a pregnant lady, she had a reconstructed bladder exstrophy

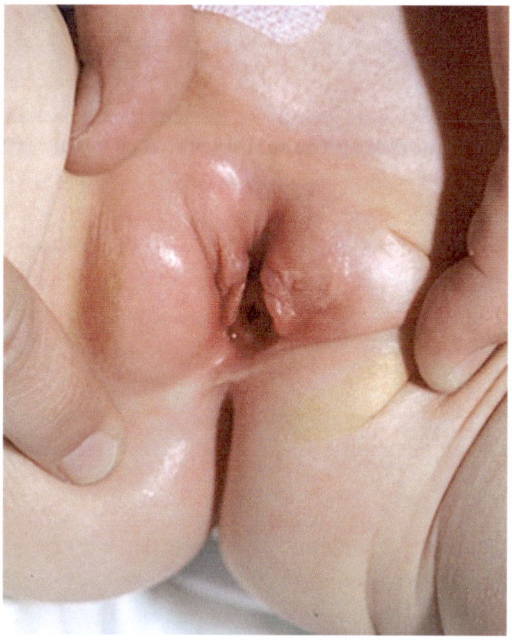

Fig. 34.17 An extremely rare case of isolated bifid clitoris without any other associated anomalies

with possible preservation of their functions (Fig. 34.16).

In addition, an case of isolated bifid clitoris without any other anomalies is an extremely rare anomaly (Fig. 34.17), but many cases are reported with an abnormally separated and short labia in females with epispadias-exstrophy complex [39]. Cases of rare syndrome of focal dermal hypoplasia or Goltz Gorlin syndrome, which is an X-linked dominant disorder affecting tissues derived from ectoderm and mesoderm, may had a bifid clitoris [40].

Modification and Mutilation (Clitoral Hood Reduction and Piercing) There are intentional and unintentional clitoral modifications, including female genital mutilation (FGM), sex reassignment surgery, and genital piercings.

In most of the world, clitoral modifications are uncommon. In some cultures, female genital mutilation (FGM) is practiced as a rite of passage into womanhood, is perceived as an improvement to the appearance of the genitalia, or is used to suppress or reduce female sexual desire and pleasure (including masturbation). FGM was performed on many children in Western countries, including previously the United States, to discourage masturbation and reduce diseases believed to relate to it.

Approximately 100–150 million women worldwide are estimated to have undergone FGM, with a daily incidence of 6000 African girls aged 4–12 years old, and two million girls per year are thought to be at risk of undergoing such a procedure. Although types I and II FGM comprise 80% of the FGM practices worldwide, the more extreme type III FGM is the most commonly performed procedure in many African countries [41].

In 2008, the World Health Assembly passed resolution WHA61.16 on the elimination of FGM, emphasizing the need for concerted action in all sectors of health, education, finance, justice and women's affairs [42].

In April 2016, the United Nations Special Rapporteur on health, Dainius Pūras, condemned this treatment as a form of female genital mutilation in the absence of symptoms or health issues warranting those procedures [43].

One modification that women often perform of their free will is to have the hood pierced and insert jewellery, both for adornment and physical pleasure. Though much less common, other women opt to have their own hood surgically trimmed or removed so as to permanently expose part or all of the clitoral glans.

Clitoral hood piercings are usually channeled in the form of vertical piercings, and, to a lesser extent, horizontal piercings. The triangle piercing is a very deep horizontal hood piercing, and is done behind the clitoris as opposed to in front of it, this piercing is highly risky with regard to damage that may occur because of intersecting nerves.

General Principles for Management of Preputial Anomalies Surgery is the treatment of choice for the anomalies affecting the clitoris and prepuce, aiming to provide an aesthetic aspect as close as possible to normal, in addition to preserving the vascular provisions and preputial innervation, which are essential conditions for sexual activity in the future. Early surgical approach to those preputial and clitoral anomalies may prevent a great deal of embarrassment for the patients and their family and it should not be postponed in favor of investigations and time consuming complementary exams.

Clitoral hoodplasty is a new provides simple, yet effective relief for women with cosmetic concerns or clitoral discomfort after previous feminizing surgery or after FGM.

Adult females with poor cosmetic outcome, loss of genital sensitivity, and associated impaired sexual function with disorders of sex development (DSD) recently have a greater awareness of the adverse long-term effects of feminizing surgery in childhood [44].

Tactile glans hypersensitivity with or without arousal associated with the full glans exposure from the absent clitoral hood is a newly recognised adverse complication of a previously performed genitoplasty.

Early surgical reduction of clitoromegaly via full or partial clitoridectomy is controversial, and intersex women exposed to such treatment have spoken of their loss of physical sensation, and loss of autonomy. In recent years, human rights institutions have criticized early surgical management of such procedures [45].

References

1. Puppo V. RE: Clitoral anatomy in nulliparous, healthy, pre-menopausal volunteers using unenhanced magnetic resonance imaging. J Urol. 2006;175:790–1.
2. Aerts L, Rubin RS, Randazzo M, Goldstein SW, CCRC, CSE, Goldstein I. Retrospective study of the prevalence and risk factors of clitoral adhesions: women's health providers should routinely examine the glans clitoris. Sex Med. 2018;6:115e122. http://creativecommons.org/licenses/by-nc-nd/4.0/
3. Malik SN, Ansar H, Shams Ul Islam M, Al Azzawi F. Acute presentation of clitoral phimosis in a 16-year-old girl. J Obstet Gynaecol. 2013;33(7):745–6.
4. Chmel R, Nováč ková M, Fait T, Zámečník L, Krejčová L, Pastor Z. Clitoral phimosis: effects on female sexual function and surgical treatment outcomes. J Sex Med. 2019;16(2):257–66.
5. Wiesmeier E, Masongsong EV, Wiley DJ. The prevalence of examiner-diagnosed clitoral hood adhesions in a population of college-aged women. J Low Genit Tract Dis. 2008;12:307–10.
6. Munarriz R, Talakoub L, Kuohung W, Gioia M, Hoag L, Flaherty E, Min K, Choi S, Goldstein I. The prevalence of phimosis of the clitoris in women presenting to the sexual dysfunction clinic: lack of correlation to disorders of desire, arousal and orgasm. J Sex Marital Ther. 2002;28(Suppl 1):181–5. https://doi.org/10.1080/00926230252851302.
7. Eva LJ. Screening and follow up of vulval skin disorders. Best Pract Res Clin Obstet Gynaecol. 2012;26(2):175–88.
8. Opipari AW Jr. Management quandary. Labial agglutination in a teenager. J Pediatr Adolesc Gynecol. 2003;16:61–2.
9. Alei G, Monarca C, Rizzo MI, Letizia P, Alei L, Scuderi N. New approach to clitoral phimosis: hoodplasty. J Gynecol Surg. 2011;27(1):25–8.
10. Powell JJ, Wojnarowska FK. Lichen sclerosus. Lancet. 1999;353:22.
11. Kunstfeld R, et al. Successful treatment of vulvar lichen sclerosus with topical tacrolimus. Arch Dermatol. 2003;139:850.
12. Flynn AN, King M, Rieff M, Krapf J, Goldstein AT. Patient satisfaction of surgical treatment of clitoral phimosis and labial adhesions caused by lichen sclerosus. Sex Med. 2015;3:251–5.
13. Sanea K, Pescovitz H. The clitoral index: a determination of clitoral size in normal girls and in girls with abnormal sexual development. J Pediatr. 1992;120(2):264–6. https://doi.org/10.1016/S0022-3476(05)80439-1.

14. Kutlu HA, Akbiyik F. Clitoral length in female newborns: a new approach to the assessment of clitoromegaly. Turk J Med Sci. 2011;41(3): 495–9.
15. Grumbach MM, Ducharme JR, Moloshok RE. On the fetal masculinizing action of certain oral progestins. J Clin Endocrinol Metabol. 1959;19(11):1369–80. https://doi.org/10.1210/jcem-19-11-1369.
16. Turcu A, Auchus R. Adrenal steroidogenesis and congenital adrenal hyperplasia. Endocrinol Metab Clin N Am. 2015;44(2):275–96.
17. Carmina E, Dewailly D, Escobar-Morreale H, Kelestimur F, et al. Non-classic congenital adrenal hyperplasia due to 21-hydroxylase deficiency revisited: an update with a special focus on adolescent and adult women. Hum Reprod Update. 2017;23(5):580–99.
18. Cui X, et al. A basic understanding of Turner syndrome: incidence, complications, diagnosis, and treatment. Intractable Rare Dis Res. 2018;7(4): 223–8.
19. Bergendi E, Plöchl E, Vlasak I, Rittinger O, Muss W. A Turner-like phenotype in a girl with an isodicentric fluorescent Y chromosome mosaicism. Klin Padiatr. 1997;209:133–6.
20. Bradbury JT, Gaensbauer F. Masculinization of the female rat by gonadotropic extracts. Proc Soc Exp Biol Med. 1939;41(1):128–31. https://doi.org/10.3181/00379727-41-10594.
21. Nelson KL, McQuillan SK, Brain P. Literature review of periclitoral cysts in the prepubertal population. J Pediatr Adolesc Gynecol. 2016;29(6):558–61. https://www.scopus.com/inward/record.uri?eid=2-s2.0-
22. Al-Shebaily MM, Qureshi VF. Malignancies in clitoris: a review of literature on etiology, diagnosis, pathology and treatment strategies. Int J Cancer Res. 2008;4:110–26. https://doi.org/10.3923/ijcr.2008.110.126.
23. Rouzi AA, Sindi O, Radhan B, Ba'aqeel H. Epidermal clitoral inclusion cyst after type I female genital mutilation. Am J Obstet Gynecol. 2001;3:185. https://doi.org/10.1067/mob.2001.117660.
24. Yannis P, Amy EW, Bertha C, Mary TJ. Preputial epidermoid cyst: an atypical case of acquired pseudoclitoromegaly. J Low Genit Tract Dis. 2010;14(4):382–6. https://doi.org/10.1097/LGT.0b013e3181d85da9.
25. Birge O, Erkan MM, Serin AN. Case report: epidermoid inclusion cyst of the clitoris as a long-term complication of female genital mutilation. J Med Case Rep. 2019;13:109.
26. Merlob P, Bahari C, Liban E, Reisner SH. Cysts of the female external genitalia in the newborn infant. Am J Obstet Gynecol. 1978;132:607–10.
27. Hirose R, Imai A, Kondo H, Itoh K, Tamaya T. A dermoid cyst of the paravaginal space. Acta Gynecol Obstet. 1991;249:39–41.
28. Palmer E. Pilonidal cyst of the clitoris. Am J Surg. 1957;93(1):133–6. https://doi.org/10.1016/0002-9610(57)90757-2.
29. Haddad HM, Jones HW. Clitoral enlargement simulating pseudohermaphroditism. J Dis Child. 1960;99:282–7.
30. Labardini MM, Kallet HA, Cerny JC. Urogenital neurofibromatosis stimulating an intersex problem. J Urol. 1968;98:627–32.
31. Rink RC, Mitchell ME. Genitourinary neurofibromatosis in childhood. J Urol. 1983;130:1176–9.
32. Chuang WY, Yeh CJ, Jung SM, Hsueh S. Plexiform schwannoma of the clitoris. APMIS. 2007;115:889–90.
33. Geramizadeh B, Anbardar MH, Shakeri S. Clitoromegaly caused by cavernous hemangioma: a rare case report and review of the literature. Urol Ann. 2012;4:175e7.
34. Gray HJ, Rendi MH, Holmes M. Painful clitoromegaly caused by rare epithelioid hemangioma. Gynecol Oncol Rep. 2013;4:60–2. https://doi.org/10.1016/j.gynor.2012.12.007.
35. Fette A. Minimal access laser therapy (malt) of genitary hemangiomas in girls. Med Surg Urol. 2014;3(145):2. https://doi.org/10.4172/2168-9857.1000145.
36. Bause H. Kryotherapie lokalisierter klassischer Hämangiome. Monatsschr Kinderheilkd. 2004;152:16–22.
37. Medina CA. Clitoral priapism: a rare condition presenting as a cause of vulvar pain. Obstet Gynecol. 2002;100(5 Pt 2):1089–91.
38. Gomes AL, et al. Clitoral anomalies not associated with disorders of sex development. J Ped Surg Case Rep. 2013;1:403e405. https://doi.org/10.1016/j.epsc.2013.11.003.
39. Sorantin E, Abou SS. Epispadias-exstrophy complex. In: Riccabona M, editor. Pediatric urogenital radiology. Medical radiology. Cham: Springer; 2018.
40. Yesodharan D, Büschenfelde UM, Kutsche K, et al. Goltz-Gorlin syndrome: revisiting the clinical spectrum. Indian J Pediatr. 2018;85:1067. https://doi.org/10.1007/s12098-018-2632-1.
41. Reisel D, Creighton SM. Long term health consequences of female genital mutilation (FGM). Maturitas. 2015;80:48–51.
42. World Health Organization (WHO), Department of Reproductive Health and Research. Eliminating female genital mutilation: an interagency statement, OHCHR, UNAIDS, UNDP, UNECA, UNESCO, UNFPA, UNHCR, UNICEF, UNIFEM, WHO. Geneva: WHO; 2008. http://www.who.int/reproductivehealth/publications/fgm/9789241596442/en/
43. Pūras D. Special Rapporteur on the right of everyone to the enjoyment of the highest attainable standard of physical and mental health. Sport and healthy lifestyles and the right to health. Report A/HRC/32/33, United Nations; 2016.
44. Wolffenbuttel KP, et al. Clitoral hoodplasty in DSD females. J Pediatr Urol. 2017;13:61.e1–5.
45. Jordan-Young RM, Sonksen PH, Karkazis K. Sex, health, and athletes. BMJ. 2014;348(28):2926. https://doi.org/10.1136/bmj.g2926.

Index

M. A. B. Fahmy, *Normal and Abnormal Prepuce*, https://doi.org/10.1007/978-3-030-37621-5

MIX
Papier aus verantwortungsvollen Quellen
Paper from responsible sources
FSC® C105338

If you have any concerns about our products, you can contact us on
ProductSafety@springernature.com

In case Publisher is established outside the EU, the EU authorized representative is:
Springer Nature Customer Service Center GmbH
Europaplatz 3, 69115 Heidelberg, Germany

Printed by Libri Plureos GmbH
in Hamburg, Germany